RENEWALS 458-4574.

DATE DUE

| SEP 30 | | | |
|--------|--|--|--|
| OCT 12 | | | |
| | | | |
| NOV 01 | | | |
| NOV 20 | | | |
| | | | |
| NOV 28 | | | |
| NOV 08 | | | |
| NOV 29 | | | |
| | | | |
| | | | |
| | | | |
| | | | |
| GAYLORD | | | PRINTED IN U.S.A. |

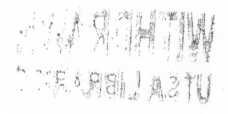

**Neurobehavioral Aspects
of Multiple Sclerosis**

# Neurobehavioral Aspects of Multiple Sclerosis

Edited by

## STEPHEN M. RAO, Ph.D.

Department of Neurology
Medical College of Wisconsin

New York   Oxford
OXFORD UNIVERSITY PRESS
1990

# Oxford University Press

Oxford   New York   Toronto
Delhi   Bombay   Calcutta   Madras   Karachi
Petaling Jaya   Singapore   Hong Kong   Tokyo
Nairobi   Dar es Salaam   Cape Town
Melbourne   Auckland

and associated companies in
Berlin   Ibadan

Library of Congress Cataloging-in-Publication Data
Neurobehavioral aspects of multiple sclerosis /
edited by Stephen M. Rao.
p.   cm.   Includes bibliographies and index.
ISBN 0-19-505400-8
1. Multiple sclerosis—Psychological aspects.   2. Multiple sclerosis—
Complications and sequelae.   3. Clinical neuropsychology.   4. Psychological
manifestations of general diseases. [DNLM:   1. Affective Disorders.
2. Cognition Disorders.   3. Multiple Sclerosis—complications.
4. Multiple Sclerosis—physiopathology.   WL 360 N494]
RC377.N48   1990   616.8′34′0019—dc20
DNLM/DLC for Library of Congress   89-16139   CIP

9 8 7 6 5 4 3 2 1
Printed in the United States of America
on acid-free paper

*This book is dedicated to persons with MS and their family members,*
*whose courage and determination are an inspiration for us all;*
*and to my family, Rebecca, Jess and Julia.*

# Preface

Multiple sclerosis (MS) is the most common nontraumatic neurological illness affecting young and middle-aged adults. This progressive white matter disease produces multiple widespread central nervous system (CNS) lesions that frequently involve the cerebral hemispheres. While the classical motor and sensory symptoms of MS have been well-defined, little scientific attention has been devoted to the study of neurobehavioral disorders in MS, at least until recently. This is surprising since Jean-Martin Charcot, the influential nineteenth century French neurologist who is credited with naming the disease, described and emphasized the neurobehavioral problems of MS patients in his Salpêtrière lectures.

During the past decade significant scientific progress has been achieved in the assessment and remediation of cognitive and affective disorders in MS. This progress has occurred as a result of major scientific contributions from neuropsychologists, psychiatrists, neurologists, neuroradiologists, neuropathologists, psychologists, and rehabilitation specialists. This book represents an attempt to provide a thought-provoking, comprehensive review of this subject from the perspective of experts in each of these disciplines. As such, the book should have appeal to an interdisciplinary audience.

The book has been divided into four parts. Part I is a background review of the neurological, neuropathological, neuroradiological, and neuropsychological features of MS. Part II presents reviews and current scientific information regarding cognitive disorders in MS—their prevalence, severity, type, course, and relationship to brain abnormalities. Practical information is also provided on how, when, and why cognitive disorders are assessed. A similar organizational approach has been used in Part III to address the neurobiological factors that influence the expression of affective disorders in MS patients. The final section, Part IV, concerns the impact of cognitive and affective disorders on activities of daily living and takes a practical approach to presenting strategies for treating these conditions.

I wish to take this opportunity to thank the contributors for their insightful and scholarly chapters. Special thanks are extended to my colleagues and collaborators, Gary Leo, Michael McQuillen, Victor Haughton, Sander Glatt, Thomas Hammeke, Linda Bernardin, Fred Unverzagt, Lee Ellington, Patricia St. Aubin-Faubert, Anne Marie Rhodes, Susan Pollard, Terri Nauertz, Stephen Ryan, and Linda Burg, who have shared with me their expertise and standards of exellence. I am also deeply appreciative of the editorial assistance and support provided by Jeffrey House and his colleagues at Oxford University Press. Support for preparation of this volume was provided by grants from the National Institutes of Health (RO1 NS22128 and K04 NS01055, Researh Career Development Award) and the National Multiple Sclerosis Society (RG 1435-A-1 and RG 2028-A-2).

*Milwaukee, WI*                                                                              S.M.R.
*November 1989*

# Contents

# Contributors

D. Frank Benson, M.D.
Augustus S. Rose Professor of Neurology
UCLA School of Medicine
Neurobehavior Unit, Brentwood Division
West Los Angeles V.A. Medical Center
Los Angeles, California

Pamela F. Cavallo, M.S.W., C.S.W.
Social Services Associate
National Multiple Sclerosis Society
New York, New York

Eileen B. Fennell, Ph.D.
Professor
Department of Clinical and Health Psychology
University of Florida
Gainesville, Florida

Christopher M. Filley, M.D.
Assistant Professor of Neurology and
  Psychiatry
University of Colorado School of Medicine
Denver, Colorado

Gary M. Franklin, M.D., M.P.H.
Assistant Professor of Neurology
University of Colorado School of Medicine
Denver, Colorado

Jordan Grafman, Ph.D.
Chief, Cognitive Neuroscience Unit
Medical Neurology Branch
National Institute of Neurological Disorders
  and Stroke
National Institutes of Health
Bethesda, Maryland

Molly Harrower, Ph.D., D.H.L.
Professor Emeritus
Department of Clinical Psychology
University of Florida
Gainesville, Florida

Robert K. Heaton, Ph.D.
Professor of Psychiatry
University of California at San Diego School
  of Medicine
San Diego, California

Nicholas G. LaRocca, Ph.D.
Associate Professor of Neurology (Psychology)
Albert Einstein College of Medicine
Bronx, New York

Irene Litvan, M.D.
Visiting Fellow
Experimental Therapeutics Branch
National Institute of Neurological Disorders
  and Stroke
National Institutes of Health
Bethesda, Maryland

Michael E. Mahler, M.D.
Assistant Professor of Neurology
UCLA School of Medicine
Neurobehavior Unit, Brentwood Division
West Los Angeles V.A. Medical Center
Los Angeles, California

Michael P. McQuillen, M.D.
Professor and Chairman
Department of Neurology
Albert B. Chandler Medical Center
University of Kentucky
Lexington, Kentucky

Sarah L. Minden, M.D.
Instructor in Psychiatry
Harvard Medical School
Department of Psychiatry, The Cambridge
  Hospital
Division of Psychiatry, Brigham and Women's
  Hospital
Boston, Massachusetts

Elisabeth Moes, Ph.D.
Instructor
Harvard Medical School
Assistant Psychologist
McLean Hospital
Belmont, Massachusetts

Lorene Nelson, M.S.
Departments of Epidemiology and Neurology
University of Washington School of Public
  Health
Seattle, Washington

Donald W. Paty, M.D., F.R.C.P.C.
Professor and Head, Division of Neurology
Director, Multiple Sclerosis Research Program
University of British Columbia
Vancouver, British Columbia, Canada

Jack H. Petajan, M.D., Ph.D.
Professor of Neurology
The University of Utah School of Medicine
Salt Lake City, Utah

Janis M. Peyser, Ph.D.
Director, Medical Psychology Program
Medical Center Hospital of Vermont
Assistant Professor of Psychiatry and
    Neurology
University of Vermont College of Medicine
Burlington, Vermont

Peter V. Rabins, M.D.
Associate Professor of Psychiatry
The Johns Hopkins University School of
    Medicine
Baltimore, Maryland

Cedric S. Raine, Ph.D., D.Sc.
Professor of Pathology (Neuropathology) and
    Neuroscience
Albert Einstein College of Medicine
Bronx, New York

Stephen M. Rao, Ph.D.
Associate Professor of Neurology and
    Psychiatry
Medical College of Wisconsin
Milwaukee, Wisconsin

Mary Eve Sanford, Ph.D.
Utah State Multiple Sclerosis Society
Salt Lake City, Utah

Randolph B. Schiffer, M.D.
Associate Professor of Neurology and
    Psychiatry
The University of Rochester Medical Center
Strong Memorial Hospital
Rochester, New York

William A. Sibley, M.D.
Professor of Neurology
University of Arizona Health Sciences Center
Tucson, Arizona

Marcia C. Smith, Ph.D.
Assistant Professor
Department of Psychology
Washington University
St. Louis, Missouri

Laetitia L. Thompson, Ph.D.
Assistant Professor of Psychiatry
University of Colorado School of Medicine
Denver, Colorado

Sharon Warren, Ph.D.
Associate Professor
Faculty of Rehabilitation Medicine
University of Alberta
Edmonton, Alberta, Canada

Ernest W. Willoughby, M.D., F.R.A.C.P.
Senior Lecturer
Department of Neurology
University of Auckland
Auckland, New Zealand

# I

# Clinicopathological Features of Multiple Sclerosis

# Introduction

MICHAEL P. McQUILLEN

The association between a loss of the fatty insulation around nerve fiber tracts in the central nervous system (CNS) and neurologic impairment of diverse types and intensity has been recognized by clinicians and pathologists for more than a century (Charcot, 1877) and, more recently, by radiologists. When that association appears in episodes involving more than one part of the nervous system at more than one time, and the patient's signs and symptoms do not suggest an alternative cause, the clinician identifies the disease as multiple sclerosis (MS).

This section provides the clinicopathological basis for understanding an illness whose neuropsychological dimensions have been all too poorly delineated to date. In Chapter 1 Sibley describes the clinical settings in which this diagnosis is made. In a small but significant proportion of patients, the time course of the illness may be chronic and even progressive. While visual symptoms (diplopia and loss of vision) and sensory complaints are common, the criteria by which disability is usually gauged focus on motor functions (Kurtzke, 1983). More recently, it has been suggested that data derived from electrophysiological (evoked potentials) and imaging techniques may suffice to identify dissemination of the disease process within the nervous system, although high false-positive rates pose a limitation for this approach (Kurtzke, 1988).

Too often, physicians have overlooked the frequency and extent of cognitive change in MS. Pathologists, on the other hand, have provided copious data from which one could readily intuit the probability of significant cognitive disturbance occurring at any stage of the disease. These data are summarized by Raine in Chapter 2 and discussed at more length in other volumes (e.g., Waksman, Reingold and

Reynolds, 1987). The thesis that MS is an autoimmune disease—an illness in which the body reacts against its own myelin or the cells, oligodendrocytes, that form myelin—has become more and more solidly grounded. Of exceeding interest and with far-reaching implications for therapy are observations indicating that remyelination can occur in the CNS.

Such observations make it all the more important that clinicians understand what the disease they are dealing with is (cf. Chapter 1 and Poser et al., 1984) and have a way of documenting in a valid, meaningful sense what is happening over time in patients with that disease. To this end, radiologists have pursued an image of the brain, most critically and most recently, with magnetic resonance imaging (MRI) techniques. In Chapter 3 Willoughby and Paty discuss these techniques in sufficient technical detail so that readers can understand the reasons for the unidentified bright objects (UBOs) commonly seen in great number in MRIs of the brains of MS patients. They call attention to the critically important observation that UBOs are neither a necessary nor a sufficient basis to make or exclude a diagnosis of MS. As they point out, there is urgent need to draw meaningful clinical correlations from the use of imaging techniques and to relate them not only to the stage of illness, but also to the effect of any proposed therapy.

In Chapter 4 Fennell and Smith provide a comprehensive description of the neuropsychological method for understanding the expression of cerebral pathology on behavior. The authors' case examples richly illustrate the range of cognitive and emotional problems that can result from this illness. Like MRI, neuropsychological testing not only can provide useful diagnostic information to the treating physician, but also can form the basis for designing and evaluating treatment programs.

That, after all, is the "reason behind the reason" for a volume such as this—to understand a problem with sufficient clarity that one may *do* something about it, not just admire it!

## REFERENCES

Charcot, J.M. (1877). *Lecons sur les maladies du systeme nervuex fautes a la Salpetriere,* recueilles et publiees par Bourneville, vol 1, 3ieme ed. Paris: V. Adriene Delahaye et Cie.

Kurtzke, J.F. (1983). Rating neurologic impairment in multiple sclerosis: An expanded disability status scale (EDSS). *Neurology, 33,* 1444–1452.

Kurtzke, J.F. (1988). Multiple sclerosis: What's in a name? *Neurology, 38,* 309–316.

Poser, C.M., Paty, D.W., Scheinberg, L., MacDonald, W.I., and Ebers, G.C., eds. (1984). *The Diagnosis of Multiple Sclerosis,* p. 253, New York: Thieme-Stratton.

Waksman, B.H., Reingold, S.C., and Reynolds, W.E. (1987). *Research on Multiple Sclerosis,* 3rd ed., p. 107, New York: Demos Publications.

# 1

# Diagnosis and Course
# of Multiple Sclerosis

WILLIAM A. SIBLEY

## DIAGNOSIS

There is no specific laboratory test for multiple sclerosis (MS). In general, it is important to document dissemination of white matter lesions in time and space in patients in the proper age range and to exclude other illnesses that might simulate the disease. To do this one relies on the following methods of gaining information (in their approximate order of importance): (1) the history, (2) the neurologic examination, (3) the magnetic resonance imaging (MRI) scan, (4) evoked potential testing, and (5) an examination of the spinal fluid.

### History

Most patients with MS fall into the age group 15–50 years, although recent data suggest that as many as 10% may have their first symptom in the sixth decade; uncommonly, too, the disease may start in children. The average age for the occurrence of initial symptoms is 29–30 years. Almost twice as many women acquire the illness, the male:female ratio varying from 1:1.5 to 1:2 in various series (Sibley et al., 1984).

The initial symptom is commonly one of the following: numbness and tingling of hands or feet, weakness of one or both legs, loss of vision in one or both eyes (retrobulbar neuritis), facial numbness, vertigo, diplopia, dysarthria, ataxia, and urinary frequency and urgency (often with incontinence). L'Hermitte's symptom is also very common: a paresthesia resembling an electrical shock which occurs with forward flexion of the head, lasting only an instant, but recurring each time with repeated head flexion, then to disappear until after a period of head rest; the sensation is most often felt in the anterior thighs, but it may occur down the spine or be referred to the arms.

A new outbreak of symptoms (exacerbation) typically lasts for at least 24–48 hours and most commonly continues for 4–12 weeks before remitting. In approximately 15% of the cases, remissions never occur and symptoms are slowly progressive from the onset; most of the latter cases include a progressive spastic paraparesis.

## Neurologic Examination

The classical neurologic examination—which includes a testing of gait, motor power, coordination, rapid succession movements, speech, skilled acts, reflexes, sensation, cranial nerve function, and mental status—should show some objective abnormality. The lesions of MS occur in the cerebral white matter in a seemingly random fashion (with the exception of a periventricular predilection). The randomness of lesion occurrence dictates that the longest white matter tracts are lesioned most frequently. Thus that portion of the corticospinal tract concerned with leg function is most frequently involved, accounting for the fact that MS is a disease of paraplegia; weakness of the arms is also common, but usually less severe. Because of corticospinal tract involvement, most moderate and advanced cases of MS have spastic weakness of the limbs, increased tendon reflexes, Babinski signs, and absent abdominal reflexes. Although there are no certain rules, the presence of symptoms for many years without some of these findings is reason to question the diagnosis.

Autonomic fibers controlling the detrusor and sphincter muscles of the bladder travel throughout the length of the neuraxis, often in close proximity to the corticospinal tracts. A spastic (though weakened) detrusor muscle frequently is seen, especially when corticospinal tract involvement is bilateral. This leads to urgency of urination and incontinence. Sometimes the urinary sphincter also becomes spastic and does not relax as the detrusor contracts (detrusor-sphincter dyssynergia) which contributes to retention of urine. The latter predisposes to an increased incidence of urinary tract bacterial infection. Patients with urinary bladder disturbances often also have sexual dysfunction: impotence in the male and anorgasmy in both sexes.

Paresthesias of numbness and tingling typically occur with lesions of the fasciculus gracilis and cuneatus (the dorsal columns of the spinal cord). L'Hermitte's symptom may occur when the dorsal columns are involved in the cervical area and the diseased area stretched by voluntary flexion of the neck. Involvement of dorsal columns is manifest in the neurologic examination by decrease or loss of position or vibratory sense, typically worse in the legs than in the arms.

Blurred vision is also a common symptom. This symptom may result from either optic neuritis or incipient diplopia; if due to the latter, the vision will clear when one eye is covered. Optic neuritis in MS is actually a demyelinated plaque in one or both optic nerves, most commonly retrobulbar. The illness is typically heralded by pain in or about the eye, is provoked by eye movement, and is associated with a decrease in visual acuity, often described as "like looking through ground glass . . . or a film negative." There is usually an associated loss of color vision in the eye, and scotomas are usually larger when tested for with a red test object.

Diplopia is usually due to a lesion of the medial longitudinal fasciculus (MLF), a paired bundle of myelinated axons running in the floor of the aqueduct of Sylvius and the fourth ventricle near the midline. The MLF actually begins high in the midbrain, runs the length of the brain stem into the upper cervical cord, and contains fibers coordinating eye movements with the vestibular system and neck muscles. When a demyelinated plaque affects the MLF between the oculomotor and abducens nucleus, on one side, there occurs the MLF syndrome: weakness or paralysis of the opposite medial rectus muscle and nystagmus of the laterally deviating eye when gaze is attempted toward the side of the MLF lesion (Figure 1–1). The finding of an MLF syndrome in a young adult is strongly suggestive of the diagnosis of MS that has at least as much specificity for the diagnosis as any current laboratory test.

Diplopia may also be due to a paralysis of the abducens nerve, commonly affected during its intrapontine course from the floor of the fourth ventricle to the ventral surface of the pons. A total oculomotor nerve palsy is rarely seen in MS.

Ataxia in MS usually correlates best with numerous lesions of the cerebellar connections in the brain stem. A lesion of the superior cerebellar peduncle produces a distinct gross intention tremor of the arms, which, when severe, produces a

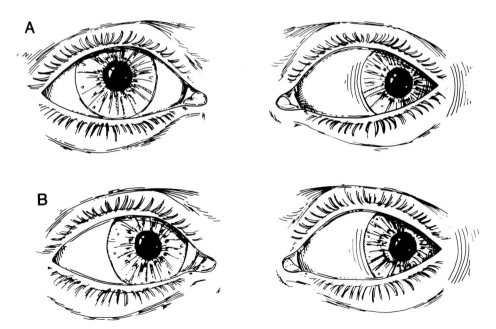

**Figure 1–1** Internuclear ophthalmoplegia due to a lesion of the medial longitudinal fasciculus (MLF). In (A) on attempted left lateral gaze there is paralysis of the right medial rectus muscle and nystagmus of the laterally deviating (left) eye. Lesser degrees of the MLF syndrome are common, as in (B), where there is only slight weakness of the right medial rectus muscle.

"wing-beating" effect on the abducted upper arm. Lesions also occur in the cerebellum itself, but they are usually less marked than in the brain stem.

Acute vertigo results from a new plaque involving the vestibular nuclei in the floor of the fourth ventricle. Vertigo is always associated with gait ataxia, but fortunately, the false sense of rotary movement usually lasts only a few days, at least in severe form. Most patients with chronic ataxia do not have vertigo.

Dysarthria most commonly results either from bilateral corticobulbar tract lesions or from bilateral lesions of the cerebellar brain-stem connections. With the former, one sees a spastic type of speech associated often with difficulty swallowing and either forced crying or forced laughter (the syndrome of pseudobulbar palsy). When the second mechanism is causative, an ataxic dysarthria with irregular emphasis (scanning speech) occurs. Mixed types of dysarthria occur frequently.

The triad of intention tremor, nystagmus, and scanning speech emphasized by Charcot as characteristic of MS is certainly common in far-advanced MS patients. It may be entirely absent, however, and is less characteristic than chronic spastic paraparesis.

A small percentage of patients develop paroxysmal symptoms: those that start suddenly and last only a few seconds, but often recurring frequently. Stabbing facial pain (trigeminal neuralgia) occurs in 5% of MS patients, and its occurrence in young adults should suggest MS. Paroxysmal dysarthria and ataxia may recur many times a day in a small number of patients, with asymptomatic periods between episodes. Painful tonic spasms of the limbs on one side of the body may occur repeatedly, often in response to postural changes. Paroxysmal weakness and sensory symptoms may also occur. Such paroxysmal symptoms typically subside after a few weeks without treatment. They often stop promptly with anticonvulsant medication, suggesting that they are dependent on neuronal discharges in the vicinity of strategically localized lesions.

### The Magnetic Resonance Imaging (MRI) Scan

The MRI scan has proven itself to be approximately 10 times more sensitive for detecting MS lesions than computerized tomography (CT) (Young, et al., 1981). MRI is currently the preferred method of imaging for the diagnosis of MS. Using a large magnet, a radio frequency stimulator, and a computer, this remarkable device is especially sensitive in detecting areas with increased water content in the brain and spinal cord. The latter occurs in a new lesions very early because of an increased permeability of the blood–brain barrier (BBB); in old demyelinated plaques the lost myelin is largely replaced by water. Since the breakdown in BBB is transitory in new lesions (a few days or weeks), such lesions may appear much larger at an early than at a later stage. Another method for distinguishing new from old lesions is by the use of gadolinium, a paramagnetic contrast agent, which passes a leaky BBB (Grossman, et al., 1986).

The MRI is useful for imaging brain-stem lesions (Figure 1–2) and can show some large lesions in the spinal cord. In many patients with clinically definite MS (CDMS), however, spinal cord lesions cannot be seen with present technology; lesions in optic nerves also are often missed.

Overall, MRI scans show more than one white matter lesion in 70–95% of

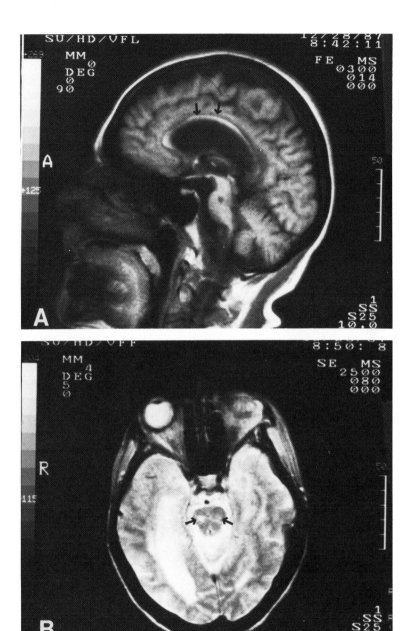

**Figure 1–2** MRI scans in a 46-year-old woman with a marked spastic paraplegia, ataxic arms, and mild cognitive deficit. (A) By the inversion recovery technique (T-1 weighting) a large lesion of the pons is evident as an area of diminished density. Note also the thinness of the corpus callosum (arrows), recently reported to be an imaging correlate of dementia in MS (Huber et al., 1987); (B) by spin-echo technique at least two more lesions of the midbrain can be seen as bright white areas.

patients with CDMS (Asbury et al., 1987). In patients with only optic neuritis or who have only a chronic progressive myelopathy, MRI scans are positive for additional lesions in approximately 60% of cases (D.W. Paty, personal communication).

While the MRI is extremely useful in detecting asymptomatic lesions in MS, under no circumstances should it be used as the sole diagnostic method, since the abnormal images are not specific for MS. Multiple scars from trauma and multiple infarcts from vasculitis (due to lupus, Behcet's disease, or periarteritis nodosa) can simulate MS on MRI scans in young people; such lesions in vasculitis are also commonly in a periventricular location (Miller et al., 1987). Unidentified bright objects (UBOs) in the white matter on $T$2-weighted (spin-echo) MRI sequences become common after the age of 60; some represent infarcts, others dilated perivascular spaces, and in some the cause remains unknown even after postmortem examination. Similar MRI white matter lesions are seen in Lyme disease and in tropical spastic paraparesis (Dalakas et al., 1988), the latter due to HTLV-1 infection and becoming increasingly common in drug addicts in the United States (Robert-Guroff et al., 1986).

## Measurement of Evoked Potentials

Because the neurologic examination may not reveal current evidence of brain stem, optic nerve, or spinal cord disease in some cases—even though the history suggests that these areas may have been involved in the past—and because present MRI technology may also miss some lesions in these areas, there is still a place for measurement of central nerve conduction velocity. Demyelinated axons cannot conduct in a rapid normal saltatory manner (from one node of Ranvier to another). Hence conduction velocity may be markedly delayed, even when this results in no neurologic deficit. The detection of such demyelinated areas may be possible only with evoked potential testing. The most commonly used tests are the visual evoked potentials, auditory evoked potentials, and somatosensory evoked potentials. Abnormally slow velocities measured by these tests can provide evidence for additional lesions, evidence which is not available by other techniques.

## Cerebrospinal Fluid (CSF) Examination

Approximately 25% of patients with clinically active MS will have a pleocytosis in the CSF, usually 5–50 white blood cells/cmm, almost all mononuclear cells. The vast majority of patients with far-advanced MS, confined to a wheelchair, have an elevation of total immunoglobulin G (IgG) fraction in the CSF; however, in early MS the number of patients having elevated IgG in the CSF averages only 10–30%.

When CSF specimens are subjected to electrophoresis on agarose gels, however, the majority of patients—both early and late—show a pattern of several bands in the IgG region. The frequency of this phenomenon in patients with CDMS is recorded in the literature as 70–90%, some laboratories finding them more frequently than others. Oligoclonal bands (OBS), in our experience, are present in about 70% of patients, certainly not in all patients. Patients with autopsy-confirmed

MS have lacked oligoclonal bands (Ebers, 1984). Neither are OBS specific for MS; they may be seen from time to time in a variety of other neurologic diseases, especially chronic infections such as syphilis and subacute panencephalitis. They may also occur occasionally without any obvious explanation.

Nevertheless, examination of the CSF may provide additional evidence for a diagnosis of MS when the diagnosis is not clear on the basis of the history, examination, MRI, and evoked potential studies.

## Diagnostic Criteria

Over two decades ago, a committee chaired by Dr. George Schumacher formulated diagnostic criteria that are still widely used (Schumacher et al., 1965). More recently, a Boston University Workshop (BUW) modified these criteria in recognition of recent technical advances (Poser et al., 1983).

The Schumacher criteria for CDMS required (1) objective abnormalities on neurologic examination, (2) examination or historical evidence of at least two separate lesions that had occurred at least 30 days apart; (3) that the symptoms and signs reflect primarily white matter involvement in patients in the proper age range, lasting at least 24 hours, and (4) that there could be no better explanation for the patient's symptoms and signs, a criterion indicating that the diagnosis be made only by a neurologist or other physician thoroughly familiar with the many other neurologic illnesses that can occasionally simulate MS.

The more recent BUW criteria are similar, but allow the second clinical lesion to be indicated by "paraclinical" evidence such as a typical MRI scan or an abnormal evoked potential test. The BUW guidelines also provide a new category of *laboratory supported definite MS:* when at least one clinical attack and examination evidence of at least one lesion are accompanied by a CSF examination showing oligoclonal bands in the IgG region. The interested reader is referred to the BUW publication, which contains many more details. Some argue that because of the nonspecificity of MRI UBOs and CSF oligoclonal bands, greatest reliance should still be given to the Schumacher criteria to avoid erroneous diagnoses of MS (Kurtzke, 1988).

With either set of diagnostic criteria, it is important to observe the requirement that evidence of new lesions be separated by at least a month: multiple white matter lesions producing similar symptoms may occur over a few days in postinfectious encephalomyelitis, a brief, nonrecurrent illness that must be distinguished from MS.

## COURSE

The variability of the course of MS is exemplified by some patients who have two or three exacerbations in a lifetime and never become disabled; at the other extreme are a few individuals who have frequent attacks, leading to death within a few months. At the present time it is impossible to predict the course any individual patient will follow. A long time after diagnosis with minimal disability often portends a benign course, but there are many exceptions. At least 20–30% of patients never become seriously disabled and continue to work productively 20–25 years after onset (Bauer and Firnhaber, 1965; MacKay and Hirano, 1967).

Most evidence suggests a strong environmental factor in the causation of MS. The exact agents responsible for the new lesions are unknown, but at least two recent studies suggest that recent viral infections are a risk factor (Sibley et al., 1985; Narod et al., 1985). One possibility is that this is a nonspecific effect of all viral infections, perhaps due to the release of gamma interferon (shown in one study to increase the frequency of exacerbations). Another possibility is that the phenomenon is a specific effect of only certain viral molecules and that the immune system mistakes peptide sequences in certain myelin proteins for virus (molecular mimicry).

In one 8-year prospective study viruslike infection was the only identifiable risk factor; it was not possible to show any adverse effect on clinical course from such things as physical trauma or stressful life events (Sibley, 1988).

About 85% of patients have a relapsing-remitting form of the disease, at least in the early years. Clinical recovery is often complete after the first attack. Among early patients a clinical exacerbation rate of 0.5–1/year is common. A recent study of a group of such patients in Vancouver, B.C., done with serial MRI scans, showed that the actual frequency of new lesions per patient was about 3/year (Willoughby et al., 1989). Thus it is apparent that only a minority of new lesions are expressed with new symptoms.

Approximately 15% of patients never have an exacerbation, but rather have slow progression of disability from the onset of disease. The majority of relapsing-remitting patients also have a slow progression of disability, because recovery is often incomplete from the disability induced by exacerbations occurring later in the illness.

The rate and manner of progression of disability has been studied by several workers (Muller, 1949; Fog, 1966; McAlpine et al., 1972). Although these studies taught us much about the natural history of MS, they were restrospective and descriptive and do not provide good guidelines to predict the course of groups of untreated patients. At the present time, with many patients receiving some type of chronic treatment, this problem is especially difficult to study.

From 1976 to 1983 we followed the course of disability in 170 patients (average follow-up 5.3 years). These patients were examined at least every three months and given Kurtzke Disability Status Scale (DSS) ratings. They received no treatment other than a short course of prednisone or ACTH for acute exacerbations. It can be seen (Table 1–1) that the annual exacerbation rate was highest in fully ambulatory patients with less disability (DSS 0–5) as was the rate of disability progression. In patients requiring aids to ambulate (DSS 6–7) and in nonambulatory patients (DSS 8–9), the rate of progression was very slow, perhaps reflecting the difficulty in clinical detection of new lesions in already badly damaged neuraxes.

Recent serial studies of a group of chronic-progressive MS cases indicate that clinical detection of disease activity is faulty in advanced patients, since the average patient with chronic-progressive MS in one series had six new MRI lesions per year, about twice as many as in those with relapsing-remitting disease (Koopmans et al., 1989). In spite of this, enough serial MRI scans have been done over a 2–3

**Table 1-1** The Mean Progress of Disability and Exacerbation Rates of 170 MS Patients at the University of Arizona Hospital Clinic during an 8-Year Period[a]

| Entry DSS[b] | No. pts. | Ann. Exac. Rate | Mean Follow-up (years) | Mean Exit DSS[b] |
|---|---|---|---|---|
| 0 | 10 | .16 | 5.5 | 0.7 |
| 1 | 22 | .50 | 5.7 | 2.3 |
| 2 | 19 | .50 | 4.3 | 3.4 |
| 3 | 18 | .39 | 4.6 | 4.1 |
| 4 | 14 | .30 | 5.0 | 5.2 |
| 5 | 12 | .30 | 6.0 | 5.8 |
| 6 | 32 | .16 | 5.0 | 6.5 |
| 7 | 28 | .17 | 5.6 | 7.7 |
| 8 | 9 | .03 | 6.2 | 8.3 |
| 9 | 6 | .02 | 6.2 | 9.2 |

[a]Mean observation period 5.3 years/patient.
[b]DSS: Kurtzke Disability Status Scale.

year period in some individual patients to know that clinical inactivity and MRI inactivity coincide at least occasionally. The implication, both for research efforts and treatment studies, of recent serial MRI studies done in groups of patients is obvious: no method of measuring activity of the MS process can be complete without repeated MRI monitoring.

## REFERENCES

Asbury, A.K., Herndon, R.M., McFarland, H.F., McDonald, W.I., McIlroy, W.J., Paty, D.W., Prineas, J.W., Scheinberg, L.C., and Wolinsky, J.S. (1987). National Multiple Sclerosis Society Working Group on Neuroimaging for the Medical Advisory Board (Editorial). *Neuroradiology, 29,* 119.

Bauer, J.J., and Firnhaber, W. (1965). Prognostic criteria in multiple sclerosis. *Ann. N.Y. Acad. Sci., 122,* 542–51.

Dalakas, M.C., Stone, G., Elder, G., Ceroni, M., Madden, D., Roman, G., Sever, J.L. (1988). Tropical spastic paraparesis: clinical, immunological, and virological studies in two patients from Martinique. *Ann. Neurol.,* 23 (Suppl. *Retroviruses in the Nervous System*).

Ebers, G.C. (1984). Cerebrospinal fluid electrophoresis in multiple sclerosis. In Poser, C. et al., eds. *The Diagnosis of Multiple Sclerosis* pp. 179–84, New York: Thieme-Stratton.

Fog, T. (1966). The course of multiple sclerosis. *Acta Neurol. Scand., 42,* 608–11.

Grossman, R.I., Gonzalez-Scarano, F., Atlas, S.W., Galetta, S., and Silberberg, D.H. (1986). Multiple sclerosis: gadolinium enhancement in MR imaging. *Radiology, 161,* 721–25.

Huber, S.J., Paulson, G.W., Shuttleworth, E.C., Chakeres, B., Clapp, L.E., Pakalnis, A., Weiss, K., and Rammohan, K. (1987). Magnetic resonance imaging correlates of dementia in multiple sclerosis. *Arch. Neurol., 44,* 732–36.

Koopmans, R.A., Li, D.K.B., Oger, J.J.F., Kastrukoff, L.F., Jardine, C., Costley, L., Hall, S., Grochowski, E.W., and Paty, D.W., (1989). Chronic progressive multiple sclerosis: serial magnetic resonance brain imaging over six months. *Ann. Neurol., 26,* 248–256.

Kurtzke, J.F. (1988). Multiple sclerosis: What's in a name? *Neurology, 38,* 309–16.

MacKay, R.P., and Hirano, A. (1967). Forms of benign multiple sclerosis. *Arch. Neurol., 17,*588–92.

McAlpine, D., Lumsden, C.E., and Acheson, E.D. (1972). Course and prognosis. In: *Multiple Sclerosis—A Reappraisal.*, p. 223, London: Churchill-Livingstone.

Miller, D.H., Ormerod, I.E.C., Gibson, A., du Boulay, E.P.G.H., Rudge, P., and McDonald, W.I. (1987). MR brain scanning in patients with vasculitis: differentiation from multiple sclerosis. *Neuroradiology,* **29,** 226–31.

Muller, R. (1949). Studies on disseminated sclerosis with special reference to symptomatology, course and prognosis. *Acta Med. Scand.,* **133** (Suppl. 222).

Narod, S., Johnson-Lussenburg, C.M., Zheng, Q., and Nelson, R. (1985). Viral infections and MS. *Lancet,* **2,** 165.

Poser, C.M., Paty, D.W., Scheinberg, L., McDonald, W.I., Davis, F.A., Ebers, G.C., Johnson, K.P., Sibley, W.A., Silberberg, D.H., and Tourtellotte, W.W. (1983). New diagnostic criteria for multiple sclerosis. *Ann. Neurol.,* **13,** 227-31.

Robert-Guroff, M., Weiss, S.H., Giron, J.A., Jennings, A.M., Ginzburg, H.M., Margolis, L.B., Blattner, W.A., and Gallo, R.C. (1986). Prevalence of antibodies to HTLV-I, -II, and III in, intravenous drug abusers from an AIDS endemic region. *J.A.M.A.,* **255,** 3133–37.

Schumacher, G.A., Beebe, G., Kibler, R.F., Kurland, L.T., Kurtzke, J.F., McDowell, F., Nagler, B., Sibley, W.A., Tourtellotte, W.W., and Willmon, T.F. (1965). Problems of experimental trials of therapy in multiple sclerosis; report by the panel on the evaluation of experimental trials of therapy in multiple sclerosis. *Ann. N.Y. Acad. Sci.,* **122,** 552-6.

Sibley, W.A., Bamford, C.R., and Clark, K. (1985). Clinical viral infections and multiple sclerosis. *Lancet,* **1,** 1313–5.

Sibley, W.A., Bamford, C.R., and Clark, K. (1984). Triggering factors in multiple sclerosis. In: C. Poser et al., eds. *Diagnosis of Multiple Sclerosis,* pp. 14–24. New York: Thieme-Stratton.

Sibley, W.A. (1988). Risk factors in multiple sclerosis—implications for pathogenesis. In: G. Serlupi Crescenzi, ed. *A Multidisciplinary Approach to Myelin Diseases.* New York: Plenum.

Willoughby, E.W., Grochowski, E., Li, D.B.K., Oger, J., Kastrukoff, L.F., and Paty, D.W. (1989). Serial magnetic resonance scanning in multiple sclerosis: a second prospective study in relapsing patients. Ann. Neurol., **25,** 43–49.

Young, I.R., Hall, A.S., Pallis, C.A., Legg, N.J., Bydder, G.M., and Steiner, R.E. (1981). Nuclear magnetic resonance imaging of the brain in multiple sclerosis. *Lancet,* **2,** 1063–6.

# 2

# Neuropathology

CEDRIC S. RAINE

Multiple sclerosis (MS) is a disease of white matter, and its major clinical manifestations are related to sensory and motor dysfunction. The disturbances in mentation that occur in some patients run the gamut from euphoria to dementia. These are probably related to massive involvement of white matter rather than gray matter, particularly in paraventricular frontal regions. This chapter deals with the salient neuropathological features of MS which render it the paradigm of the human demyelinating diseases (see Table 2–1). Except for brief mention of other members of the group, the present analysis does not dwell on differences among the group since these aspects have been covered elsewhere in extensive detail (Roizin et al., 1982; Allen, 1984; Raine, 1984a, 1985a). Clinically, MS is an enigmatic disease, and its accurate diagnosis is often a lengthy process fraught with pitfalls. It is not unusual for definitive diagnosis to come from the final autopsy report. MS is an intriguing neurologic entity with clinical and pathological manifestations that can be attributed to the destruction of a single membrane unique to nervous tissue, myelin, and of the cell that elaborates it, the oligodendrocyte. Neuropathologically, MS stands alone, in that no other disease displays a lesion with the same degree of selectivity in the destructive process.

From the pathological standpoint, the inseparable association between inflammation and lesion activity has been instrumental to the view that myelin loss in MS may result from an immunologic attack precipitated by sensitization either to myelin or to an infectious agent sequestered within the central nervous system (CNS). The recognition that enlargement of the zones of myelin depletion correlates with periods of clinical activity and occurs against a backdrop of waves of

**Table 2-1**   Classification of the Demyelinating Diseases

*Central nervous system (CNS)*
1. Chronic MS
2. Variants of MS
      Acute MS (Marburg type)
      Neuromyelitis optica (Devic's)
      Concentric sclerosis (Balo's)
3. Acute disseminated encephalomyelitis
      Postinfectious encephalomyelitis
      Postimmunization encephalomyelitis
4. Acute hemorrhagic leukoencephalopathy
5. Progressive multifocal leukoencephalopathy

*Peripheral nervous system (PNS)*
6. Idiopathic polyneuritis
7. Diphtheric neuropathy

cellular infiltration (e.g., Adams and Kubik, 1952), now well documented immunocytochemically (Traugott et al., 1983a,b; Booss et al., 1983; Hauser et al., 1983), has led to innovative therapeutic rationales for clinical intervention.

The following paragraphs provide an update of the appearance and genesis of the MS plaque and perhaps help clarify some of the hitherto unexplained facets of lesion development.

## DEFINITION AND CLASSIFICATION

*Demyelination* is a term reserved by neuropathologists for the MS group of conditions (i.e., the acquired inflammatory and infectious diseases of myelin, see Raine, 1984a) and refers to the selective loss of myelin from white matter, leaving axons denuded but intact. The process almost invariably occurs as the result of an inflammatory event and culminates with the formation of demyelinated foci, plaques, which in the brain of an MS patient reach grossly visible diameters, sometimes 2–3 cm wide and several centimeters long. The basic histologic hallmark of the condition is a perivascular cuff of inflammatory cells surrounded by a rim of demyelination. It is believed that by the fusion of many such foci, the demyelinated plaque is formed. The historical nosology of demyelination is given in greater detail elsewhere (e.g., Raine, 1985a).

While no consensus currently exists among neuropathologists as to what constitute the classification constraints of the diseases in which myelin loss is a feature (namely, the hereditary, metabolic, and toxic diseases of myelin, Raine 1984a), the members of the group of which MS is the archetype are usually regarded as the true demyelinating diseases.

With only a few exceptions the common denominator of the demyelinated plaque is myelin and oligodendroglial cells loss. Inflammation, fibrillary astrogliosis (scarring), relative sparing of axons, and fibrosis of vessels are common and occur in varying degrees. These features are best seen in MS which, in general, stands apart from all other members of the group in terms of its chronicity and variation in clinical presentation (acute, chronic, relapsing-remitting, and progressive). Its variant forms tend to be more acute and display a higher mortality. The clinical aspects of the various forms of MS are covered in detail earlier in this volume (see Introduction and Chapter 1).

## MYELIN—THE TARGET

White matter, the battlefield of the CNS myelin diseases, is white because it is made up of millions of nerve fibers, each of which is covered (insulated) by multiple lengths (internodes) of myelin. Each myelin sheath is formed from layers of compacted oligodendroglial cell membrane (myelin) which is unusually rich in lipids (70% lipid, 30% protein) and which serves to separate the axon functionally and to expedite impulses along the fibers by saltatory conduction (Ritchie, 1984). Myelin is the major structural component of normal white matter (Figure 2–1). It accounts for about 25% of the dry weight of the brain. Each sheath is elaborated around a segment of axon by the spiral wrapping and flattening of a cell process from an oligodendrocyte (Figures 2–2 and 2–3) which forms an internode of myelin, being demarcated at either end by a node of Ranvier. The onset and cessation of myelination are believed to be orchestrated by neuronal signals (see Raine, 1984b).

Myelin possesses a number of unique components that can be used experimentally as immunogens to induce its own selective, immune-mediated destruction or to produce specific antibodies against itself which can then be used as experimental

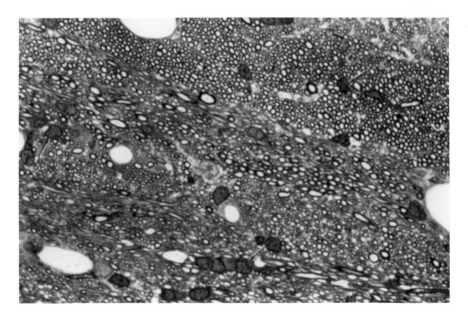

**Figure 2-1** An area of normal white matter consists mainly of myelinated nerve fibers (black rings), mostly in cross section. Interfascicular oligodendrocytes (densely staining cells at arrows), an occasional astrocyte (pale staining nucleus and cytoplasm at *) and a few blood vessels (clear spaces) are also present. One-micron epoxy section, stained with toluidine blue. × 650. (From Raine, 1985a; with permission.)

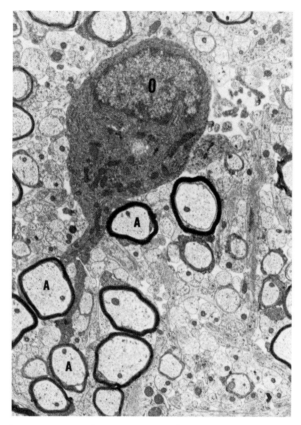

**Figure 2–2** An electron micrograph from an area of developing white matter shows an oligodendrocyte (0) connected to myelin sheaths around three axons (A) by bridges of cytoplasm. Elsewhere in the field, nerve fibers at different stages of myelination can be seen as well as many yet to be invested by oligodendroglial cytoplasm. × 8000.

probes in the analysis of myelin and myelination. By possessing unique, potent antigens, myelin renders the CNS highly vulnerable to autoimmune-mediated processes. For example, there is the distinct possibility that whenever the blood–brain barrier (BBB) is breached (e.g., by trauma), the immunologic privilege of the CNS is lost, and cells of the immune system enter, fail to recognize constitutive components of the CNS (from which they have been previously sequestered), and mount an immunologic attack on the tissue. The ability of the experimentalist to create a pattern of myelin pathology similar to that observed in MS in animals by sensitization to myelin antigens (or by the injection of lymphocytes recognizing myelin antigens) has led to suggestions that MS is an autoimmune disease (see Raine, 1985b). The nature of the putative antigen in MS remains to be elucidated, however.

Aligned often in rows among bundles of myelinated axons are interfascicular oligodendrocytes, the cells responsible for CNS myelination. Oligodendrocytes are heavily outnumbered by the myelin sheaths they produce, and it has been estimated that each cell is capable of elaborating and maintaining between 30 and 50

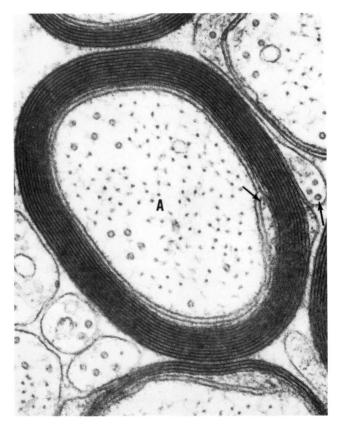

**Figure 2-3** A high-power view of a myelinated nerve fiber shows a spirally-wrapped myelin sheath around an axon (A) containing microtubules and cross-bridged neurofilaments. The inner and outer tongues of oligodendroglial cytoplasm (the beginning and end of the myelin membrane) are also apparent (arrows). The myelin period is about 11 nm between each pair of major dense lines. For further details on the process of myelination, see Raine 1984b and 1985c. × 75,000.

internodes (segments) of sheath. This 1:30–1:50 ratio means that each oligodendrocyte must make and support 1000–3000 times its own cell membrane at considerable distances from the cell soma (Raine, 1985c). Most myelin-specific components also occur in oligodendrocytes, albeit in lower concentration. Thus the cell body is also a potential target for immunologic attack. Separating and penetrating the bundles of myelinated nerve fibers in the CNS are astrocytes, which are the second glial cell type and the major supporting and structural elements of gray and white matter and the cells that react to injury by proliferating and synthesizing glial fibrils. This fibrillary astrogliosis leads to a state of sclerosis (scarring), a pathological hallmark of the MS plaque. Astrocytes in gray matter (protoplasmic astrocytes) and white matter (fibrous astrocytes) usually form a barrier to or, in special cases, a route of entry for molecules passing from the bloodstream or meninges into the white matter parenchyma. The layer of astrocytes separating white matter from the meninges and blood vessels is known as the *glia limitans*. Completing the components that make up white matter are the microglia, the resident macrophages of the CNS which are of mesodermal (hematogenous) origin, and blood vessels. The manner in which these structural components (oligodendrocytes, astrocytes, microglia, and blood vessels) interact with the cells of the immune system appears to determine the pathogenesis of the demyelinated lesion.

## THE CLASSIC (CHRONIC) LESION

Macroscopic examination of the MS brain usually reveals no superficial abnormalities, and the brain weight is unremarkable. Areas where white matter forms the surface of the CNS, such as optic nerve, brain stem and spinal cord, however, frequently display atrophy and patches of gray discoloration (demyelination). Coronal section of the brain reveals large plaques varying in appearance, texture, size, shape, number, and topography (Figure 2–4). Variations among these parameters sometimes reflect lesion age and activity, inasmuch as pink, soft lesions are recent and active, while gray, glassy regions are typically older. Lesion location in MS defies clinical and anatomical explanation. It is frequently found at autopsy that the degree of involvement exceeds by far that which might have been anticipated from the clinical history. MS has on many occasions only been diagnosed at autopsy in the total absence of clinical history—so-called benign multiple sclerosis.

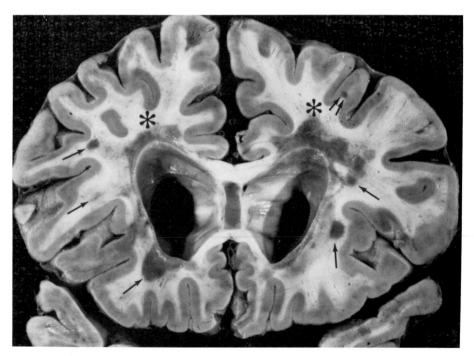

**Figure 2–4**  Coronal section of the brain from a case of chronic MS. Multiple, disseminated plaques of demyelination (arrows) occur throughout the white matter. Note the predominance of paraventricular involvement, particularly the "Wetterwinkel" zones (*). A small lesion at the top of the gyrus is also evident (double arrow, upper right). Plaques can also be seen deeper and more frontally along the roof of the ventricles. (From Raine, 1985a; with permission.)

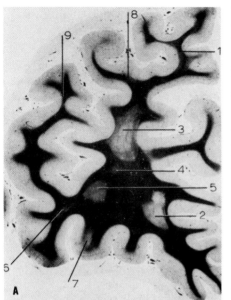
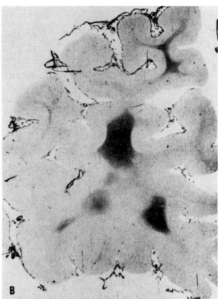

**Figure 2–5** Cerebral MS plaques (numbered 1–9) are shown in (A) stained for myelin and in (B) for gliofibrils. The different ages and degree of demyelinated lesions in (A) correlate with the extent of the fibrillary gliosis in (B). (From Raine, 1985a; with permission.)

While no area of vulnerability can be consistently identified in MS, there is a tendency for paraventricular white matter to be involved, and such lesions are often centered on subependymal vessels. One common paraventricular area of involvement is the angle between the caudate nucleus and the corpus callosum— the so-called Wetterwinkel or storm center of Steiner (see Raine, 1985a). Small lesions commonly occur at the tips of gyri where they may spill over into nearby gray matter (perhaps accounting for some of the disturbances in mentation), which also contains myelinated fibers. No region of the neuraxis is spared, and the disease can strike gray and white matter structures alike, that is, wherever myelinated axons are found. Optic nerve, chiasm, optic tract, and spinal cord lesions are very common in MS, and there are suggestions that these may originate in relation to subpial vessels. As is the case elsewhere in the CNS, brain and spinal cord lesions demonstrate no regularity or symmetry (features which distinguish MS from some of the metabolic disorders of myelin that are typified by large symmetrical lesions) and disregard functional and anatomical boundaries.

From the microscopic standpoint, it is difficult to better some of the descriptions of earlier neuropathologists like Dawson (1916), who perceived that the lesion of chronic MS is frequently centered on a small vein from which the disease process appears to spread. Myelin staining of a chronic lesion reveals the demyelinated area to be sharply demarcated from adjacent white matter, giving it a punched-out appearance (Greenfield and King, 1936; Lumsden, 1970; Raine, 1985a). It is accepted that the sharpness of the plaque contour equates with chronicity and that the demyelinated area will, in adjacent sections, be matched by robust fibrillary astrogliosis (Figure 2–5)—the so-called isomorphic gliosis of the older literature.

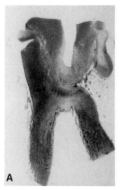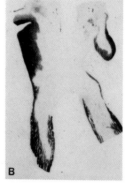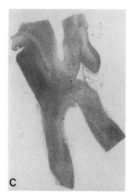

**Figure 2-6**   Adjacent sections of a lesion involving the optic chiasm in a case of chronic MS are stained by H + E in (A), a myelin stain in (B), and an axon stain in (C), to show the relative sparing of axons. (From Raine, 1985a; with permission.)

Axon stains confirm the relative sparing of axons (Figure 2–6), particularly at the periphery of the lesion, although deeper (older) areas show fiber depletion that increases with the age of the lesion. Axons in chronically demyelinated lesions display shrinkage, and severe loss of axons is associated only in about 10% of all MS cases studied (Greenfield and King, 1936). Consistent with its lack of regard for anatomic boundaries, areas of involvement in MS can vary from one level to another—for example, the spinal cord. Related to the loss of myelin and the intense fibrillary astrogliosis, atrophy or shrinkage of affected regions is not uncommon.

Most chronic silent lesions have an overall acellular appearance, being made up in large part of a network of fibrous astrocytes, a major contributor to the color and texture of the lesion. Astroglial cell bodies are often hypertrophic and sometimes multinucleated. They give rise to twiglike cell processes which are generally loose and open in cerebral white matter lesions but tightly packed in spinal cord and optic nerve lesions. This astroglial network invests demyelinated axons as they traverse the plaque (Figure 2–7). At the perimeter of lesions, axons abruptly lose their myelin sheaths. Hypertrophic astrocytes and fibrillary astrogliosis often spill over into the adjacent myelinated white matter.

Oligodendrocytes are almost invariably absent from deeper areas of chronic lesions, although about the margins, oligodendroglial hyperplasia and myelin regeneration are not uncommon. Microglial cells are present as foamy cells that stain positively with lipid stains. These macrophages have other synonyms such as fat granule cells, compound granular corpuscles, foamy cells, histiocytes, and Gitter cells. They occur scattered among demyelinated axons, are sometimes related to blood vessels (Figure 2–8), and are diffusely spread throughout the adjacent myelinated white matter. They are also involved in myelin phagocytosis, discussed in the next section.

Blood vessels in MS plaques display a wide spectrum of changes, usually a reflection of prior inflammatory activity. The most common change is a nonspecific increase in the space between the endothelial cells of the vessel wall and the glia limitans of the CNS parenchyma—the Virchow-Robin space. This space becomes hyalinized and fibrotic subsequent to inflammation, when it accumulates

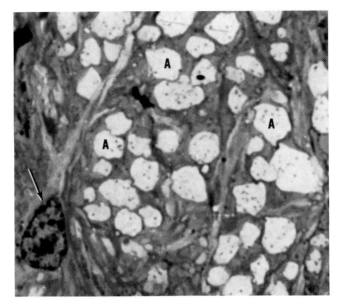

**Figure 2-7**  A light micrograph of a spinal cord lesion shows a group of demyelinated axons (A) in cross section embedded in a matrix of fibrillary gliosis. The body of a fibrous astrocyte (arrow) is also seen. One-micron epoxy section; toluidine blue stain. × 1100.

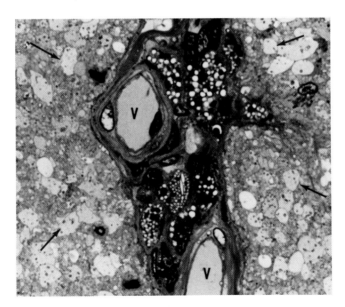

**Figure 2-8**  An area of spinal cord demyelination contains many naked axons (arrows) and a vessel (lumen at V) surrounded by a cuff of cells, most of which are foamy macrophages. A few plasma cells are also present. One-micron epoxy section, toluidine blue stain. × 400.

collagen and fibroblasts. Often, the Virchow-Robin space also contains collections of lipid-laden microglial cells, perhaps en route to the bloodstream (Figure 2–8). In active chronic lesions, the Virchow-Robin space becomes filled with lymphocytes, monocytes, and plasma cells. The glia limitans is often thickened, shows intense fibrillary gliosis, and is scalloped.

It is unlikely that a chronic MS lesion is ever pathologically silent. Close scrutiny with immunocytochemical probes invariably reveals the occasional parenchymal T cell, plasma cells around blood vessels, scattered foamy macrophages, and a small amount of myelin breakdown at the interface between plaque and adjacent white matter. The cells have been quantitated and characterized by different techniques (e.g., electron microscopy, Prineas and Wright, 1978; immunocytochemistry, Traugott et al., 1983b). The consensus is that in chronic "established" lesions, plasma cells predominate, T cells are present but in small numbers, macrophages (monocytes) occur but are difficult to distinguish from microglial cells, and a rare mast cell is not unusual. Polymorphonuclear leukocytes are never seen.

## CHRONIC ACTIVE AND ACUTE MS LESIONS

Chronic active MS lesions refer to established plaques within or around which inflammatory activity, myelin phagocytosis, and lesion extension are in evidence. Extracellular edema occurs and a shelving edge of lipid-filled macrophages separates the established plaque from adjacent, unaffected white matter (Adams, 1983). Some oligodendroglial hyperplasia is occasionally seen. The lesion retains a punched-out appearance, but the margin is less distinct than that of a chronic silent lesion. Occasionally, a finger of demyelinative activity extends from the plaque as a sleeve around the perivascular space of a blood vessel.

Acute MS lesions typify the rare form of MS, acute MS, which has a rapid onset, short duration, and a frequently fatal outcome. The clinical history is typically weeks to months after onset of neurologic signs. The term *acute MS,* often mistakenly ascribed to a period of activity in chronic-relapsing MS, is reserved for this condition. Fresh lesions occurring in previously unaffected white matter in chronic MS overlap histologically with acute MS lesions. Acute MS lesions are grossly visible and pink at autopsy; display a topography typical of chronic MS plaques; are intensely cellular, edematous, and filled with foamy macrophages; and have an indistinct margin. In life, the condition is difficult to differentiate from acute disseminated encephalomyelitis (ADE) such as postinfectious encephalomyelitis, but the typical MS lesion topography distinguishes it from ADE (ADE lesions are almost invariably microscopic, perivascular, and subpial; see Alvord, 1985).

It might sometimes be difficult to recognize CNS elements in acute MS lesions, because the inflammatory process disrupts the tissue architecture (Prineas and Raine, 1976). Hypertrophic astrocytes and fibers undergoing demyelination can be demonstrated, however. Small lymphocytes and macrophages occupy the Virchow-Robin spaces of blood vessels and permeate the parenchyma. Polymorphonuclear cells are not seen. The lesion margin is not sharp but merges gradually with the adjacent white matter. Some of the many small nuclei at the margin of the lesion may belong to hyperplastic oligodendrocytes, because it is known that these cells can proliferate during periods of active disease (Raine et al., 1981).

## PATHOGENESIS OF THE MS LESION

The development of the MS plaque attends a loss of immunologic privilege within the CNS, a breach in the BBB (normally impermeable except for small molecules), infiltration of the tissue by cells and products of the immune system, destruction of target antigen, and formation of a scar. While the antecedent provocateur of these events still evades researchers, it is generally believed to be a childhood viral infection that leads to autosensitization to myelin antigens. Of the several viruses linked to MS, a paramyxovirus of the measles type is the most often implicated. It would appear from the literature that separate but closely related roles are played in lesion genesis by T cells and immunoglobulin, that T cells are the initial crusaders, but that once the lesion is established, it appears to become more a site for immunoglobulin synthesis than a T cell depot. The demonstration of the intra-CNS synthesis of immunoglobulin G (IgG) (Tourtellotte et al., 1984), the localization of IgG and plasma cells within lesions (Esiri et al., 1976; Prineas and Raine, 1976), the presence of oligoclonal IgG in the CSF (Ebers, 1984), and the ability for MS serum to cause demyelination in vitro (see Raine, 1984c) suggest a pathogenetic role for antibody in MS, albeit later than that of T cells.

The presence of patterns of cellular infiltration within the acute MS lesion, which are very similar to those seen in animals sensitized for experimental allergic encephalomyelitis (EAE, a T cell–mediated autoimmune condition), has traditionally provided a major link between MS and allergic or autoimmune models. It was not until 1983, however, that T cells were unequivocally demonstrated with monoclonal antibodies in MS plaques (Traugott et al., 1983a,b). Moreover, identified subsets of T cells were discernible within MS lesions of different ages, as discussed below.

Precisely what precipitates the invasion of the normally sequestered CNS by cells of the immune system has been the subject of much research in recent years. Evidence is burgeoning that active disease correlates with the appearance in the CNS of transplantation antigens, molecules normally not expressed by nervous tissue, on the lining of blood vessels and on astrocytes (Traugott et al., 1985b). These observations correlate with the known propensity of endothelial cells and astrocytes to express class II major histocompatibility complex (MHC) molecules in vitro, a phenomenon that can be up-regulated by the cytokine, interferon (Burger et al., 1981; Pober et al., 1983). Since class II MHC (Ia) are associated with antigen presentation [helper T cells only recognize antigen on the surface of antigen presenting cells (APCs) in the context of Ia], this raises the possibility that these cells might function as APCs during plaque formation.

Thus the following hypothetical scenario, which is supported by several lines of indirect evidence, represents the present working hypothesis for MS lesion formation. As a result of an intercurrent viral infection or another stressful event, lymphokines (e.g., interferon gamma) are released into the circulation and cause system-wide (including CNS) up-regulation of Ia molecule expression on endothelial cells. Within the CNS, the endothelial Ia becomes associated with circulating fragments of myelin basic protein (demonstrated by several workers, e.g., Whitaker, 1984). This Ia/antigen complex is recognized by appropriately sensitized T cells that attach to the vessel wall, release lymphokines, and recruit, in a nonantigen-specific fashion, other T cells to the site. These cells then secrete soluble mediators that cause a breach in the vessel wall, and cells enter the CNS. Monocytes and B cells are then recruited by the CD4 cascade and antibody synthesis, and target cell damage occurs. The cessation of each wave of inflammatory events might be the result of some feedback mechanism that causes down-regulation of Ia expression. Astrocytic expression of Ia appears to follow that of endothelial cells and may be related to lesion extension and later events.

Thus the initial inflammatory events are believed to be orchestrated by T cells (Traugott et al., 1983a,b; Booss et al., 1983; Hauser et al., 1984). In this process, CD4+ T cells have been interpreted to have a primary role, entering the CNS and migrating to the white matter parenchyma, where they interact with Ia-expressing APCs (microglial cells, the endogenous macrophages of CNS tissue, see Figure 2–9). The latter presumably process and present myelin antigens. CD8+ T cells, which are claimed by some to appear later, are restricted more to perivascular spaces at the perimeter of the (resolving?) lesion and might down-regulate the CD4 response. Evidence from longitudinal studies of EAE in the guinea pig, mouse, and rat has shown similar sequences of events (Sobel et al., 1983, 1987; Traugott et al., 1985a, 1986; Matsumoto and Fujiwara, 1987). Established, silent chronic MS lesions reveal few T cells (Traugott et al., 1983a,b), B cells are common (Prineas and Wright, 1978), and Ia expression is seen at low levels on the occasional microglial cell.

In the process of myelin breakdown, microglial cells are major participants. Within lesions displaying active inflammation and myelin breakdown they express Ia and are associated with lymphocytes (Figure 2–9). Myelin becomes dissociated from nerve fibers, either while in contact with a microglial cell which internalizes directly the debris into lysosomal vacuoles (Figure 2–10) or as extracellular droplets (Figure 2–11) which are then phagocytosed by microglial cells. Presumably, therefore, soluble mediators of as yet unknown origin and specificity (antibody/complement, cytokines, proteolytic enzymes) are responsible for the lysis of the myelin from the sheath, and the microglial cell phagocytoses the damaged membrane material. In addition to the phagocytosis of large droplets of myelin, smaller fragments also become attached to the surface of macrophages at structures known as clathrin-coated pits, a common site for receptor-mediated uptake of material in a number of cell systems (Pastan and Willingham, 1981). From these points of attachment, the myelin debris is selectively internalized by the macrophage (Figure 2–12) (Prineas and Connell, 1978; Epstein et al., 1983). Recently, it has been shown that IgG serves as a ligand in this receptor-mediated phagocytosis of myelin, presumably by Fc receptors (Moore and Raine, 1988).

Astrocytes respond very early during plaque formation by becoming hypertrophic and then, as the period of infiltration and tissue breakdown subsides, they undergo fibrillary astrogliosis and may develop multiple nuclei. In addition, they have also been shown to express Ia molecules (Traugott et al., 1985b) and to par-

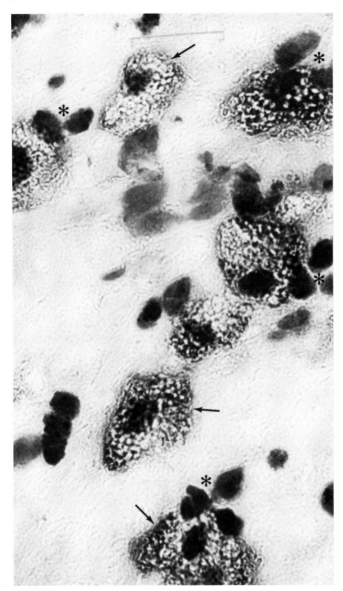

**Figure 2–9**  An active chronic MS lesion is stained with an anti-Ia monoclonal antibody and coun-
terstained with hematoxylin. Ia-positive foamy microglial cells are seen (arrows), some of which
are associated with groups of small nuclei, probably belonging to T cells (*). × 1000. (From Traugott et al. 1983b; with permission.)

ticipate in myelin and oligodendrocyte degradation (Raine, 1983; Raine and
Scheinberg, 1988). Therefore, like the microglial cell, the astrocyte is both a potential phagocyte and an orchestrator of immunologic events. Similar activity by
astrocytes might have been inferred from observations on these cells in vitro (Fontana et al., 1984).

In most considerations of the genesis of MS lesions, oligodendrocytes have

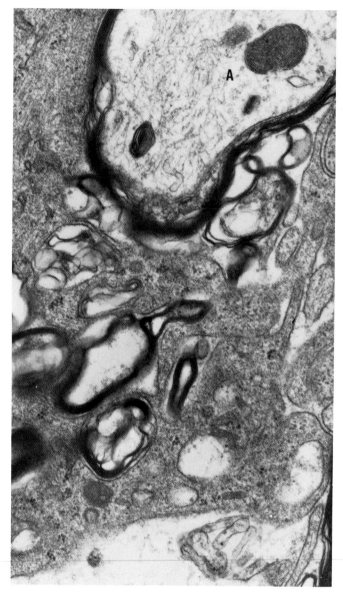

**Figure 2-10**  Fingers of cytoplasm from a microglial cell invest a myelinated fiber (axon at A) and are engaged in the internalization of myelin debris as it is lysed from the myelin sheath above. ×37,000.

played a central role. Their selective depletion from MS lesions gave rise to the oligodendrogliolysis theory of Lumsden (1955), a theory that was later reincarnated by reports on anti-oligodendrocyte antibodies and on oligodendrocytes sharing antigens with suppressor T cells (Abramsky et al., 1977; Oger et al., 1982) which implied primary, selective damage to oligodendrocytes in MS. Subsequent works from other groups were unable to confirm these reports (see Raine, 1983). Indeed,

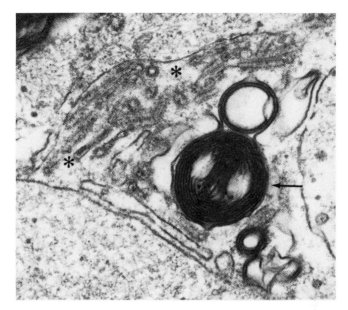

**Figure 2-11** Within the extracellular space of an active chronic lesion, myelin debris is seen, some of which (arrow) has retained its typical lamellar pattern and some of which has been transformed into rodlike profiles (*). × 55,000.

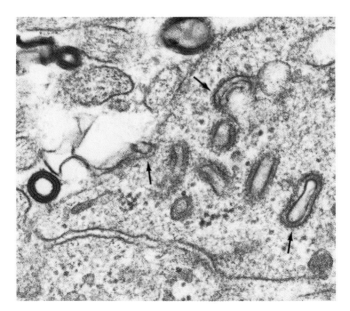

**Figure 2-12** Myelin debris is seen in the process of being internalized by a microglial cell after its attachment to a coated pit on the surface of the cell (arrows). Lamellar myelin debris also lies in the extracellular space (above and left). × 55,000.

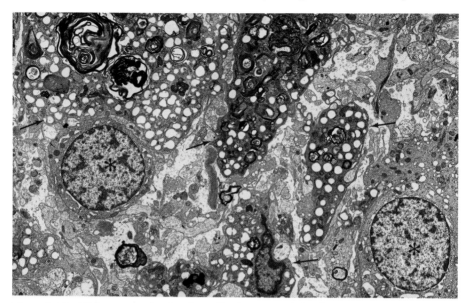

**Figure 2-13**  With an area of active demyelination, microglial cells (arrows) are filled with lipid droplets and myelin debris. Two oligodendrocytes (*) have survived the destruction. Several small-diameter, naked axons and processes from fibrous astrocytes can be seen in the neuropil. × 5600. (From Raine, 1985a; with permission).

there are numerous reports demonstrating that myelin is the primary target, that oligodendrocytes survive the initial period of myelination, and that these cells are capable of surviving and proliferating (Figure 2-13) (Raine et al., 1981; Ibrahim and Adams, 1963; Raine and Traugott, 1985). Oligodendrocytes in active MS lesions have recently been shown not to express Ia and are therefore probably not involved as APCS (Lee and Raine, in press).

## REMYELINATION

In most classical pictures of the neuropathology of MS, little canvas is given to the topic of myelin regeneration (remyelination). This omission was probably due to three factors. First was the belief that the CNS was incapable of remyelination, a view held with some dogmatism until quite recently (Lumsden, 1970). Second, what was probably remyelination was a lesion termed a *Markschattenherde* by Schlesinger (1910), which today is known as a *shadow plaque* or a well-demarcated area of myelin thinning. Within such lesions (Figure 2-14) myelin breakdown products and macrophage activity are rare, and there is only mild fibrillary gliosis; see Raine (1985a). Third, the technology and experimental background data at that time were insufficient to distinguish remyelination from incomplete demyelination; see Raine and Traugott (1985).

Remyelination was first documented in MS by Suzuki et al. (1969) and has since been documented on numerous occasions; see Prineas (1985). Interestingly, its presence does not always follow lesion quiescence, and several reports have

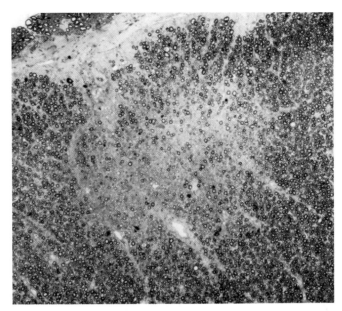

**Figure 2–14** A shadow plaque lies within an anterior column of the spinal cord from a case of chronic MS. The myelin pallor is related to the existence of many thinly myelinated (remyelinated) nerve fibers. × 160.

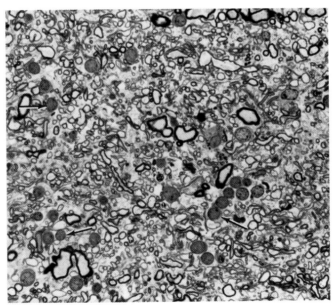

**Figure 2–15** At the periphery of a silent chronic MS plaque, a rim of remyelinated fibers (note the disproportionately thin myelin sheaths) and many proliferated oligodendrocytes (arrows) are seen. Unaffected fibers, discernible by the thicker myelin sheaths, are also present. × 400.

noted appearances typical of remyelinative activity in the midst of ongoing myelin breakdown (Raine et al., 1981; Prineas et al., 1984; Prineas, 1985). This seems to suggest that during lesion extension, there might occur *pari passu* transient, abortive myelin repair, perhaps effected by oligodendrocytes stimulated by the presence of myelin breakdown products or soluble mediators of the immune system. Sometimes, a broad zone of remyelination containing supernumerary (presumably, proliferated) oligodendrocytes (oligodendroglial hyperplasia) borders a chronically demyelinated lesion (Figure 2–15). Such an appearance suggests some degree of permanence, since macrophage activity is negligible or absent. The failure for the vast majority of involved CNS tissue to remyelinate in MS is probably related to the cumulative effects of multiple insults to the tissue, leading to the demise and disapperance of oligodendrocytes. Nevertheless, that the CNS in MS is capable of myelin regeneration should be taken as a positive indicator in future therapeutic rationales.


## EXPERIMENTAL MODELS

While researchers are acutely aware of the possibility that the myelin damage in MS may be a nonspecific event resulting from the destruction of an "innocent bystander" membrane by soluble mediators secreted by cells involved in an unrelated immunologic attack (e.g., against a virus), the ability to produce similar pathology in animals by specific sensitization to myelin has led us to focus on autoimmunity as the modus operandi in MS. Support for an autoimmune process in MS has almost exclusively come from the EAE model, first introduced by Rivers and Schwentker (1935) as a result of work on postrabies immunization encephalomyelitis, a form of ADE. Because this condition bears striking resemblances to acute MS, a link between chronic MS and EAE was established. The literature on EAE is too overwhelming for this chapter; see Raine (1976, 1984c, 1985), Paterson (1977), and Alvord et al. (1984).

Of particular relevance to this chapter are the several forms of chronic relapsing EAE which have been applied to structural, immunologic, and therapeutic questions in MS (see Raine, 1976, 1983, 1984, 1985b; Alvord et al., 1984). These models involve the inoculation of an animal with CNS myelin products or with cells sensitized against myelin components. In this regard, the EAE models differ from the situation in MS in that the causative agent and time of exposure are known. Nevertheless, the clinical course of some of these chronic forms and the subsequent pathology (e.g., primary demyelination, gliosis, receptor-mediated phagocytosis of myelin, and remyelination) are highly reminiscent of MS in terms of scale and inflammatory activity, although their location in EAE tends to be more subpial than paraventricular and disseminated, similar to that seen in ADE. Viral models of demyelination exist that also share clinical and pathological features in common with MS. These include natural conditions such as canine distemper encephalomyelitis (Wisniewski et al., 1972) and laboratory models such as mouse hepatitis virus encephalomyelitis (Lampert et al., 1973) and Theiler's virus encephalomyelitis (Dal Canto and Rabinowitz, 1982). The latter have provided useful paradigms for the dissection of viral-host contributions to lesion pathogenesis.

Several therapeutic insights for MS have emerged from the autoimmune models of demyelination. For example, the effects of antiinflammatory drugs, steroids, endocrine-blocking agents, vasoactive drugs, synthetic peptides with actions comparable to myelin sequences, immunoglobulin, irradiation, vaccination, adoptive transfer of tolerance, stress, and myelin components have all been tested in EAE; see Raine (1985b). The recent advent of monoclonal antibody technology now affords more novel applications of the EAE model to the selective depletion of lymphocyte subpopulations and immune system molecules in attempts to stem the progression of disease in the CNS. Similar trials have also been conducted on MS subjects but without dramatic results to date (Morimoto et al., 1987). Thus while MS lacks a spontaneous animal analog, the availability of different forms of acute and chronic-relapsing EAE in a broad range of genetically varied laboratory species provides a valuable adjunct in our search for agents to modulate or arrest the course of this devastating condition of the human CNS.

## ACKNOWLEDGMENTS

I thank Drs. G.R.W. Moore, L.C. Scheinberg, W.T. Norton, C.F. Brosnan, and M.B. Borstein for valuable collaboration; Everett Swanson, Miriam Pakingan, and Howard Finch for expert technical assistance; and Michele Briggs for careful preparation of the manuscript. Supported in part by RG 1001-F-6 from the National Multiple Sclerosis Society and NS 08952, NS 07098, and NS 11920 from the USPHS.

## REFERENCES

Abramsky, O., Lisak, R.P., Silberberg, D.H., and Pleasure, D.E. (1977). Antibodies to oligodendroglia in patients with multiple sclerosis. *N. Engl. J. Med.,* **297,** 1207–81.

Adams, C.W.M. (1983). The general pathology of multiple sclerosis: Morphological and chemical aspects of the lesions. In: J.F. Hallpike, C.W.M. Adams, and W.W. Tourtellotte, eds., *Multiple Sclerosis,* pp. 203–40. London: Chapman and Hall.

Adams, R.D., and Kubik, C.S. (1952). The morbid anatomy of the demyelinative diseases. *Am. J. Med.,* **12,** 510–46.

Allen, I.V. (1944). Demyelinating Diseases. (1984). In: J.H. Adams, J.A.N. Corsellis, and L.W. Duchen, eds., *Greenfield's Neuropathology,* 4th ed., pp. 338–84. New York: Wiley.

Alvord, E.C. (1985). Disseminated encephalomyelitis: its variations in form and their relationships to other diseases of the nervous system. In: J.C. Koetsier, ed., *Handbook of Clinical Neurology,* vol. 3(47), *Demyelinating Diseases,* pp. 467–502. Amsterdam: Elsevier.

Alvord, E.C., Kies, M.W., and Suckling, A.F. (eds.) (1984). *Experimental Allergic Encephalomyelitis: A Useful Model for Multiple Sclerosis.* New York: Liss.

Booss, J., Esiri, M., Tourtellotte, W.W., and Mason, D.Y. (1983). Immunohistological analysis of T lymphocyte subsets in the central nervous system in chronic progressive multiple sclerosis. *J Neurol. Sci.,* **62,** 219–32.

Burger, D.R., Ford, D., Vetto, R.M., Hamblin, A., Goldstein, A., Hubbard, M., and Dumonde, D.C. (1981). Endothelial cell presentation of antigen to human T cells. *Human Immunol.,* **3,** 209–30.

Dal Canto, M.C., and Rabinowitz, S.G. (1982). Experimental models of virus-induced demyelination of the central nervous system. *Ann. Neurol.,* **11**, 109–27.

Dawson, J.W. (1916). The histology of disseminated sclerosis. *Transactions of the Royal Society of Edinburgh,* **50**, 517–740.

Ebers, G.C. (1984). Oligoclonal banding in MS. In: L.C. Scheinberg and C.S. Raine, eds., *Multiple Sclerosis: Experimental and Clinical Aspects, Ann. N.Y. Acad. Sci.,* **436**, 206–12.

Epstein, L.G., Prineas, J.W., and Raine, C.S. (1983). Attachment of myelin to coated pits on macrophages in experimental allergic encephalomyelitis. *J. Neurol. Sci.,* **61**, 341–8.

Esiri, M.M., Taylor, C.R., and Mason, D.Y. (1976). Application of an immunoperoxidase method to a study of the central nervous system: Preliminary findings in a study of human formalin-fixed material. *Neuropath. App. Neurobiol.,* **2**, 233–46.

Fontana, A., Fierz, W., and Wekerle, H. (1984). Astrocytes present myelin basic protein to encephalitogenic T cell lines. *Nature* (London), **307**, 273–76.

Greenfield, J.G., and King, L.S. (1936). Observations on the histopathology of the cerebral lesions in disseminated sclerosis. *Brain,* **59**, 445–58.

Hauser, S.L., Bhan, A.K., Gilles, F.H., Hoban, C.J., Reinherz, E.L., Schlossman, S.F., and Weiner, H.L. (1983). Immunohistochemical staining of human brain with monoclonal antibodies that identify lymphocytes, monocytes and the Ia antigen. *J. Neuroimmunol.,* **5**, 197–205.

Ibraham, M.Z.M., and Adams, C.W.M. (1963). The relationship between enzyme activity and neuroglia in plaques of multiple sclerosis. *J. Neurol. Neurosurg. Psychiat.,* **26**, 101–10.

Lampert, P.W., Sims, J.K., and Kniazeff, A.J. (1973). Mechanism of demyelination in JHM virus encephalomyelitis. *Acta Neuropath.,* **24**, 76–85.

Lee, S.C., and Raine, C. S. (in press). Multiple sclerosis: Oligodendrocytes in active lesions do not express class II MHC molecules. *J. Neuroimmunol.*

Lumsden, C.E. (1955). In: D. McAlpine, N.D. Compston, and C.E. Lumsden, eds., *Multiple Sclerosis,* p. 231. Edinburgh: Livingstone.

Lumsden, C.E. (1970). The neuropathology of multiple sclerosis. In: P.J. Vinken and G.W. Bruyn, eds., *Handbook of Clinical Neurology,* vol. 9, pp. 217–309. Amsterdam: North Holland.

Matsumoto, Y., and Fujiwara, M. (1987). The immunopathology of adoptively transferred experimental allergic encephalomyelitis (EAE) in Lewis rats, Part 1. Immunohistochemical examination of developing lesions of EAE. *J.Neurol. Sci.,* **77**, 35–47.

Matsumoto, Y., Hara, N., Tanaka, R., and Fujiwara, M. (1986). Immunohistochemical analysis of the rat central nervous system during experimental allergic encephalomyelitis, with special reference to Ia-positive cells with dendritic morphology. *J. Immunol.,* **136**, 3668–76.

Moore, G.R.W., and Raine, C.S. (1988). Immunogold localization and analysis of IgG in acute experimental allergic encephalomyelitis. Lab. Invest., **59**, 641–48.

Morimoto, C., Hafler, D.A., Weiner, H.L., Letvin, N.L., Hagan, M., Daley, J., and Schloddman, S.F. (1987). Selective losses of the suppressor/inducer T cell subsets in progressive multiple sclerosis. *N. Eng. J. Med.,* **316**, 67–72.

Oger, J., Szuchet, S., Antel, J.P., and Arnason, B.G.W. (1982). A monoclonal antibody against human T suppressor lymphocytes binds specifically to the surface of cultured oligodendrocytes. *Nature* (London), **295**, 66–68.

Pastan, I.H., and Willingham, M.C. (1981). Journey to the center of the cell: role of the receptosome. *Science,* **214**, 504–09.

Paterson, P.Y. (1977). Autoimmune neurological diseases: Experimental animal systems and implications for multiple sclerosis. In: N. Talal, ed., *Autoimmunity: Genetic, Immunologic, Virologic and Clinical Aspects.*, pp. 643–92. New York: Academic Press.

Pober, J.S., Gimbrone, M.A., Cotran, R.S., Reiss, S., Burakoff, J., Fiers, W., and Aults, A. (1983). Ia expression by vascular endothelium is inducible by activated T cells and by human γ-interferon. *J. Exp. Med.,* **157,** 1339–53.

Prineas, J. (1985). The neuropathology of multiple sclerosis. In: J.C. Koetsier, ed., *Handbook of Clinical Neurology,* vol. 3(47), Demyelinating Diseases, pp. 213–57. Amsterdam: Elsevier.

Prineas, J.W., and Connell, F. (1978). The fine structure of chronically active multiple sclerosis plaques. *Neurology, 28,* 68–75.

Prineas, J.W., and Connell, F. (1979). Remyelination in multiple sclerosis. *Ann. Neurol.,* **5,** 22–31.

Prineas, J.W., Kwon, E.E., Cho, R.S., and Sharer, L.R. (1984). Continual breakdown and regeneration of myelin in progressive multiple sclerosis plaques. In: *Multiple Sclerosis: Experimental and Clinical Aspects,* L.C. Scheinberg and C.S. Raine, eds., *Ann. N.Y Acad. Sci.,* **436,** 11–32.

Prineas, J.W., and Raine, C.S. (1976). Electron microscopy and immunoperoxidase studies of early multiple sclerosis lesions. *Neurology* (Minneapolis), **26**(Supp), 29–32.

Prineas, J.W., and Wright, R.G. (1978). Macrophages, lymphocytes, and plasma cells in the perivascular compartment in chronic multiple sclerosis. *Lab. Invest.,* **38,** 409–21.

Raine, C.S. (1976). Experimental allergic encephalomyelitis and related conditions. In: H.M. Zimmerman, ed., *Progress in Neuropathology,* vol. 3, pp. 225–51. New York: Grune and Stratton.

Raine, C.S. (1983). Multiple sclerosis and chronic EAE: Comparative ultrastructural neuropathology. In: J.F. Hallpike, C.W.M. Adams, and W.W. Tourtellotte, eds., *Multiple Sclerosis.*, pp. 413–60. London: Chapman and Hall.

Raine, C.S. (1984a). The neuropathology of myelin diseases. In: P. Morell, ed., *Myelin,* 2nd ed., pp. 259–310. New York: Plenum.

Raine, C.S. (1984b). The morphology of myelin and myelination. In: P. Morell, ed., *Myelin,* 2nd ed., pp. 1–50. New York: Plenum.

Raine, C.S. (1984c). Biology of Disease. The analysis of autoimmune demyelination: Its impact upon multiple sclerosis. *Lab. Invest.,* **50,** 608–35.

Raine, C.S. (1985a). Demyelinating Diseases. In: R.L. Davis and D.M. Robertson, eds., *Textbook of Neuropathology,* pp. 468–547. Baltimore: Williams and Wilkins.

Raine, C.S. (1985b). Experimental allergic encephalomyelitis and experimental allergic neuritis. In: J.C. Koetsier, ed., *Handbook of Clinical Neurology,* vol. 3(47), Demyelinating Diseases, pp. 429–66. Amsterdam: Elsevier.

Raine, C.S. (1985c). Oligodendrocytes and central nervous system myelin. In: R.C. Davis, and D.M. Robertson, eds., *Textbook of Neuropathology,* pp. 92–116. Baltimore: Williams and Wilkins.

Raine, C.S., and Scheinberg, L.C. (1988). On the immunopathology of plaque development and repair in multiple sclerosis. *J. Neuroimmunol.,* **20,** 189–201.

Raine, C.S., Scheinberg, L.C., and Waltz, J.M. (1981). Multiple Sclerosis: Oligodendrocyte survival and proliferation in an active, established lesion. *Lab. Invest.,* **45,** 534–46.

Raine, C.S., and Traugott, U. (1985). Remyelination in chronic relapsing experimental allergic encephalomyelitis and multiple sclerosis. In: M. Adachi, A. Hirano, and S. Aronson, eds., *Current Trends in Neuroscience,* vol. 3, Pathology of the Myelinated Axon, pp. 229–75. New York: Igaku-Shoin.

Ritchie, J.M. (1984). Physiological basis of conduction in myelinated nerve fibers In: P. Morell, ed., *Myelin,* 2nd ed., pp. 117–46. New York: Plenum.

Rivers, T.M. and Schwentker, F.F. (1935). Encephalomyelitis accompanied by myelin destruction experimentally produced in monkeys. *J. Exp. Med.,* **61,** 689–702.

Roizin, L., Haymaker, W., and D'Amelio, F. (1982). Disease states involving the white matter of the central nervous system. In: W. Haymaker and R.D. Adams, eds., *Histology and Histopathology of the Nervous System,* pp. 1276–1489. Springfield Ill.: Thomas.

Schlesinger, H. (1910). Zur Frage der akuten multiplen Sklerose und der Enzephalomyelitis disseminata im Kindesalter. *Arch. Neurol. Inst. Wien,* **17,** 410–32.

Sobel, R.A., Blanchette, B.W., Bhan, A.K., and Colvin, R.B. (1984). The immunopathology of experimental allergic encephalomyelitis. II. Endothelial cells. Ia increases prior to inflammatory cell infiltration. *J. Immunol.,* **132,** 2402–7.

Sobel, R.A., Natale, B.A., and Schneeberger, E.E. (1987). The immunopathology of acute experimental allergic encephalomyelitis. IV. An ultrastructural immunocytochemical study of class II major histocompatibility complex molecule (Ia) expression. *J. Neuropath. Exp. Neurol.,* **46,** 239–49.

Suzuki, K., Andrews, J.M., Waltz, J.M., and Terry, R.D. (1969). Ultrastructural studies of multiple sclerosis. *Lab. Invest.,* **20,** 444–54.

Tourtellotte, W.W., Walsh, M.J., Baumhefner, R.W., Staugaitis, S.M., and Shapshak, P. (1984). The current status of multiple sclerosis intra-blood-brain-barrier IgG synthesis. In: *Multiple Sclerosis: Experimental and Clinical Aspects.* L.C. Scheinberg, and C.S. Raine, eds., *Ann. N.Y. Acad. Sci.,* **436,** 52–67.

Traugott, U., McFarlin, D.E., and Raine, C.S. (1986). Immunopathology of the lesion in chronic relapsing experimental autoimmune encephalomyelitis in the mouse. *Cell. Immunol.,* **99,** 395–410.

Traugott, U., Raine, C.S., and McFarlin, D.E. (1985a). Acute experimental allergic encephalomyelitis in the mouse: Immunopathology of the developing lesion. *Cell. Immunol.,* **91,** 240–54.

Traugott, U., Reinherz, E.L., and Raine, C.S. (1983a). Multiple Sclerosis: Distribution of T cell subsets within active chronic lesions. *Science,* **219,** 308–10.

Traugott, U., Reinherz, E.L., and Raine C.S. (1983b). Multiple sclerosis: Distribution of T cells, T cells subsets and Ia-positive macrophages in lesions of different ages. *J. Neuroimmunol.,* **4,** 201–21.

Traugott, U., Scheinberg, L.C., and Raine, C.S. (1985b). On the presence of Ia-positive endothelial cells and astrocytes in multiple sclerosis lesions and its relevance to antigen presentation. *J. Neuroimmunol.,* **8,** 1–14.

Whitaker, J.N. (1984). Indicators of disease activity in multiple sclerosis: Studies of myelin basic protein-like materials. In: *Multiple Sclerosis: Experimental and Clinical Aspects,* L.C. Scheinberg and C.S. Raine, eds., *Ann. N.Y. Acad. Sci.,* **436,** 140–150.

Wisniewski, H., Raine, C.S., and Kay, W.J. (1972). Observations on viral demyelinating encephalomyelitis—canine distemper. *Lab. Invest.,* **26,** 589–99.

# 3

# Brain Imaging in Multiple Sclerosis

ERNEST W. WILLOUGHBY AND DONALD W. PATY

The most valuable techniques for imaging the brain in multiple sclerosis (MS) are x-ray computed tomography (CT) and magnetic resonance imaging (MRI). Their place in imaging the spinal cord is more limited, and myelography remains valuable for the exclusion of other causes of lesions of the spinal cord. Older techniques such as air encephalography and standard radionuclide (isotope) brain scanning were never very useful in the diagnosis of MS and are now, in effect, obsolete. Positron emission tomography (PET), which makes use of the radiation generated when positrons from administrated radionuclides are absorbed in tissue, remains a research tool in the study of cerebral metabolism and blood flow. Studies with PET have been carried out in MS patients by several groups, but have not yet provided any new insights into the pathological process (Brooks et al., 1984; Herscovitch et al., 1984; Sheremata et al., 1984; Frey et al., 1987).

## CT SCANNING (X-RAY)

Although computed tomographic techniques are also used in MRI scanning, the abbreviation CT is usually limited to x-ray CT scanning. Since the first reports of low-density lesions in CT brain scans in MS patients in the mid-1970s (Gyldensted, 1976; Warren et al., 1976; Cala et al., 1978), the yield of positive brain scans has increased considerably with the development of high-resolution scanners and the use of delayed scanning after high-dose intravenous contrast agents. The limited value of CT scanning of the spinal cord results from low resolution in that area and

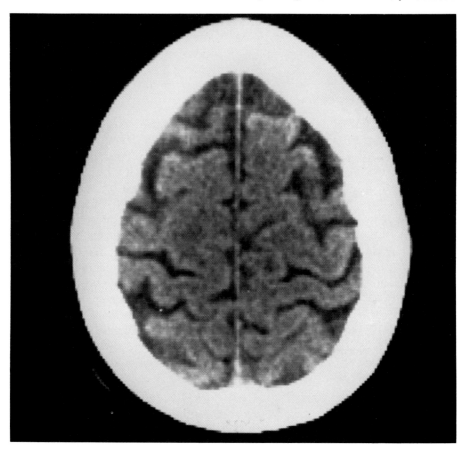

**Figure 3–1**  Atrophy in MS. This is a noncontrast CT on an MS patient showing appearance of cortical atrophy. Note how the sulci (dark) areas are large.

the length of time taken to gather information from a series of axial slices of the cord. CT scans of the brain stem and cerebellum also are often of poor quality, largely because of artifacts induced by the surrounding bone.

## Unenhanced CT Brain Scanning

Unenhanced CT brain scans in MS may show focal low-density lesions and evidence of generalized atrophy with associated ventricular dilatation (Figure 3–1). These abnormalities often coexist.

Cerebral atrophy reflects extensive loss of cerebral tissue and is usually most obvious in severe disease of long duration. It has been reported in a high proportion of patients (Gyldensted, 1976; Loizou et al., 1982), but reports using higher-resolution scanners have demonstrated that in some cases apparent enlargement of the ventricles is due to areas of low density in the periventricular white matter (Ormerod et al., 1986c).

Focal lesions of low density on unenhanced CT scans may be isolated but are typically multiple in established disease. They are most obvious in the white matter of the cerebral hemispheres, particularly in the periventricular regions. The low-density lesions may enlarge or contract on repeat CT scans over time, but the age of such lesions on a single, unenhanced scan cannot be readily determined.

## Contrast Enhancement in CT Scanning

More information is obtained from scans taken after administering intravenous iodine-containing contrast agents which leak into cerebral tissue at sites of break-down of the blood–brain barrier. Enhancing focal lesions in MS were first reported by Wuthrich et al. (1976) and Cole and Ross (1977), and multiple enhancing lesions were later shown in some patients, particularly during clinically active phases of the disease (Aita et al., 1978; Harding et al., 1978; Lane et al., 1978; Lebow et al., 1978; Sears et al., 1978; Lidegaard et al., 1983; Ebers et al., 1984; Barrett et al., 1985; Morimoto et al., 1985; Vliegenthart et al., 1985). Contrast enhancement may be homogeneous in the affected area or ringlike around the periphery of the lesion (Fig. 3–2). It may occur in an area of low density or in an area that appears normal on an unenhanced scan. A potential trap, if only an enhanced scan is carried out, is the occasional slight enhancement of a low-density area to render it indistinguishable from the surrounding normal brain.

The technique of delayed CT scanning one hour after high doses of intravenous contrast was first shown by Vinuela et al. (1982) to increase significantly the yield of enhancing lesions in MS patients over that obtained with scans taken immediately after a conventional dose of intravenous contrast. Later studies by Spiegel et al. (1985) showed that both the high dose of contrast and the hour's delay were important in increasing the number of detectable lesions. With this technique the proportion of patients showing one or more enhancing brain lesions on CT during phases of clinically active disease is of the order of 50–80% (depending on patient selection), with the frequency of positive scans diminishing in groups of patients without evidence of clinical activity (Vinuela et al., 1982; Ebers et al., 1984; Spiegel et al., 1985; unpublished Vancouver MS Clinic data).

## Pathological Correlation in CT Scanning

The focal low-density lesions in the white matter on unenhanced CT scans undoubtedly represent the pathological areas of inflammatory demyelination. Their distribution on CT corresponds to the pathological distribution of the typical demyelinated plaques, and confirmation has been obtained at autopsy and on cerebral biopsy (Warren et al., 1976; Sagar et al., 1982; Wippold and Cuetter, 1982).

It would be expected that contrast enhancement would occur in areas of acute inflammatory demyelination during acute attacks of MS rather than in chronic demyelinated plaques, and characteristic pathological changes have been found on biopsy of the enhancing lesion (Haughton et al., 1980; Marano et al., 1980; Nelson et al., 1981; Sagar et al., 1982; Wang et al., 1983). Autopsies of patients previously shown during life to have had enhancing lesions on CT brain scan have also confirmed the presence of typical areas of inflammatory demyelination (Lebow et al., 1978; van der Velden et al., 1979; Ebers et al., 1984; Latack et al., 1984). Repeat CT scans have shown resolution of the contrast enhancement (Cole and Ross,

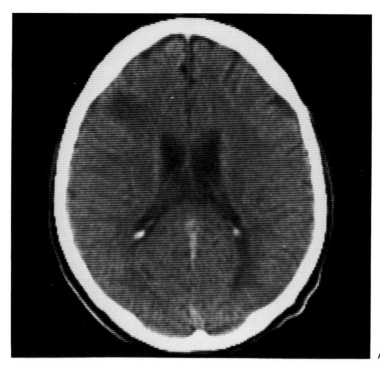

A

**Figure 3-2**   CT scans in MS. Note focal low-density lesion in the right frontal area of scan A. HVD
scan (B) shows enhancement in the margin of that low-density area. C shows a markedly positive
HVD CT scan of a patient with multiple enhancing lesions.

1977; Aita et al., 1978; Harding et al, 1978; Sears et al, 1978; Weinstein et al, 1978;
Morariu et al., 1980), and there is evidence that this may occur more rapidly after
treatment with steroids, particularly if administered intravenously (Lodder et al.,
1983; Troiano et al., 1984).

It should be noted that the low-density and contrast-enhancing lesions on the
CT brain scan, whether single or multiple, are not specific for the demyelinating
lesions of MS. The same appearances are produced by a number of pathological
processes, and demyelinating lesions that enhance with contrast may look very
much like cerebral tumors (van der Velden et al., 1979; Nelson et al., 1981; Rieth
et al., 1981; Abbott et al., 1982; Sagar et al., 1982; Wang et al., 1983). Multiple low-
density lesions with or without contrast enhancement in the appropriate clinical
setting are highly suggestive of MS, as are large lesions with diffuse, ringlike
enhancement but with relatively little evidence of associated mass effect or surrounding cerebral edema in relation to their size. Resolution of the contrast
enhancement on repeat scans is also characteristic of MS.

## MAGNETIC RESONANCE IMAGING

By convention, the original title of nuclear magnetic resonance (NMR) imaging has
been shortened by dropping of the first word. Magnetic resonance imaging (MRI)

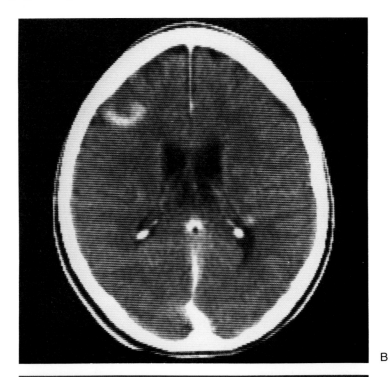

B

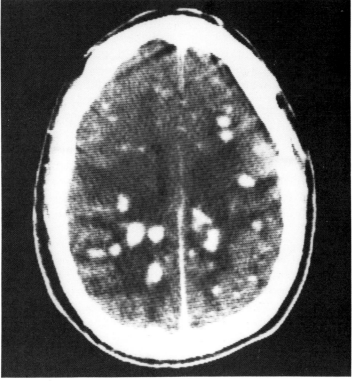

C

makes use of low-energy, low-frequency radio waves, which are in a different part of the electromagnetic spectrum from the high-energy, high-frequency x-rays used in conventional CT imaging. Thus while imaging in CT depends on absorption by the tissue of ionizing radiation, MRI is based on an interaction between radio waves and hydrogen nuclei in the tissue in the presence of a strong external magnetic field. The intensity or density of each segment of the image (picture element or pixel intensity) depends largely on the density of the tissue electrons in x-ray CT and on the density of mobile hydrogen nuclei (protons) modified by their chemical environment in MRI.

The basis of the MRI scanner is a large, cylindrical magnet, which creates a strong, evenly distributed magnetic field into which the patient is placed. The most widely used scanners of high-field strength make use of superconducting cryo-magnets cooled by liquid helium. These now provide static magnetic field strengths of 1.5 T, compared with field strengths of 0.15–0.3 T of older units. In general, higher field strengths increase the signal-to-noise ratio and produce sharper images. Separate coils in the magnet produce superimposed linear gradients on the main magnetic field. These alter the resonant frequency of protons in different parts of the field and allow spatial localization of the MRI signals to the tissue slice of interest. An appropriately tuned transmitter applies pulses of radio frequency waves, and the resulting signals from the tissue are detected by receiver coils.

## Principles of MRI Scanning

Useful brief reviews of the principles of MRI are provided by Fullerton (1982) and Bradley et al. (1985) and more detailed reviews by Young (1984) and Valk et al. (1985). Tissue protons with their single spinning electron act as tiny bar magnets, although not all atomic nuclei have this property. Those that do have an odd number of protons and/or neutrons, so that other common atoms in organic tissue such as $C_{12}$ or $O_{16}$ are not of importance in MRI. Because of its abundance, the proton is the main determinant of clinical MRI scanning.

Under normal circumstances tissue protons are randomly aligned, because the earth's magnetic field is too weak to influence them significantly. When placed in a strong external magnetic field (as in an MRI scanner) the protons align their magnetic fields with the external field in the same way that a compass needle aligns itself with the earth's magnetic field. This alignment fluctuates, however, in that each of the individual proton magnetic fields rotates or wobbles (precesses) about the direction of the external field, much as a slowly spinning top wobbles about the direction of the earth's gravitational field. The aligned protons themselves create a net magnetic field, which is directed longitudinally along the external field. The precession of individual protons is random or out of phase, so that there is no net magnetic field directed in a transverse direction across the external field.

In MRI the aligned protons are perturbed by short pulses of radio frequency waves. Some of this energy is absorbed by tissue protons if it is of the appropriate resonant frequency, which depends on the position of the proton in the gradient of the external magnetic field. The excited protons then return to their former state and release absorbed energy as radio waves, which are analyzed by computer to produce the MRI.

The radio frequency pulses have two effects on the aligned protons in the tissue slice under study. First, they alter the direction of the net longitudinal magnetic field (usually flipping it 90 or 180 degrees) thereby reducing the magnetic vector directed along the external field. Second, they cause aligned protons for a brief period to wobble or precess in phase, which causes the net longitudinal vector to rotate or precess about its original direction and thereby produce net magnetization also in the transverse direction across the external field.

The recovery of the protons to their state of equilibrium after the radio frequency pulse is described in terms of the return of these magnetic vectors (longitudinal and transverse) to their former state as the $T_1$ and $T_2$ relaxation times. $T_1$ is a measure of the time taken for the net magnetic vector in the longitudinal direction to return to its initial value. This is determined by thermal interactions between the resonating protons and other nuclei in the tissue or lattice and is therefore also known as the longitudinal or spin-lattice relaxation time. $T_2$ is a measure of the time taken for the precessing protons to again lose phase with one another. This is determined by interactions between the spinning protons. As dephasing occurs, the net transverse magnetization is lost, and $T_2$ is therefore also known as the *spin-spin* or *transverse relaxation time.* $T_2$ is always shorter than $T_1$ in solid tissue.

## Clinical MRI

The MRI is the result of a complex interaction between repeated sequences of radio frequency pulses and intermittently activated magnetic field gradients. The key to the increased information contained in the MRI compared with a CT image is its dependence not only on the density of tissue nuclei but also on the tissue $T_1$ and $T_2$ relaxation times (and also on tissue blood flow). This is of relevance because the changes of $T_1$ and $T_2$ in abnormal tissue in disorders such as MS are relatively much greater than changes in proton density. Different pulse sequences are used that emphasize the effect of either $T_1$ or $T_2$ and produce images that differ considerably in character. The most commonly used are the inversion recovery (IR) sequence which is dependent largely on $T_1$ ($T_1$ weighted) and the spin-echo (SE) sequence which emphasizes $T_2$ ($T_2$ weighted).

The IR sequence consists of an initial inverting pulse of radio frequency waves that flip the original net longitudinal magnetic vector in the brain slice of interest 180 degrees so that it is directed in the opposite direction along the external magnetic field. As the vector returns to its equilibrium position (at a rate characterized by the $T_1$ relaxation time), a second radio frequency pulse flips it 90 degrees to its original direction so that it is directed across the external field. It is the second pulse that allows measurement of the return of the longitudinal vector to equilibrium. The 180-degree and 90-degree pulses of the IR sequence are separated by an interval known as the inversion time.

The SE sequence consists of an initial 90-degree radio frequency pulse followed by a 180-degree pulse. The echo time is the time between the first of the pair of pulses and the receipt of a signal (or spin echo). Both SE and IR scans are formed from averaged signals from a series of repeated pulse sequences, each of which is separated by an interval known as the repetition time.

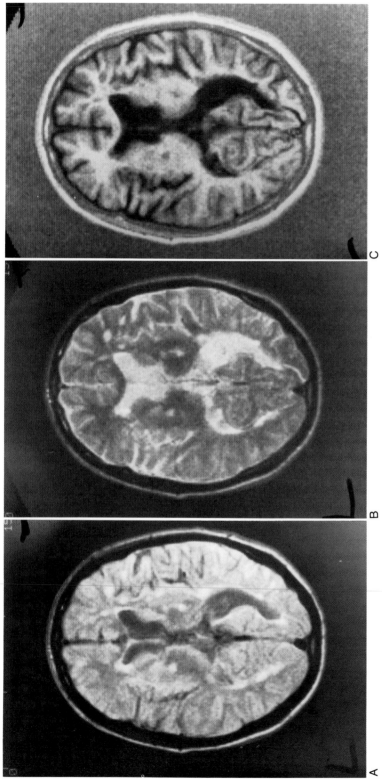

**Figure 3–3** A typical MRI appearance in MS. A is the SE 40 sequence, B the SE 120 sequence, and C the IR 400 sequence. Note how the MS lesions are bright on SE and dark on IR. The SE 120 sequence makes the CSF light so that it is difficult to distinguish CSF from MS lesions.

A     B     C

The inversion time, echo time, and repetition time are all parameters that can be adjusted in MRI. They have a major influence on the contrast between different tissues and in the distinction of pathological from normal tissue in different circumstances.

IR scans show anatomical detail in the brain well, with a clear distinction between gray and white matter. SE scans, which have less contrast between gray and white matter, distinguish more clearly, however, between normal and abnormal cerebral tissue, and in our experience this is the most reliable technique for demonstrating cerebral lesions in MS as long as adjustment is made to maintain contrast between the cerebral ventricles (dark) and the cerebral white matter (gray). Patches of demyelination have prolonged $T_1$ and $T_2$ and show up as black areas on IR scans and as white areas on SE scans (Figure 3–3).

## MRI Versus CT Scanning

Since the first reports by Young et al. (1981) and Bydder et al. (1982) it has been clear that MRI scanning is more sensitive than CT in detecting subclinical lesions in the brain in MS (Figure 3–4). Those early studies with the IR technique have been confirmed in later reports, which in most instances have indicated that the SE technique is the most useful one in MS (Lukes et al., 1983; Runge et al., 1984; Kirshner et al., 1985; Sheldon et al., 1985; Simon et al., 1986). Virtually all lesions on CT scans are readily demonstrated on MRI scans, which in most cases also show extra lesions not seen on CT. This results from the superior resolution by MRI of small plaques that are nonenhancing on CT and the improved visualization on MRI of structures in the posterior fossa, where there is often considerable artefact on CT induced by the surrounding bone.

In many cases the demonstration of extra lesions on an MRI scan is not of much consequence from a diagnostic point of view, particularly in patients with clinically definite MS. In patients with suspected MS, however, where a definite diagnosis cannot be made clinically, MRI scanning increases the diagnostic yield over CT (of cases confirmed by typical scan abnormalities) about three- to fivefold (Gebarski et al., 1985; Paty et al., 1988).

An advantage of MRI scanning over CT is the ability to produce scans directly in axial, sagittal, or coronal planes (Figure 3–5). This can be very helpful in assessing the extent of many structural lesions of the brain, although in practice in the diagnosis of MS we have found the standard axial slices to be the most useful.

A further advantage of MRI scanning is that it can be carried out repeatedly without known risk to the patient, while the numbers of repeat CT scans are limited by the problems produced by ionizing radiation. MRI also does not carry the hazards, albeit rare, of injecting iodine-containing contrast materials necessary for CT in the diagnosis of MS. A potential advantage of CT is that it requires less time for scanning, but although it is true that a single CT scan occupies less machine time, the most sensitive procedure for the diagnosis of MS requires a preceding intravenous infusion of contrast followed by a delay of one hour before the scan.

Apart from being less expensive and more widely available, CT does have one important advantage over MRI in MS patients, in that it shows a difference in a single study between chronic, established MS lesions and new, acute, inflammatory

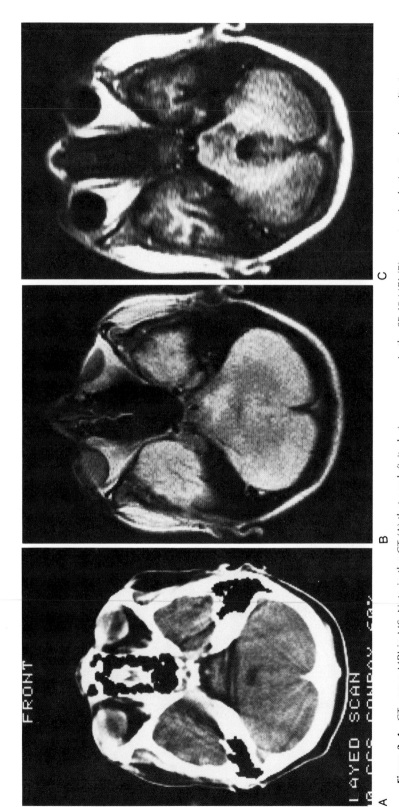

**Figure 3-4** CT versus MRI in MS. Note in the CT (A) that no definite lesions are seen. In the SE 40 MRI (B) an extensive brain-stem abnormality is seen. The IR 400 sequence (C) shows the MS lesions (dark) even better than does the SE sequence.

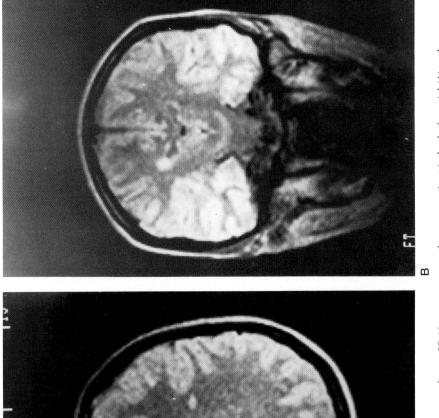

**Figure 3–5** MRI in two planes. SE 40 sequences on the same patient in both the axial (A) and coronal (B) planes. The large lesion in the right hemisphere can be seen in both planes.

lesions. The latter are distinguished on CT by contrast enhancement, while on standard MRI scans using either SE or IR techniques old and new lesions have essentially the same appearance, as MRI does not readily separate edematous cerebral tissue from other tissue abnormalities. On the face of it, this is suprising, as water is a rich source of protons, but the effects of the increased density of protons with increased tissue hydration tend to be balanced by associated complex interactions that lead to reductions in $T_1$ and $T_2$ in the tissue. Because all the lesions seen on CT are virtually always also seen on MRI, this is not a practical problem in the diagnosis of MS. The ability to distinguish old from new lesions is of value in the correlation of lesions on scans with new clinical symptoms or signs, however, and is potentially of considerable use in following treatment.

## Contrast Enhancement in MRI

The usual iodine-containing contrast materials used in CT scanning are not of value in MRI, but a number of other compounds are potentially useful. These are all paramagnetic substances with one or more unpaired electrons that cause them to interact with tissue protons in a manner that leads to shortening of both $T_1$ and $T_2$ relaxation times, a process known as proton relaxation enhancement. The three main types of paramagnetic compounds are oxides of nitrogen, molecular oxygen, and elements of the transitional and rare-earth type. Only gadolinium from the latter group has been used clinically.

Gadolinium is injected intravenously in a stable, nontoxic, chelated form as gadolinium-DTPA which leaks into the brain where the blood-brain barrier is damaged. It produces contrast enhancement on MRI of cerebral tumors with the edges of the tumor enhancing more than the surrounding edematous cerebral tissue, as is also the case with enhancement on CT (Carr et al., 1984; Claussen et al., 1985). Two reports from the same group of gadolinium-enhanced MRI scanning in MS patients (Grossman et al., 1986; Gonzalez-Scarano et al., 1987) showed that all the lesions that enhanced on CT also enhanced on MRI, most clearly on the $T_1$-weighted images. Many additional enhancing lesions were also seen on MRI.

These studies indicate that this technique may be of considerable value in separating old from new MS lesions and may be more sensitive than contrast-enhanced CT in this respect also. Another advantage is that relatively small volumes of gadolinium are needed, and it is probable that it will prove to be less hazardous in large-scale use than iodine-containing contrast agents. At present, gadolinium-DTPA is limited in availability.

## Pathological Correlations in MRI Scanning

Pathological confirmation of changes seen on MRI scans in MS have been limited to date. This is at least partly because the characteristic changes in MS were recognized soon after MRI scanning was introduced, and biopsies of demyelinating lesions in patients premortem have not been reported. Pathological correlations in postmortem studies in eight MS patients by Stewart et al. (1984, 1986) showed that MRI scans taken immediately after death were similar to scans taken during life and accurately indicated the extent of the areas of demyelination defined pathologically. These studies, which were carried out in patients with chronic MS of long standing, also showed that the patches of demyelination were still visible on SE sequence MRI scans taken after the brain was fixed in formalin. IR sequence scans on fixed cerebral tissue did not demonstrate the MS plaques as clearly.

The change in the MRI signal in MS is probably due to increased tissue water in the acute inflammatory lesions and to astrocytosis in chronic demyelinated lesions. Loss of myelin in itself is probably not an important factor, as myelin in normal brain does not contribute significantly to the MRI signal (Pykett and Rosen, 1983). The factors contributing to changes in $T_1$ and $T_2$ in MS lesions of all ages are undoubtedly complex, however. We have noted inhomogeneities in the MRI signal in different parts of the same lesion, as reported by Drayer & Barrett (1984), and some demyelinated lesions exhibit pathologically a mixture of chronic gliosis and more acute inflammatory change.

These data are supported by pathological and MRI studies in animals with experimental allergic encephalomyelitis (EAE), an animal model of acute inflammatory demyelinating disease (Stewart et al., 1985; Karlik et al., 1984, 1986; Noseworthy et al., 1985, 1986). The acute lesions are seen on MRI scans during life and immediately postmortem but disappear after fixation of the brain in formalin. The chronic gliotic lesions in established MS appear to be more stable on fixation with respect to their influence on MRI. The in vitro studies by Karlik et al. (1986) in EAE in rodents indicated that changes in MRI in acute inflammatory lesions in the spinal cord vary over time, with early alterations in $T_1$ and $T_2$ which tend to return toward normal when the cellular inflammatory infiltrate is heavy. These results were obtained by direct measurement of $T_1$ and $T_2$ by magnetic resonance spectroscopy without imaging, however, and it is not clear how they relate to changes in MRI obtained in vivo.

It should be noted that, as with CT, the changes on MRI are not specific for MS. Patchy lesions in the white matter of the cerebral hemispheres and irregular or smooth periventricular lesions are also seen in a variety of other disorders, including diffuse cerebrovascular disease, postirradiation cerebral damage, and some infections (Bradley et al., 1984; Ormerod et al., 1984, 1986c; Frytak et al., 1985). Similar isolated white matter lesions or smooth lesions along the cerebral ventricles are occasionally seen in otherwise healthy persons, particularly in the elderly (Bradley, 1984). Their usual significance has not been determined, but a number of different disturbances may lead to the appearance of lesions of that sort. It is worth noting, however, that clinically unrecognized MS does occur. Gilbert and Sadler (1983) reported evidence of unsuspected MS in 5 of 2450 brains examined on routine postmortem.

## Clinical Correlations in MRI Scanning

Studies of the relationship between the abnormality seen on MRI scans of the brain and the patient's clinical state have considered two main aspects: (1) the correlation of individual lesions with specific symptoms and signs and (2) the correlation of the total extent of brain involvement with the degree of overall neurologic impairment or disability suffered by the patient.

There have been a number of reports that episodes with new neurologic signs on examination can be related to lesions in appropriate areas in the brain on MRI. This has been shown particularly in the brain stem, where clinical localization of lesions is frequently more precise than in the cerebral hemispheres (Beck et al., 1982; Bogousslavsky et al., 1986; Constantino et al., 1986; Ormerod et al., 1986b). These and other studies, however, have made it clear that most of the cerebral lesions seen on MRI scans are asymptomatic (Jackson et al., 1985; Sheldon et al., 1985; Jacobs et al., 1986a). The explanation is that most of these lesions occur in parts of the brain that are clinically silent, at least as far as can be determined on standard neurologic examination of motor and sensory function in the cranial nerves and limbs. How these cerebral lesions relate to impairment of higher mental function is discussed elsewhere in this volume. The frequent occurrence of asymptomatic cerebral lesions has been particularly striking in prospective serial MRI scans in patients with MS (discussed later).

The converse also occurs, namely, the appearance of new symptoms and signs that localize a lesion to a part of the brain stem where no changes are seen on the MRI scan. The probable explanation is that pathological lesions too small to be clearly seen on MRI scans can produce neurologic dysfunction, especially in the brain stem, where many important nuclei and tracts are concentrated in small areas. In our experience this occurs in up to 50% of new brain-stem lesions in MS, but Ormerod et al. (1986b) report a higher yield of positive MRI scans in this situation, using a scanner of high field strength (0.5 T).

Although, in general, patients with more severe progressive MS tend to have evidence of more extensive disease on MRI brain scans than patients with more benign disease (Koopmans et al., 1989a), the correlation between disease extent on MRI and neurologic impairment in most reports is not particularly good (Kirshner et al., 1985; Sheldon et al., 1985; Edwards et al., 1986a; Reese et al., 1986; Baumhefner et al., 1986; Stewart et al., 1986). This is not surprising, as on the one hand much of the neurologic disability in MS results from spinal cord lesions, and on the other hand, many of the cerebral lesions seen on MRI are asymptomatic. The cerebral changes that seem to correlate best with overall clinical disability are extensive confluent periventricular lesions (Edwards et al., 1986; Koopmans et al., 1989a). Baumhefner et al. (1986) have reported a correlation between the extent of the cerebral lesions on MR and evidence of active inflammation in the brain and spinal cord, as judged by increased cerebrospinal fluid (CSF) immunoglobulin G levels.

## Quantitative Measurement of Lesions on MRI Scans

The studies correlating the total "load" of disease shown on MRI with the patient's overall clinical state have been associated with efforts to standardize the quantitative measurement of the extent of the MRI lesions. Runge et al. (1984), Kirshner et al. (1985), and Edwards et al. (1986a) used semi-quantitative visual methods, while Paty et al. (1985) have developed a computer-assisted method of determining the total area of lesions in a series of MRI slices. After decoding the computer tape from the MRI machine, the MRI of each axial slice is projected onto a graphics display monitor. Each lesion is outlined using a track ball–controlled cursor connected to a Vax computer. An experienced technician can carry out this process with good reproducibility (a coefficient of variation on repeat measurements of about 6%).

As a measure of the volume of diseased tissue, this is clearly a compromise because of the volume-averaging effects of MRI changes in the 10-mm-thick slices, but the technique has proved useful in repeat studies in the same patients in trials of treatment (Paty et al., 1986; Palmer et al., 1986) and in assessing the relationship between disease extent and psychiatric symptoms (Honer et al., 1987). The demyelinated plaques are often irregular in shape and frequently confluent, so that relatively small changes in the position of the patient's head can produce considerable changes in the appearance of the lesions in contiguous slices. We have found that quantitative measurement of an area gives a more consistent measure of disease extent in repeat studies than simply counting the number of individual lesions seen on the series of slices.

## Quantitative Measurement of $T_1$ and $T_2$ Relaxation Times

As noted, the standard MRI taken with SE or IR sequences depends on the density of protons as well as the tissue $T_1$ and $T_2$ relaxation times. By combining data from two scans taken of the same slice of brain using different techniques it is possible to calculate approximate quantitative values for $T_1$ and $T_2$ in any area of interest. Thus images based on quantitative $T_1$ values can be formed by combining data either from an IR plus an SE sequence or from two SE sequences carried out at different repetition times. Quantitative $T_2$ images can be calculated from two SE sequences taken using different echo times. In practice, the necessary data can be accumulated by doing an IR scan and a multiecho scan that simultaneously obtains the two SE sequences with different echo times.

Technical and theoretical considerations potentially limit the reliability of quantitative values for $T_1$ and $T_2$ using these techniques (Bradley et al., 1985) but there have been several reports that accurate and reproducible results can be obtained (Kjos et al., 1985a,b; Johnson et al., 1987). It is possible that $T_1$ and $T_2$ values may give more information about some pathological processes than can be obtained from standard SE and IR scans.

In MS the main issue is the separation of new lesions from old lesions, with the possibility that inflammatory lesions of different ages may be separable. Of particular interest in this respect is the study by Barnes et al. (1987) of two different types of experimental cerebral edema in cats. On SE and IR scans it was not possible to distinguish vasogenic edema (with high protein content) from cytotoxic edema (with low protein content). The patterns of the increase in $T_1$ and $T_2$ were characteristic for each type of edema, however, with $T_1$ and $T_2$ increasing to a similar degree in vasogenic edema and $T_2$ increasing twice as much as $T_1$ in cytotoxic edema. Ormerod et al. (1986b) have reported that acute MS lesions have longer $T_1$ and $T_2$ values than chronic lesions, but the place of these measurements in routine patient assessment has yet to be established.

Lacomis et al. (1986) reported that plaque-free white matter in the cerebral hemispheres in MS patients had longer $T_1$ values than white matter in normal persons. This is of interest, because there have been suggestions in the past that the myelin in MS patients may have a basic abnormality that makes it more likely to

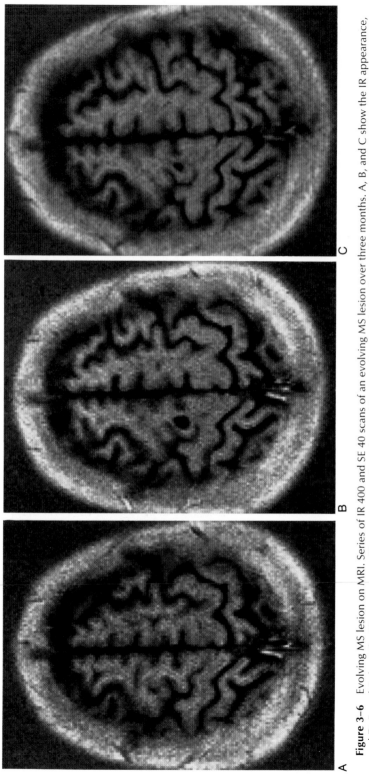

**Figure 3–6** Evolving MS lesion on MRI. Series of IR 400 and SE 40 scans of an evolving MS lesion over three months. A, B, and C show the IR appearance, and D, E, and F show the SE appearance. These are approximately monthly scans showing the evolution of a new lesion appearing in the high vertex white matter of the right hemisphere. Note how the lesion enlarges over time and then decreases in size.

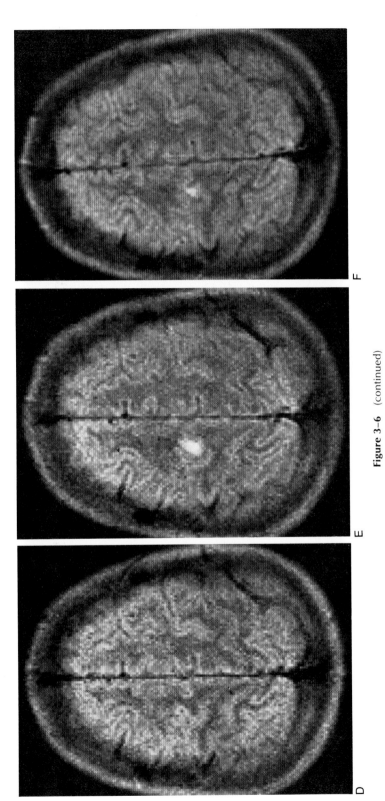

**Figure 3–6** (continued)

break down. We have not found any differences, however, in $T_1$ or $T_2$ values between plaque-free white matter in 9 mildly affected MS patients and 15 aged-matched normal subjects (Willoughby et al., 1989). A likely explanation for the discrepancy is the inclusion of unrecognized small demyelinated plaques in the "plaque-free" white matter in the earlier study, which made use of a relatively low-resolution resistive magnet.

## Prospective Serial MRI Scan in MS

Repeat MRI scans in several MS patients were reported by Johnson et al. (1984) and Li et al. (1984a) to show that some cerebral lesions diminished in size with time while others increased and that new lesions appeared without accompanying symptoms. A series of three prospective studies has now been carried out at the University of British Columbia, where MRI brain scans were done regularly at two- to four-week intervals for up to six months in a total of 24 patients with either relapsing-remitting or chronic-progressive disease (Paty et al., 1986a; Willoughby et al., 1989; Koopmans et al., 1989b). For this sort of study, careful repositioning of the patient in the machine is necessary for each scan, a process that requires considerable patience on the part of both patient and technician.

New lesions appeared in 19 of 24 patients, with up to 23 occurring in some patients over the course of the study (Figure 3–6). The new lesions were found apparently at random in all parts of the white matter or the cerebral hemispheres and cerebellum and had a characteristic temporal profile. They appeared suddenly and expanded to reach a maximum size in four to six weeks before decreasing again more gradually over a further six to ten weeks, usually leaving a small residual abnormal area. It was striking that different lesions were often in different phases of evolution at the same time in individual patients.

Only four of the patients suffered new symptoms or signs during these studies, and none of the new lesions on MRI scans could be correlated with the clinical episodes. In general, new MRI lesions occurred with 5–10 times the frequency of new clinical episodes. On average, their rate of development ranged from 2.5 per patient per year in mildly affected patients with relapsing-remitting disease to 6 per patient per year in chronic-progressive disease of long standing.

The pathological nature of the expanding and contracting new lesions is uncertain, but local breakdown of the blood–brain barrier with fluid extravasation with or without acute inflammation is likely. Almost certainly the lesions correspond to the transient contrast-enhancing lesion seen on CT scans. There is no doubt that acute lesions of this type may be associated with typical symptoms and signs of an acute attack of MS if they are in an appropriate area of the brain. As it happens, most of them arise in clinically silent areas and are not recognized except on MRI scans.

It is possible that the expanding and contracting new lesions actually represent the primary or basic lesion in MS, in which case it is likely that the characteristic chronic demyelinated plaques are the residua of numerous lesions of that sort occurring over many years. In any event, the MRI studies indicate that MS is a much more active disease process than has previously been recognized in patients with clinically stable disease. They also indicate that the same fluctuating process continues as actively (if not more so) in patients who have entered a slowly progressive phase of the disease as defined clinically. This suggests that there is not, in fact, a fundamental change in the nature of the disease in the chronic-progressive phase.

## SUMMARY

MRI is now well established as the most useful scanning technique in the diagnosis of MS. CT brain scanning was a major step forward in the 1970s, however, before the development of MRI scanning in the 1980s, and it still has an important place when access to MRI scanning is limited.

MRI brain scanning has an important place in supporting a diagnosis of MS by showing characteristic multiple asymptomatic cerebral lesions in patients presenting with an isolated spinal cord lesion or optic neuritis or in patients with neurologic symptoms but no clear-cut signs of organic neurologic disease. While early confirmation of a diagnosis of MS has as yet no important therapeutic implications, it may be of considerable value in epidemiological studies (Ebers et al., 1986; McFarland et al., 1985). Important cautions, however, are that multiple white matter lesions on MRI are not specific for MS and that a normal MRI scan does not exclude the diagnosis of MS (Paty et al., 1986b).

The ability to carry out repeated MRI scans without hazard to the patient has led to better understanding of disease activity in early relapsing-remitting and late chronic-progressive disease, and the use of gadolinium-enhanced scanning and perhaps the quantitative measurement of $T_1$ and $T_2$ relaxation times have the potential to provide new insights by distinguishing lesions at different phases of development. Studies relating disease activity to changes in immune function will be strengthened considerably by serial MRI scanning (Kastrukoff et al., 1986; Oger et al., 1988).

One of the most promising applications of MRI scanning in MS is in the assessment of the effects of treatment. At present this has to be judged by changes in the patient's neurologic state, which it is now clear is a very inexact measure of disease activity. The serial studies of MRI scanning to date suggest that regular scans at approximatley six-week intervals would detect most new asymptomatic cerebral lesions and allow earlier rejection of ineffective therapy in trials of treatment.

## ACKNOWLEDGMENT

The studies described in this chapter were supported by the Canadian Medical Research Council, the B.C. Health Care Research Foundation, The MS Society of Canada, the Kroc Foundation, and the Jacob W. Cohen Fund for Research in MS. We would like to thank our colleagues at the University of British Columbia for all their help with these studies, and also the neurologists of British Columbia for their cooperation in referring and following the patients.

# REFERENCES

Abbott, R.J., Howe, J.G., Currie, S., and Holland, I. (1982). Multiple sclerosis plaque mimicking tumour on computed tomography. *Br. Med. J.,* **285,** 1616–17.

Aita, J.F., Bennett, D.R., Anderson, R.E., and Ziter, F. (1978). Cranial CT appearance of acute multiple sclerosis. *Neurology,* **28,** 251–55.

Barnes, D., McDonald, W.I., Johnson, G., Tofts, P.S., and Landon, D.N. (1987). Quantitative nuclear magnetic resonance imaging: Characterisation of experimental cerebral oedema. *J. Neurol. Neurosurg. Psychiat.,* **50,** 125–33.

Barrett, L., Drayer, B., and Shin, C. (1985). High-resolution computed tomography in multiple sclerosis. *Ann. Neurol.,* **17,** 33–38.

Baumhefner, R.W., Tourtellotte, W.W., Ellison, G., Myers, L., Syndulko, K., Cohen, S.N., Shapshak, P., Osborne, M., and Waluch, V. (1986). Multiple sclerosis: Correlation of magnetic resonance imaging (MRI) with clinical disability, quantitative evaluation of neurologic function (QENF), evoked potential and intra-blood-brain-barrier (BBB) IgG synthesis. *Neurology,* **36**(Suppl 1), 283.

Beck, R.W., Savino, P.J., Schatz, N.J., Smith, C.H., and Sergott, R.C. (1982). Plaque causing homonymous hemianopsia in multiple sclerosis identified by computed tomography. *Am. J. Ophthal.,* **94,** 229–34.

Bogousslavsky, J., Fox, A.J., Carey, L.S., Vinitski, S., Bass, B., Noseworthy, J.H., Ebers, G.C., and Barnett, H.J.M. (1986). Correlates of brain-stem oculomotor disorders in multiple sclerosis: Magnetic resonance imaging. *Arch. Neurol.,* **43,** 460–63.

Bradley, W.G. (1984). Patchy periventricular white matter lesions in the elderly: A common observation during NMR imaging. Non-invasive medical imaging. *Non-Invasive Medical Imaging,* **1,** 35–41.

Bradley, W.G., Edy, W.R., and Hasso, A.N. (1985). *Magnetic Resonance Imaging of the Brain, Head, and Neck: A Text Atlas.* Rockville, Md.: Aspin Systems Corporation.

Bradley, W.G., Waluch, V., Wycoff, R.R., and Yadley, R.A. (1984). Differential diagnosis of periventricular abnormalities in NMRI of brain. In: *Program and Book of Abstracts of the Society of Magnetic Resonance in Medicine, Third Annual Meeting.* San Francisco, The Society of Magnetic Resonance in Medicine. pp. 81–2.

Brooks, D.J., Leenders, K.L., Head, G., Marshall, J., Legg, N.J., and Jones, T. (1984). Studies on regional cerebral oxygen utilisation and cognitive function in multiple sclerosis. *J. Neurol. Neurosurg. Psychiat.,* **47,** 1182–91.

Bydder, G.M., Steiner, R.E., Young, I.R., and Hall, A.S., Thomas, D.J., Marshall, J., Pallis, C.A., and Legg, N.J. (1982). Clinical NMR imaging of the brain: 140 cases. *AJR,* **139,** 215–36.

Cala, L.A., Mastaglia, F.L., and Black, J.L. (1978). Computerized tomography of brain and optic nerve in multiple sclerosis. *J. Neurol. Sci.,* **36,** 411–26.

Carr, D.H., Brown, J., Bydder, G.M., Weinmann, H.J., Speck, U., Thomas, D.J., and Young, I.R. (1984). Intravenous chelated gadolinium as a contrast agent in NMR imaging of cerebral tumours. *Lancet,* **1,** 484–86.

Claussen, C., Laniado, M., Schorner, W., Niendorf, H.P., Weinmann, H.J., Fiegler, W., and Felix, R. (1985). Gadolinium-DTPA in MR imaging of glioblastomas and intracranial metastases. *AJNR,* **6,** 669–74.

Cole, M., and Ross, R.J. (1977). Plaque of multiple sclerosis seen on computerized tranaxial tomogram. *Neurology,* **27,** 890–91.

Costantino, A., Black, S.E., Carr, T., Nicholson, R.L., and Noseworthy, J.H. (1986). Dorsal midbrain syndrome in multiple sclerosis with magnetic resonance imaging correlation. *Can. J. Neurol. Sci.,* **13,** 62–5.

Crisp, D.T., Kleiner, J.E., DeFillip, G.J., Greenstein, J.I., Liu, T.H., and Sommers, D. (1985).

Clinical correlations with magnetic resonance imaging in multiple sclerosis. *Neurology*, **35**(Suppl 1), 137.

Dryer, B.P., and Barrett, L. (1984). Magnetic resonance imaging and CT scanning in multiple sclerosis. *Ann. N.Y. Acad. Sci.*, **436**, 294–313.

Ebers, G.C., Vinuela, F.V., Feasby, T., and Bass, B. (1984). Multifocal CT enhancement in MS. *Neurology*, **34**, 341–46.

Ebers, G.C., Dennis, M.D., Bulman, E., Sadovnick, A.D., Paty, D.W., Warren, S., Hader, W., Murray, J., Seland, P., Duquette, P., Grey, T., Nelson, R., Nicolle, M., and Brunet, D. (1986). A population-based study of multiple sclerosis in twins. *N. Engl. J. Med.*, **315**, 1638–42.

Edwards, M.K., Farlow, M.R., and Stevens, J.C. (1986a). Multiple sclerosis: MRI and clinical correlation. *AJR*, **147**, 571–74.

Edwards, M.K., Farlow, M.R., and Stevens, J.C. (1986b). Cranial MR in spinal cord MS: Diagnosing patients with isolated spinal cord symptoms. *AJNR*, **7**, 1003–5.

Frey, K.A., Wieland, D.M., Brown, L.E., Rogers, W.L., Agranoff, B.W., and Pate, B. (in press). Development of a tomographic myelin scan. *Ann. Neurol.*.

Frytak, S., Franklin, E., O'Neill, B., Lee, R.E., Creagan, E.T., and Trautman, J.C. (1985). Magnetic resonance imaging for neurotoxicity in long-term survivors of carcinoma. *Mayo Clin. Proc.*, **60**, 803–12.

Fullerton, G.D. (1982). Basic concepts for nuclear magnetic resonance imaging. *Magnetic Resonance Imaging*, **1**, 39–55.

Gebarski, S.S., Gabrielsen, T.O., Gilman, S., Knake, J.E., Latack, J.T., and Aisen, A.M. (1985). The initial diagnosis of multiple sclerosis: clinical impact of magnetic resonance imaging. *Ann. Neurol.*, **17**, 469–74.

Gilbert, J.J., and Sadler, M. (1983). Unsuspected multiple sclerosis. *Arch. Neurol.*, **40**, 533–36.

Gyldensted, C. (1976b). Computer tomography of the cerebrum in multiple sclerosis. *Neuroradiology*, **12**, 33–42.

Gonzalez-Scarano, F., Grossman, R.I., Galetta, S., Atlas, S.W., and Silberberg, D.H. (1987). Multiple sclerosis disease activity correlates with gadolinium-enhanced magnetic resonance imaging. *Ann. Neurol.*, **21**, 300–6.

Grossman, R.I., Gonzalez-Scarano, F., Atlas, S.W., Galetta, S., and Silberberg, D.H. (1986). Multiple sclerosis: Gadolinium enhancement in MR imaging. *Radiology*, **161**, 721–25.

Gyldensted, C. (1976). Computer tomography of the cerebrum in multiple sclerosis. *Neuroradiology*, **12**, 33–42.

Harding, A.E., Radue, E.W., and Whiteley, A.M. (1978). Contrast-enhanced lesions on computerised tomography in multiple sclerosis. *J. Neurol. Neurosurg. Psychiat.*, **41**, 754–58.

Haughton, V., Schmidt, J., Syvertsen, A., Khatri, B., Ho, K.C., and Wilson, C. (1980). Detection of demyelinated plaques with xenon-enhanced computed tomography. *Neuroradiology*, **20**, 181–83.

Herscovitch, P., Trotter, J.L., Lemann, W., and Raichle, M.E. (1984). Positron emission tomography (PET) in active MS: Demonstration of demyelination and diaschisis. *Neurology*, **34** (Suppl 1), 78.

Hershey, L.A., Gado, M.H., and Trotter, J.L. (1979). Computerized tomography in the diagnostic evaluation of multiple sclerosis. *Ann. Neurol.*, **5**, 32–9.

Honer, W.G., Hurwitz, T., Li, D.K.B., Palmer, M., and Paty, D.W. (1987). Temporal lobe involvement in multiple sclerosis patients with psychiatric disorders. *Arch. Neurol.*, **44**, 187–90.

Hyman, R.A., Blankfein, R.J., Pitman, E.R., Naidich, J.B., and McGeachie, R.E. (1979).

Computed tomography: Regression of periventricular enhancing lesions in multiple sclerosis. *Comput. Tomogr.,* **3,** 93–6.

Isaac, C., Li, D.K.B., Genton, M., Jardine, C., Grochowski, E., Palmer, M., Kastrukoff, L.F., Oger, J., and Paty, D.W. (1988). Multiple sclerosis: A serial study using MRI in relapsing patients. *Neurology,* **38,** 1511–15.

Jackson, J.A., Leake, D.R., Schneiders, N.J., Rolak, L.A., Kelley, G.R., Ford, J.J., Appel, S.H., and Bryan, R.N. (1985). Magnetic resonance imaging in multiple sclerosis: Results in 32 cases. *AJNR,* **6,** 171–76.

Jacobs, L., Kinkel, P.R., and Kinkel, W.R. (1986a). Silent brain lesions in patients with isolated idiopathic optic neuritis. A clinical and nuclear magnetic resonance imaging study. *Arch. Neurol.,* **43,** 452–55.

Jacobs, L., Kinkel, W.R., Polachini, I., and Kinkel, R.P. (1986b). Correlations of nuclear magnetic resonance imaging, computerized tomography, and clinical profiles in multiple sclerosis. *Neurology,* **36,** 27–34.

Johnson, G., Ormerod, I.E.C., Barnes, D., Tofts, P.S., and MacManus, D. (1987). *Br. J. Radiol.,* **60,** 143–53.

Johnson, M.A., Li, D.K.B., Bryant, D.J., and Payne, J.A. (1984). Magnetic resonance imaging: Serial observations in multiple sclerosis. *AJNR,* **5,** 495–99.

Joseph, R., Pullicino, P., Goldberg, C.D.S., and Rose, F.C. (1985). Bilateral pontine gaze palsy. *Arch. Neurol.,* **42,** 93–4.

Karlik, S.J., Noseworthy, J., and Gilbert, J.J. (1984). Nuclear magnetic resonance (NMR) spectroscopy studies in experimental allergic encephalomyelitis (EAE). *Society of Magnetic Resonance in Medicine, Scientific Program 3rd Annual Meeting,* p. 399.

Karlik, S.J., Strejan, G., Gilbert, J.J., and Noseworthy, J.H. (1986). NMR studies in experimental allergic encephalomyelitis (EAE): Normalization of $T_1$ and $T_2$ with parenchymal cellular infiltration. *Neurology,* **36,** 1112–14.

Kastrukoff, L.F., Oger, J., and Paty, D.W. (1986). Multiple sclerosis: Correlation of peripheral blood lymphocyte phenotype and natural killer cell activity with disease assessed clinically and by MRI. *Ann. Neurol.,* **20,** 164.

Kinkel, W.R., Jacobs, L., Polachini, I., and Kinkel, R.P. (1984). Computerized tomography (CT) and nuclear magnetic resonance (NMR) in multiple sclerosis (MS): A comparative study. *Neurology,* **34** (Suppl 1), 136.

Kirshner, H.S., Tsai, S.I., Runge, V.M., and Price, A.C. (1985). Magnetic resonance imaging and other techniques in the diagnosis of multiple sclerosis. *Arch. Neurol.,* **42,** 859–63.

Kjos, B.O., Ehman, R.L., Brant-Zawadzki, M., Kelly, W.M., Norman, D., and Newton, T.H. (1985a). Reproducibility of relaxation times and spin density calculated from routine MR imaging sequences: Clinical study of the CNS. *AJNR,* **6,** 271–76.

Kjos, B.O., Ehman, R.L., and Brant-Zawadzki, M. (1985b). Reproducibility of $T_1$ and $T_2$ relaxation times calculated from routine MR imaging sequences: Phantom study. *AJNR,* **6,** 277–83.

Koopmans, R.A., Li, D.K.B., Grochowski, E., Cutler, P.J., and Paty, D.W. (1989a). Benign versus chronic progressive multiple sclerosis: Magnetic resonance imaging features. *Ann. Neurol.,* **25,** 74–81.

Koopmans, R.A., Li, D.K.B., Oger, J.J.F., Kastrukoff, L.F., Jardine, C., Costleg, L., Hall, S., Groschowski, E.W., and Paty, D.W., (1989b). Chronic progressive multiple sclerosis: Serial magnetic resonance imaging over six months. *Ann. Neurol.,* **26,** 248–56.

Lacomis, D., Osbakken, M., and Gross, G. (1986). Spin-lattice relaxation ($T_1$) times of cerebral white matter in multiple sclerosis. *Magnetic Resonance in Medicine,* **3,** 194–202.

Lane, B., Carroll, B.A., and Pedley, T.A. (1978). Computerized cranial tomography in cerebral diseases of white matter. *Neurology,* **28,** 534–44.

Latack, J.T., Gabrielsen, T.O., Knake, J.E., Gebarski, S.S., and Dorovini-Zis, K. (1984).

Computed tomography of spinal cord necrosis from multiple sclerosis. *AJNR,* **5,** 485–87.

Lebow, S., Anderson, D.C., Mastri, A., and Larson, D. (1978). Acute multiple sclerosis with contrast-enhancing plaques. *Arch. Neurol.,* **35,** 435–39.

Li, D., Mayo, J., Fache, S., Robertson, W.D., and Paty, D., and Genton, M. (1984a). Early experience in nuclear magnetic resonance imaging of multiple sclerosis. *Ann. N.Y. Acad. Sci.,* **436,** 483–86.

Li, D., Mayo, J., Fache, S., Robertson, W., Kastrukoff, L.F., Oger, J., and Paty, D.W. (1984b). Lack of correlation between clinical manifestations and lesions in MS as seen by NMR. *Neurology,* **34** (Suppl 1), 136.

Lidegaard, O., Gyldensted, C., Juhler, M., and Zeeberg, I. (1983). CT findings in acute MS. *Acta Neurol. Scand.,* **68,** 77–83.

Lodder, J., de Weerd, A.W., Koetsier, J.C., and van der Lugt, P.J.M. (1983). Computed tomography in acute cerebral multiple sclerosis. *Arch. Neurol.,* **40,** 320–22.

Loizou, L.A., Rolfe, E.B., and Hewazy, H. (1982). Cranial computed tomography in the diagnosis of multiple sclerosis. *J. Neurol. Neursurg. Psychiat.,* **45,** 905–12.

Lukes, S.A., Crooks, L.E. Aminoff, M.J., Kaufman, L., Panitch, H.S., Mills, C., and Norman, D. (1983). Nuclear magnetic resonance imaging in multiple sclerosis. *Ann. Neurol.,* **13,** 592–601.

McFarland, H.F., Patronas, N.J., McFarlin, D.E., Mandler, R.N., Beall, S.S., Cross, A.H., Goodman, A., and Krebs, H. (1985). Studies of multiple sclerosis in twins using nuclear magnetic resonance. *Neurology,* **5** (Suppl 1), 137.

Marano, G.D., Goodwin, C.A., and Ko, J.P. (1980). Atypical contrast enhancement in computerized tomography of demyelinating disease. *Arch. Neurol.,* **37,** 523–24.

Matias-Guiu, J., Sanz, M., Gili, J., Mollins, A., Bonaventura, I., and Capdevila, A. (1986). Correlation of MRI with the clinical status of patients with multiple sclerosis. *Neurology,* **36,** 1626.

Mills, C.M., Crooks, L.E., Kaufman, L., and Brant-Zawadzki, M. (1984). Cerebral abnormalities: Use of calculated $T_1$ and $T_2$ magnetic resonance images for diagnosis. *Radiology,* **150,** 87–94.

Morariu, M.A., Wilkins, D.E., and Patel, S. (1980). Multiple sclerosis and serial computerized tomography (Delayed contrast enhancement of acute and early lesions). *Arch. Neurol.,* **37,** 189–90.

Morimoto, T., Nagao, H., Sano, N., Habara, S., Takahashi, M., Matsuda, H., Beppu, K., and Shoda, T. (1985). A case of multiple sclerosis with multi-ring-like and butterfly-like enhancement on computerized tomography. *Brain Dev.,* **7,** 43–45.

Nelson, M.J., Miller, S.L., McLain, L.W. Jr., and Gold, L.H.A. (1981). Multiple sclerosis: Large plaque causing mass effect and ring sign. *J. Comput. Assist. Tomogr.,* **5,** 892–94.

Noseworthy, J.H., Strejan, G., Gilbert, J.J., and Karlick, S. (1985). Comparison of in vitro nuclear magnetic resonance (NMR) properties and histopathology in experimental allergic encephalomyelitis (EAE). *Neurology,* **35** (Suppl 1), 259.

Noseworthy, J.H., O'Brien, J.T., Gilbert, J.J., and Karlick, S.J. (1986). Nuclear magnetic resonance (NMR) changes in experimental allergic encephalomyelitis (EAE) precede clinical and pathological events. *Can. J. Neurol. Sci.,* **13,** 162.

Oger, J., Willoughby, E., and Paty, D. (1987). Serial studies of relapsing multiple sclerosis: Reduced IgG secretion in vitro and reduced suppressor cell function correlate with disease activity as recognised by magnetic resonance imaging. *Ann. Neurol.,* **22,** 152.

Oger, J., Kastrukoff, L. F., Li, D.K.B., and Paty, D.W., (1988). Multiple sclerosis: In relapsing patients, immune functions vary with disease activity as assesed by MRI. *Neurology,* **38,** 1739–44.

Ormerod, I.E.C., du Boulay, E.P.G.H., Callanan, M.M., Johnson, G., Logsdail, S.J., Moseley, I.S., Rudge, P., Roberts, R.C., McDonald, W.I., Halliday, A.M., Kendall, B.E., MacManus, D.G., Ron, M.A., and Zilkha, K.J. (1984). NMR in multiple sclerosis and cerebral vascular disease. *Lancet,* **2,** 1334–35.

Ormerod, I.E.C., McDonald, W.I., doBoulay, G.H., Kendall, B.E., Moseley, I.F., Halliday, A.M., Kakigi, R., Kriss, A., and Peringer, E. (1986a). Disseminated lesions at presentation in patients with optic neuritis. *J. Neurol. Neurosurg. Psychiat.,* **49,** 124–27.

Ormerod, I.E.C., Bronstein, A., Rudge, P., Johnson, G., MacManus, D., Halliday, A.M., Barratt, H., du Boulay, E.P.G.H., Kendal, B.E., Moseley, I.F., Jones, S.J., Kriss, A., and Peringer, E. (1986b). Magnetic resonance imaging in clinically isolated lesions of the brain stem. *J. Neurol. Neurosurg. Psychiat.,* **49,** 737–43.

Ormerod, I.E.C., Du Boulay, G.H., and McDonald, W.I. (1986c). Imaging of multiple sclerosis. In: W.I. McDonald, and D.H. Silberberg, eds. *Multiple Sclerosis,* pp. 11–36. London: Butterworth.

Palmer, M.R., Bergstrom, M., Grochowski, E., Apted, C., Li, D.K., Genton, M., Hashimoto, S.A., and Paty, D.W. (1986). Magnetic resonance imaging (MRI) in multiple sclerosis (MS): Quantitative changes in the size of lesions over 6 months in the placebo limb of a therapeutic trial. *Can. J. Neurol. Sci.,* **13,** 168.

Paty, D.W., Bergstrom, M., Palmer, M., MacFadyen, J., and Li, D. (1985). A quantitative magnetic resonance image of the multiple sclerosis brain. *Neurology,* **35** (Suppl 1), 137.

Paty, D.W., Isaac, C.D., Grochowski, E., Palmer, M.R., Oger, J., Kastrukoff, L.F., Nord, B., Genton, M., Jardine, C., and Li, D.K. (1986a). Magnetic resonance imaging (MRI) in multiple sclerosis (MS): A serial study in relapsing and remitting patients with quantitative measurements of lesion size. *Neurology,* **36** (Suppl 1), 177.

Paty, D.W., Asbury, A.K., Herndon, R.M., McFarland, H.F., McDonald, W.I., McIlroy, W.J., Prineas, J.W., Scheinberg, L.C., and Wolinsky, J.S. (1986b). Use of magnetic resonance imaging in the diagnosis of multiple sclerosis: Policy statement. *Neurology,* **36,** 1575.

Paty, D.W., Hashimoto, S.A., Hooge, J., Eisen, A., Eisen, K., Purves, S., Brandejs, V., Robertson, W.D., and Li, D.K. (1988). Magnetic resonance imaging (MRI) in multiple sclerosis (MS): A prospective evaluation of usefulness in diagnosis. *Neurology,* **38,** 180–85.

Pykett, I.L., and Rosen, B. (1983). Nuclear magnetic resonance: In vivo proton chemical shift imaging. *Radiology,* **149,** 197–210.

Reese, L., Carr, T.J., Nicholson, R.L., and Lepp, E.K. (1986). Magnetic resonance imaging for detecting lesions of multiple sclerosis: comparison with computed tomography and clinical assessment. *Can. Med. Assoc. J.,* **135,** 639–43.

Rieth, K.G., Di Chiro, G., Cromwell, L.D., McKeever, P.E., Kornblith, P.L., Kufta, C.V., and Pleet, A.B. (1981). Primary demyelinating disease simulating glioma of the corpus callosum: Report of three cases. *J. Neurosurg.,* **55,** 620–4.

Robertson, W.D., Li, D., Mayo, J., and Paty, D. (1984). Clinical versus magnetic resonance imaging: Diagnosis of multiple sclerosis: *Ann. Neurol.,* **16,** 140.

Runge, V.M., Price, A.C., Kirshner, H.S., Allen, J.H., Partain, C.L., and James, A.E., Jr. (1984). Magnetic resonance imaging of multiple sclerosis: A study of pulse-technique efficacy. *AJR,* **143,** 1015–26.

Sagar, H.J., Warlow, C.P., Sheldon, P.W.E., and Esiri, M.M. (1982). Multiple sclerosis with clinical and radiological features of cerebral tumour. *J. Neurol. Neurosurg. Psychiat.,* **45,** 802–8.

Scotti, G., Scialfa, G., Biondi, A., Landoni, L., Caputo, D., and Cazzuloo, C.L. (1986). Magnetic resonance in multiple sclerosis. *Neuroradiology,* **28,** 319–23.

Sears, E.S., Tindall, R.S.A., and Zarnow, H. (1978). Active multiple sclerosis. *Arch. Neurol.,* **35,** 426–34.

Sears, E.S., McCammon, A., Bigelow, R., and Hayman, L.A. (1982). Maximizing the harvest of contrast enhancing lesions in multiple sclerosis. *Neurology,* **32,** 815–20.

Sheldon, J.J., Siddharthan, R., Tobias, J., Sheremata, W.A., Soila, K., and Viamonte, M., Jr. (1985). MR imaging of multiple sclerosis: Comparison with clinical and CT examinations in 74 patients. *AJR,* **145,** 957–64.

Sheremata, W.A., Sevush, S., Knigh, D., and Ziajka, P. (1984). Altered cerebral metabolism in MS. *Neurology,* **34** (Suppl 1), 118.

Simon, J.H., Holtas, S.L., Schiffer, R.B., Rudick, R.A., Herndon, R.M., Kido, D.K., and Utz, R. (1986). Corpus callosum and subcallosal-periventricular lesions in multiple sclerosis: Detection with MR. *Radiology,* **160,** 363–67.

Spiegel, S.M., Vinuela, F., Fox, A.J., and Pelz, D.M. (1985). CT of multiple sclerosis. Reassessment of delayed scanning with high doses of contrast material. *AJR,* **145,** 497–500.

Stewart, W.A., Hall, L.D., Berry, K., and Paty, D.W. (1984). Correlation between NMR scan and brain slice: Data in multiple sclerosis: *Lancet,* **2,** 412.

Stewart, W.A., Alvord, E.C., Hruby, S., Hall, L.D., and Paty, D.W. (1985). Early detection of experimental allergic encephalomyelitis by magnetic resonance imaging. *Lancet,* **2,** 898.

Stewart, W.A., Hall, L.D., Berry, K., Churg, A., Oger, J., Hashimoto, S.A., and Paty, D.W. (1986). Magnetic resonance imaging (MRI) in multiple sclerosis (MS): Pathological correlation studies in eight cases. *Neurology,* **36** (Suppl 1), 320.

Troiano, R., Hafstein, M., Ruderman, Dowling, P., and Cook, S. (1984). Effect of high-dose intravenous steroid administration on contrast-enhancing computed tomographic scan lesions in multiple sclerosis. *Ann. Neurol.,* **15,** 257–63.

Valk, J., MacLean, C., and Algra, P.R. (1985). *Basic Principles of Nuclear Magnetic Resonance Imaging.* Amsterdam, Elsevier.

van der Velden, M., Bots, G.T.A.M., and Endtz, L.J. (1979). Cranial CT in multiple sclerosis showing a mass effect. *Surg. Neurol.,* **12,** 307–10.

Vinuela, F.V., Fox, A.J., Debrun, G.M., Feasby, T.E., and Ebers, G.C. (1982). New perspectives in computed tomography of multiple sclerosis. *AJR,* **139,** 123–27.

Vliegenthart, W.E., Sanders, E.A.C.M., Bruyn, G.W., and Vielvoye, G.J. (1985). An unusual CT-scan appearance in multiple sclerosis. *J. Neurol. Sci.,* **71,** 129–34.

Wang, A.M., Morris, J.H., Hickey, W.F., Hammerschlag, S.B., O'Reilly, G.V., and Rumbaugh, C.L. (1983). Unusual CT patterns of multiple sclerosis. *AJNR,* **4,** 47–50.

Warren, K.G., Ball, M.J., Paty, D.W., and Banna, M. (1976). Computer tomography in disseminated sclerosis. *Can. J. Neurol. Sci.,* **3,** 211–16.

Weinstein, M.A., Lederman, R.J., Rothner, A.D., Duchesneau, P.M., and Norman, D. (1978). Interval computed tomography in multiple sclerosis. *Radiology,* **129,** 689–94.

Weisberg, L. (1981). Contrast enhancement visualized by computerized tomography in acute multiple sclerosis. *Comp. Tomogr.,* **5,** 293–300.

Willoughby, E.W., Grochowski, E., Li, D.K.B., Oger, J., Kastrukoff, L.F., and Paty, D.W. (1989). Serial magnetic resonance scanning in multiple sclerosis: A second prospective study in relapsing patients. *Ann. Neurol.,* **25,** 43–49.

Wippold, F.J., and Cuetter, A.C. (1982). Computed tomography in multiple sclerosis: Case report with radiologic-pathologic correlation *Military Med.,* **147,** 68–9.

Wuthrich, R., Gigli, H., Wiggli, U., Muller, H.R., Elke, M., and Hunig, R. (1976). CT scanning in demyelinating diseases. In: W. Lanksch, and E. Kafner, eds., *Cranial Computerized Tomography,* pp. 239–243. New York, Springer-Verlag.

Young, I.R., Hall, A.S., Pallis, C.A., Bydder, G.M., Legg, N.J., and Steiner, R.E. (1981). Nuclear magnetic resonance imaging of the brain in multiple sclerosis. *Lancet,* **2,** 1063–66.

Young, S.W. (1984). *Nuclear Magnetic Resonance Imaging: Basic Principles.* New York: Raven Press.

# 4

# Neuropsychological Assessment

EILEEN B. FENNELL AND MARCIA C. SMITH

Since the early description of intellectual, emotional and memory problems in patients with multiple sclerosis (Charcot, 1877), a variety of cognitive and affective changes have been reported in these patients. Depending on the type of examination rendered (e.g., brief mental status exam versus comprehensive neuropsychological examination), estimates of cognitive dysfunction accompanying multiple sclerosis (MS) have ranged from 30% to greater than 50% of the patients examined (Peyser and Poser, 1986; Rao, 1986; Trimble and Grant, 1982). In this chapter we present a brief review of the research describing the neuropsychological deficits that have been observed among MS patients. Then we describe the methods used by our neuropsychology service to determine the presence or absence of higher cortical dysfunction. Finally, we present two recently evaluated cases to describe the clinical performance of these patients as well as to demonstrate how the findings from a neuropsychological examination can be meaningfully conveyed to the patient and the consulting physician.

## NEUROPSYCHOLOGICAL DYSFUNCTION IN MULTIPLE SCLEROSIS

A variety of changes in higher brain functions have been described in clinical case reports and in research with MS patients. Changes have been reported in broad areas of neuropsychological functions, including intellect, memory, visuospatial/ visuomotor performance, motor speed and dexterity, sensation, executive functions, and emotional/affective behavior. Three different kinds of studies have contributed to these observations: (1) the *clinical case study,* in which a particular type of dysfunction is described to demonstrate an aspect of the clinical diagnosis and/ or course of the disease; (2) *between-group comparison studies,* in which the performance of a group of patients with MS is compared with that of a contrast group, typically normals, but occasionally also patients with other types of neurologic or affective illnesses; and, (3) *within-group comparison studies,* in which patients with different clinical courses (e.g., relapsing-remitting versus chronic-progressive) or different degrees of disability are compared with each other.

Typically, these studies measure aspects of the patient's performance at a single point in time. There have been relatively few longitudinal studies of patients with MS (see Chapter 8). Thus the clinician who is asked to evaluate a patient with MS often must compare findings in this individual case with the data derived from cross-sectional studies of groups of patients who may differ along several dimensions. These dimensions include age of onset, presenting symptomatology, progression of symptoms and course of disease, state of remission at the time of examination, current medications, degree of associated physical disability (Kurtzke, 1970; Poser et al., 1983), and reason for referral (Peyser and Poser, 1986).

In addition, the individual patient may have undergone a variety of neurodiagnostic procedures, including the neurologic examination, studies of cerebral spinal fluid (CSF), electroencephalographic (EEG) and evoked potential studies, CT scanning, and the more recently developed magnetic resonance imaging (MRI) (Cutler et al., 1986; Stevens et al., 1986). Information from these diagnostic procedures has only recently been correlated with neuropsychological test findings in studies of MS patients (see Chapter 7). Such information could lead to improved understanding of brain–behavior relationships in MS and provide more accurate predictions of neurobehavioral outcome for the individual patient.

Excellent reviews of the symptoms, course, and neuropathological and neuroimaging findings in MS are presented in other chapters and are not repeated here. In the following sections, we present a brief review of the different neuropsychological deficits that have been described in the clinical research on MS. The discussion is divided into sections on intellectual functions, memory, visuospatial/visuoperceptual/visuoconstructional deficits, language disorder, executive functions, and affective disorder.

## Intellectual Functions

Studies of the performance of MS patients on standardized group or individually administered intelligence tests generally report full scale IQ scores within the average range (90–110), with verbal IQ scores typically greater than performance scores. Reported verbal-performance discrepancies range between 9 and 15 points in individual studies (Matthews et al., 1970; Goldstein and Shelley, 1974; Ivnik, 1978a,b; Marsh, 1980; Heaton et al., 1985). This disparity is usually attributed to MS-related sensorimotor deficits, which preferentially affect the timed aspects of the performance subtests. Alternatively, the verbal subtests may be more resistant to the effects of brain disease than the performance subtests (Lezak, 1983).

Studies that attempt to address the issue of longitudinal decline of intellectual functioning in MS have produced somewhat inconsistent results and are marred by methodological deficiencies. These deficiencies include the lack of a control group, small sample size, failure to control for education, and differences in follow-up time ranging from six months (Canter, 1951) to periods of up to five years (see Chapter 8). It is likely that declines in intellectual functioning are related to the course of the disease, with chronic-progressive patients being at greater risk than relapsing-remitting patients (Heaton et al., 1985), although definitive studies on this issue have not been reported. Whether longitudinal declines in intellectual functions are correlated with the rate of progression of physical disability is unclear, although cross-sectional studies have not found such a relationship (Heaton et al., 1985; Rao et al., 1985; Rao et al., 1987).

## Memory Functions

Memory disorder is frequently reported in studies of MS patients, but only recently has it been systematically evaluated (Huber et al., 1987; Litvan et al., 1988a; Peyser and Poser, 1986; Rao, 1986). A variety of memory measures have been used, including tests of attention span (e.g., digit span), story recall (immediate and delayed), verbal list learning, free verbal memory after interference conditions, recall of geometric stimuli (immediate and delayed), memory for tonal sequences, and composite memory measures [e.g., Wechsler Memory Scale (WMS)]. Recent reviews (Rao, 1986; Chapter 6) suggest that while memory impairment is frequently observed in MS, the type (i.e., verbal versus nonverbal; recall versus recognition), severity, and pattern of the disorder are quite variable. In general, span memory is unaffected, as is short-term recognition memory. Verbal memory tests that involve more complex material or require acquisition of a supraspan list of related or unrelated items are more likely to reveal impairment (Huber et al., 1987; Litvan et al., 1988b). MS patients show a greater than expected loss of information over time, significant buildup of proactive interference with repeated presentations, and a reduced curve of learning on word list tests. Thus tasks that tap recall of new verbal information over a time delay or that assess the efficiency of learning/ retrieval strategies may be affected preferentially in MS, particularly for patients with chronic-progressive courses (Heaton et al., 1985).

Nonverbal memory is typically assessed by having the patient draw a geometric design from memory. Nonverbal memory findings may be confounded in MS patients with significant sensorimotor impairment. Whether similar differences between recognition and recall of nonverbal materials are also present in some MS patients is still unclear, because of limited data characterizing the nonverbal learning deficits among these patients.

At present, the memory disorder in MS has been characterized as representing deficits in retrieval from long-term storage. This pattern is not unlike the clinical picture observed in patients with lesions affecting frontal-subcortical pathways (Heilman and Valenstein, 1985).

## Visuoperceptual, Visuospatial, Visuoconstructional Functions

Most studies of MS patients infer the presence of dysfunction in visuoperceptual or visuospatial functions from the observation of performance deficits on tests of general intelligence. Unfortunately, solutions to problems on these subtests frequently require input from multiple brain functional systems requiring visual perception, visuospatial analysis, executive functions, memory, and speed of motor output (Lezak, 1983). In addition, constructional requirements of some of the subtests (e.g., Block Design, Object Assembly, Digit Symbol) further confound the ability to separate input deficiencies (i.e., perceptual difficulties) from output problems (i.e., motor speed and planning). Use of "purer" measures of visuoperceptual functions, which do not require a motor output (e.g., the Visuospatial Subtest from Thurstone's Test of Primary Mental Abilities; Thurstone and Thurstone, 1962), has not been reported in the research to date, although such an approach is not infrequently used in a comprehensive clinical assessment battery (Lezak, 1983). In the clinical cases to be described later in this chapter, we administered Raven's Standard Progressive Matrices (Raven, 1960) to determine the visual spatial processing capabilities of patients when a motor output is removed. A recent study determined that the first three subtests depend more heavily on perceptual than reasoning abilities (Mings, 1987). As we shall demonstrate, use of other tests of visual analysis such as the Hooper Test of Visual Organization (Hooper, 1958) coupled with the complex figure of Rey (Lezak, 1983) allows the clinician a broader comparison of subcomponents of visuospatial and visuoconstructional functions.

In a recent study Casey and Fennell (1985) reported that significant deficiencies in copying the Rey-Osterreith figure were observed in 41 chronic MS patients, despite above-average verbal IQs. While lower scores were obtained by patients with greater physical disability, the authors interpreted that these constructional deficits resulted from deficiencies of planning and execution, as commonly observed in frontal lobe dysfunction, rather than from pure sensorimotor defects. Support for this interpretation was obtained from the significant correlations between the patients' performances on measures of visuoconstructional tasks and those of frontal lobe integrity. If these observations are supported in future studies, it would suggest that the performance deficits observed on broad-band measures, such as intelligence tests, may need to be reinterpreted to reflect primary deficits in planning and execution.

## Language Disorder

Disorders of language expression and/or comprehension are rarely reported in MS (for reviews, see Peyser and Poser, 1986; Rao, 1986). Research employing comprehensive neuropsychological assessment of MS patients may include a screening test for aphasic symptoms, but performance is reported in terms of number rather than type of errors (Heaton et al., 1985). Thus while chronic-progressive patients perform worse than relapsing-remitting patients and normal controls, the type of errors committed by these patients is unclear. An earlier study, employing the more classical neurologic assessment of language functions (reading, comprehension, and written language) found evidence of reading and writing (spelling) deficiencies in a large group of MS patients (Jambor, 1969). While other investigators have suggested that more classical aphasic disorders or other disconnection syndromes may be observed in some MS patients (Huber et al., 1987; Rao, 1986), the nature of the language disorder, if present, is still open to description and investigation. The reports of impaired verbal fluency (Heaton et al., 1985; Casey and Fennell, 1985) may need to be interpreted in the context of general problems of behavioral fluency related to frontal-subcortical dysfunction rather than as an aspect of language disorder in the absence of frank symptoms of aphasia.

## Executive Functions

Deficiencies in concept formation, abstract reasoning, behavioral fluency, and planning and organizational skills have been part of the clinical literature in MS since its earliest descriptions (Peyser and Poser, 1986; Rao, 1986; Trimble and Grant, 1982). Most recent studies that have examined MS patients for conceptual or abstract reasoning deficits have employed tests such as the Category Test from the Halstead-Reitan Battery (HRB) (Boll, 1981) or the Wisconsin Card Sorting Test (Grant and Berg, 1960). In general, MS patients, particularly chronic-progressive patients, perform worse than normal controls do (Rao et al., 1987; Heaton et al., 1985; Casey and Fennell, 1985; Elpern et al., 1984) and score within the same range as brain-damaged control groups (Matthews et al., 1970; Goldstein and Shelly, 1974). On the Wisconsin Card Sorting Test, chronic-progressive patients have been found to commit a greater number of perseverative errors and to need more trials to achieve the first category than relapsing-remitting patients (Casey and Fennell, 1985; Rao et al., 1987).

Behavioral fluency measures such as verbal, motor, or design fluency have also been reported in a limited number of studies (Casey and Fennell, 1985; Heaton et al., 1985; Huber et al., 1987). In general, MS patients appear to be slowed relative to norms, and this slowing is present across a variety of modalities, supporting the suggestion that prefrontal cortex and its subcortical connections can sometimes be involved in these patients (Rao, 1986).

As suggested earlier, the problems with visuoconstructional tasks observed in some MS patients may reflect a deficit in planning and organizational skills related to dysfunction of the frontal systems. Specific studies of the planning and organizational capacities of MS patients are clearly needed in the future, and the relationship between deficits in these areas to deficits in other higher-order executive functions needs to be better described in large groups of different types of MS patients.

It should be noted also that problems of fatigue and difficulties in arousal and sustained attention reported in some MS patients may be related to the frontal-subcortical system dysfunctions (Rao, 1986). Previous studies employing continuous performance tasks (Casey and Fennell, 1985; Elsass and Zeeberg, 1983) have yielded mixed results. In the former study, no group differences were observed between mild and severely physically impaired MS patients, nor did they differ from norms on an auditory continuous performance measure. In the latter study, MS patients demonstrated delayed reaction times compared with nonneurologic patient controls on a continuous simple reaction time measure. Since a choice reaction time task was not included, however, it is difficult to determine how much higher-order factors versus motor speed accounted for these findings. Finally, differences in testing modality, that is, by comparing visual to auditory continuous performance measures, have not been examined in MS patients. Clearly, more research in this area is needed to assist the clinician in evaluating the impact of deficits in arousal, activation and other attentional functions on the performance of MS patients.

## Emotional/Affective Functions

Early studies of MS patients described a number of different emotional and affective disturbances in these patients. Emotional blunting, emotional lability, apathy, depression, irritability, and, more rarely, psychosis were described (Trimble and Grant, 1982). It has become increasingly clear, however, that there is no single type of emotional disturbance observed in MS patients (Peyser and Poser, 1986). Emotional symptoms also do not appear to be clearly related to the length of illness, but they may be related to the relative degree of cerebral versus spinal involvement (Schiffer et al., 1983), with cerebral patients at higher risk for major depression.

Symptoms of emotional disorder may be elicited through clinical interview, formal psychiatric diagnostic schedules, self-report measures, and ratings by others. In a recent review of emotional disorder in MS, Devins and Seland (1987) caution that the overlap of physical symptoms of the disease with items indexed to psychopathology on personality measures such as the Minnesota Multiphasic Personality Inventory (MMPI) (Hathaway and McKinley, 1951) or the General Health Questionnaire (Goldberg, 1972) may lead to inflated estimates of psychopathology in these patients. The authors critically reviewed 10 recent studies and concluded that there is little empirical evidence to support the assertions that depression is a direct symptom of the disease process or that stress enhances the depressive symptoms in MS patients. Rather, depression is viewed as a response to the functional limitations imposed by the disease activity in the MS patient. Such a conclusion may be somewhat premature, however, since recent studies, not cited in their review, have found correlations between affective state and brain imaging (see the chapters in Part III of this volume and Honer et al., 1987).

Current clinical approaches to treating depression in MS patients (Schiffer, 1987) argue for subtyping of depressive disorders according to Research Diagnostic criteria prior to prescribing specific treatments, including pharmacotherapy. In clinical practice, however, clinicians will continue to employ self-report measures (MMPI) along with the patient's subjective complaint to document the degree of depressive symptomatology in these patients. It would be helpful, therefore, to compare the profile of an individual patient to published profiles of MS patients (e.g., Peyser et al., 1980) rather than to rely solely on an analysis of T-score elevations. Other self-report inventories, designed to assess both cognitive and neurovegetative symptoms of depression, may also prove helpful in assessing mood disturbance in MS (i.e., Beck Depression Scale, Beck et al., 1988; Profile of Mood States, Educational and Industrial Testing Service, 1971).

Euphoria and psychosis are two of the more dramatic emotional symptoms associated with MS. They have also been described as side effects of steroid treatments (Trimble and Grant, 1982). The majority of studies examining these symptoms occurred prior to the mid-1970s, and there has been relatively little recent research activity (Peyser and Poser, 1986). This probably reflects the difficulty in developing quantitative measures of euphoria as well as the relative rarity of psychosis in this disorder. Most of the recent studies have emphasized the symptoms of depression and anxiety as prominent emotional correlates of MS. Rao (1986) suggests that even when the primary focus of an evaluation is on cognitive symptoms, one should evaluate for the presence of emotional complaints in the clinical examination of the MS patient.

The question of fluctuating emotional complaints during the course of the illness is an important one that clearly needs further research, particularly as part of a longitudinal study. In our experience, tests designed for repeated assessment such as the Profile of Mood States (Educational and Industral Testing Service, 1971) may be more useful indices of weekly or monthly emotional complaints than more traditional clinical instruments such as the MMPI (Hathaway and McKinley, 1951) or the State-Trait anxiety scales (Speilberger et al., 1970).

Finally, the relationship between affective complaints and cognitive dysfunction has yet to be experimentally evaluated in MS patients. More studies of the effects of depression, anxiety, and apathy on neuropsychological performance of MS patients are needed. The degree to which depression and/or anxiety selectively impairs neuropsychological test scores has been examined in psychiatric patients (Yozawitz, 1986; Heilman and Satz, 1983) but remains to be carefully documented in neurologic disorders such as MS that may be accompanied by affective disturbance.

In the following section, we briefly describe the comprehensive neuropsychological test battery employed at the University of Florida. Following this description, we report the results of examinations of two MS patients to illustrate how such a comprehensive assessment can be used to reveal cognitive and emotional problems in these patients. Finally, we discuss the implications of neuropsychological dysfunction for the patients' ability to engage in everyday activities.

## CLINICAL EXAMINATION OF THE MS PATIENT: CASE EXAMPLES

A list of tests commonly used for neuropsychological evaluations at the University of Florida is presented in Table 4–1. This list represents a sampling of the tests that typically comprise a "flexible battery." The choice of instruments may vary considerably, depending on the referral question and the nature of the patient's difficulties. The particular tests listed in Table 4–1 were administered to the MS patients presented in this chapter, with the goal of examining a broad range of functions. It is beyond the scope of this chapter to provide a description of the individual tests included in this battery; the interested reader is referred to Lezak's (1983) compendium of neuropsychological assessment instruments or to the specific test references cited in Table 4–1.

The following summaries of clinical neuropsychological evaluations illustrate the types of subtle and overt dysfunctions often experienced by patients with MS.

*Case Example One: Patient J.M.*
J.M. was a 29-year-old, right-handed housewife, who had completed four years of college. She had worked prior to the birth of her only child, but was presently unemployed. The original diagnosis of MS was made five years prior to the present examination. Her first symptoms were diplopia, whole body paresthesias, vertigo, nausea, and vomiting.

**Table 4-1**  University of Florida Neuropsychological Battery

A. Global cognitive function
  1. Composite intellectual functions
    a. Wechsler Adult Intelligence Test-Revised (WAIS-R; Wechsler, 1981)
  2. Conceptual reasoning
    a. Progressive Matrices (Raven, 1960)
    b. California Proverb Test (Delis et al., 1988)


B. Executive Functions
  1. Attention, concentration, and mental control
    a. Digit Span and Arithmetic (WAIS-R)
    b. Mental Control from Wechsler Memory Scale (WMS; Wechsler and Stone, 1945) or
       Wechsler Memory Scale-Revised (WMS-R; Wechsler, 1987)
    c. Visual Memory Span (WMS-R)
  2. Executive Control
    a. Wisconsin Card Sorting Test (Grant and Berg, 1960; Heaton, 1981)
    b. Trail-Making Test (Reitan, 1958)
    c. Stroop Color Interference Test (Stroop, 1935)
    d. Word List Generation (Spreen and Benton, 1969)
  3. Organization and Planning
    a. Cancellation Test (Mesulam and Weintraub, unpublished)
    b. Rey-Osterreith Complex Figure Test (Osterreith, 1944)—copy
    c. Draw-A-Clock (Goodglass and Kaplan, 1983)
  4. Simple and Complex Motor Function
    a. Finger Tapping Test (Reitan and Davison, 1974)
    b. Grooved Pegboard (Reitan and Davison, 1974)
    c. Digit Symbol (WAIS-R)
    d. Symbol Copy (Kaplan, unpublished)
    e. Go-No Go Paradigm (Luria, 1966)
    f. Reciprocal Motor Programs (Luria, 1966)
    g. Alternating Sequences: 3-Step Motor Programs (Luria, 1966)
    h. Alternating Graphomotor Sequences (Luria, 1966)


C. Language and Related Abilities
  1. Composite Aphasia Testing
    a. Western Aphasia Battery (WAB; Kertesz, 1979)
    b. Boston Diagnostic Aphasia Examination (BDAE; Goodglass and Kaplan, 1983)
  2. Naming
    a. Boston Naming Test (Kaplan et al., 1983)
    b. Finger Gnosis (Goodglass and Kaplan, 1983)


D. Visuoperceptual, Visuospatial, and Visuoconstructional Functions
  1. Perception
    a. Picture Completion (WAIS-R)
    b. Hooper Visual Organization Test (Hooper, 1958)
    c. Benton Test of Facial Recognition (Benton and Van Allen, 1973; short form: Levin et
       al., 1975)
    d. USA Map and Drawings from Boston Spatial-Quantitative Battery (Goodglass and
       Kaplan, 1983)
    e. Florida Map (Fennell, unpublished)
  2. Construction
    a. Block Design (WAIS-R)
    b. Object Assembly (WAIS-R)
    c. Rey-Osterreith Complex Figure Test (Osterreith, 1944)—copy

E. Learning and Memory
  1. Composite Memory Testing (WMS or WMS-R)
  2. Verbal Memory Functions
     a. Logical Memory (WMS or WMS-R)
     b. Paired Associates (WMS or WMS-R)
     c. California Verbal Learning Test (CVLT; Delis et al., 1983)
     d. Auditory Consonant Trigrams (Peterson and Peterson, 1956)
  3. Nonverbal Memory Functions
     a. Visual Reproduction (WMS or WMS-R)
     b. Visual Paired Associates (WMS-R)
     c. Figural Memory (WMS-R)
     d. Rey-Osterreith Complex Figure Test (Osterreith, 1944)—memory
     e. Milner Facial Recognition Test (Milner, 1968)
     f. Continuous Visual Memory Test (Trahan and Larrabee, 1984)
     g. Benton Visual Retention Test (Benton, 1974)

F. Personality Screening
   Minnesota Multiphasic Personality Inventory (Hathaway and McKinley, 1951)

---

A lumbar puncture at that time was normal except for one oligoclonal band and elevated myelin basic protein. Her symptoms gradually resolved during an otherwise uncomplicated pregnancy. Two months after she delivered a healthy baby, she developed right-sided weakness and trouble walking. A CT scan demonstrated a large oval contrast-enhancing lesion extending from the lateral ventricles to include both limbs of the left internal capsule. Visual evoked responses were consistent with a left retrochiasmic lesion, while brain stem auditory evoked responses were normal. Repeat lumbar puncture revealed cerebrospinal fluid containing a glucose of 52 with no oligoclonal bands. A neurologic examination revealed mild dysarthria of speech, right-sided spasticity with normal strength, and dysmetria in all extremities.

During the neuropsychological evaluation, both J.M. and her husband denied that she was showing evidence of cognitive difficulties. No marital problems were described. J.M. noted difficulty in writing and walking because of spasticity in her right arm and leg, sensory changes on the right side, slurred speech, fatigue, and drowsiness. These symptoms generally did not affect her ability to carry out household and child care tasks, except for the compromises attendant to fatigue and drowsiness which mostly affected her energy level in caring for her child. Medication at the time of testing included Norpramine and Lioresal.

Throughout the evaluation, J.M. was alert, friendly, and cooperative. Her spontaneous speech was fluent and prosodic, despite mild dysarthria, with no word-finding difficulties or paraphasias noted. She did not appear to be depressed, and her affect was appropriate to the situation.

On intellectual testing with the WAIS-R, J.M. achieved full scale, verbal, and performance IQs of 94, 96, and 92, respectively. In light of her educational background, these scores were felt to reflect a decline from premorbid levels of functioning. Particularly low scores were observed on the Digit Span, Object Assembly, and Digit Symbol subtests, suggesting problems with attention, visuoconstructional abilities, and psychomotor speed, respectively. The latter task may have been negatively influenced by her primary motor difficulties in light of the slowness she demonstrated on a task of simple symbol copying.

On more specific cognitive test measures, J.M. performed normally on measures of conceptual reasoning (Raven's Progressive Matrices, California Proverbs Test). On measures of executive control, however, her performance was more variable. While she completed all six categories of the Wisconsin Card Sorting Test in 107 cards, a slightly below-normal performance, she exhibited mild slowing on Part B of the Trial-Making Test and on the color/word interference condition of the Stroop Test. Furthermore, her ability to generate words from phonemic categories ("verbal fluency") was at the twenty-second percentile, with several perservative responses.

On tests of organization and planning, J.M.'s approach to relatively unstructured tasks was relatively unsystematic. For example, J.M.'s productions of the Rey-Osterreith Complex Figure revealed a segmented, disorganized approach for both copy and memory conditions. This approach is illustrated in Figure 4–1, which shows the sequence of her pencil strokes. A similar lack of planning was evident in her drawing of a clock, in which the numbers were unevenly spaced, and on the California Verbal Learning Test, in which she did not spontaneously make use of the inherent semantic organization of the material to facilitate encoding and subsequent retrieval of information.

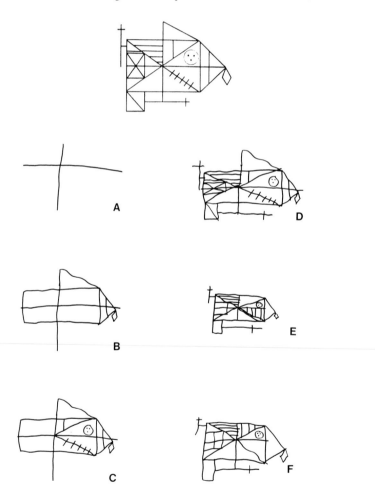

**Figure 4–1**  Rey-Osterreith Complex Figure Test for patient J.M. Top, stimulus figure; (A,B,C) partial productions by J.M. showing sequence of copy; (D) final copy; (E) immediate recall; (F) delayed recall.

Assessment of simple motor functions, as reflected by the Finger Tapping and Grooved Pegboard tests, revealed problems with speed and coordination of the right hand. Measures of complex motor functions (Go-No Go, Reciprocal Motor Programs, Alternating Sequences, and Alternating Graphomotor Sequences) were performed normally, suggesting an absence of problems in inhibiting, alternating, or switching motor programs.

Formal language testing with the Western Aphasia Battery, the Boston Naming Test, and the Finger Gnosis Test was performed flawlessly. Likewise, her performance on measures of visuoperception (Picture Completion on the WAIS-R, Hooper Visual Organization Test, Benton Facial Recognition Test, Map of the USA and Florida Test) and visuoconstruction (Block Design on the WAIS-R, Rey-Osterreith) was intact, despite disorganization in the planning and execution of visuoconstructional tasks (see above).

J.M.'s immediate and delayed memory for verbal and visuospatial information was within normal limits on the WMS (memory quotient = 116), Rey-Osterreith Complex Figure and Milner Facial Recognition Test. On the California Verbal Learning Test, J.M. demonstrated a normal learning curve, but she exhibited perseverative responses and semantically related intrusions. Mild impairment was noted in the decay of information from short-term memory on the Auditory Consonant Trigrams.

Personality testing with the MMPI (Welsh code: 132-6809/47:5# KL/F) indicated that J.M. saw herself as well adjusted and capable, perhaps at times to the point of denying or minimizing her difficulties. These personality features were generally consistent with behavioral observations.

## Summary of J.M.'s Neuropsychological Evaluation

J.M.'s basic executive, language, visuospatial, and memory functions were within normal limits. In contrast, she displayed mild but pervasive deficits in organizational and planning skills, mild perseveration, abnormal interference from distraction, and cognitive slowing. In addition, she exhibited motor slowing and incoordination of her right, dominant upper extremity.

*Case Example Two: Patient C.A.*
C.A. was a 39-year-old, college-educated, right-handed woman whose diagnosis of MS was made just four months prior to our examination. Over the previous several years, she had on different occasions experienced dizziness, whole-body paresthesias, fatigue, and difficulties with coordination in both hands. A neurologic examination two years prior to diagnosis revealed slight reflex asymmetries and a right peripheral facial paralysis. Reexamination at the time of diagnosis additionally showed difficulty with tandem gait, a left Babinski response, and an equivocal response on the right. An MRI scan revealed multiple areas of white matter abnormality, particularly in the periventricular region in both hemispheres (see Figure 4–2). In addition, she had been experiencing frequent back pains for many years, as well as depression associated with premenstrual syndrome.

During the present examination, C.A. acknowledged feelings of weakness, edginess, emotional lability, and depression. She stated that she had to concentrate with great effort to complete tasks. Like J.M., C.A. denied significant memory problems, but admitted that she does not presently engage in activities that would tax her memory, having quit her job as a supervisor in a medical facility several months earlier because of fatigue. The patient reported that some of her emotional complaints were related to stress associated with dissolution of a long-term relationship and to the lack of meaningful employment because of her disease.

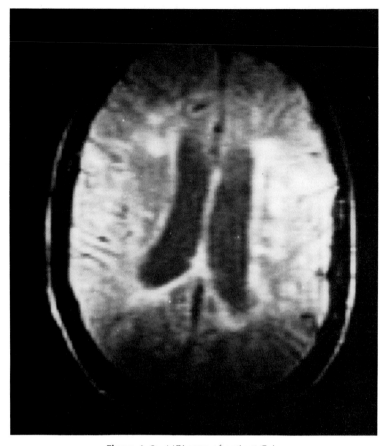

**Figure 4–2**  MRI scan of patient C.A.

C.A. was initially very guarded and skeptical regarding the usefulness of testing, but she became more relaxed and cooperative when the purpose of testing was discussed with her. She fatigued easily, which at times appeared to affect her ability to concentrate. C.A. was affectively labile during the evaluation, expressing a broad range of emotions from laughing to crying. She appeared socially disinhibited and did not seem to be concerned about the image she was projecting.

On the WAIS-R, C.A. achieved a full scale IQ of 93, which is at the low end of the average range. As a college graduate, this score was felt to be 10–20 points below premorbid levels. Furthermore, a 22-IQ-point difference was observed between her verbal (verbal IQ = 103) and nonverbal (performance IQ = 81) abilities. Analysis of subtest scores indicated that C.A. performed significantly worse on tasks requiring active concentration (e.g., digit recall, mental arithmetic), psychomotor speed, and manipulation of novel, visuospatial information. On the latter, C.A. did not demonstrate gross visuoconstructional deficits; rather, her test scores were penalized because of motor slowness and incoordination.

On measures of executive control, C.A.'s performance on the Wisconsin Card Sorting Test was normal, while word list generation was moderately impaired for letters, but normal for semantic categories. Both Trails A and B were impaired because of motor slowness and scanning problems. Tests of organization and planning were performed with some difficulty. She displayed poor planning in drawing a clock, with unequal spacing between numbers and one number placed outside the boundary of the clock face. In contrast, her ability to copy the Rey-Osterreith Figure was fairly well organized (see Figure 4–3).

Simple motor functions were performed slowly and with reduced fine motor dexterity. In addition, C.A. displayed echopraxic errors on reciprocal motor programs, disinhibition on go-no go sequences, impaired sequence learning of three unrelated hand positions, and perseverations on alternating graphomotor sequences (i.e., repetitive sequences of alternating m's and n's).

Language and visuoperceptual testing was performed without difficulty.

On memory testing, C.A. obtained a memory quotient of 92 on the WMS, which was consistent with her current level of intellectual functioning. While her immediate and delayed recall of the WMS prose stories was normal, she demonstrated difficulty in learning the low-association words on Paired Associates. Additionally, she showed a flat

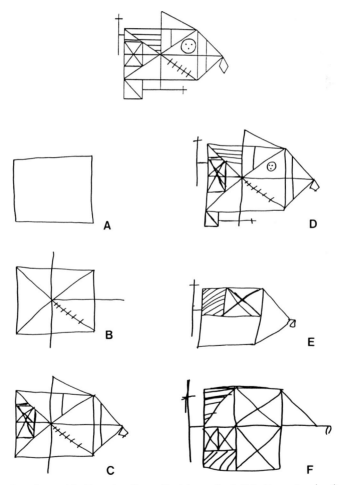

**Figure 4–3** Rey-Osterreith Complex Figure Test for patient C.A. Top, stimulus figure; (A,B,C) partial productions by J.M. showing sequence of copy; (D) final copy; (E) immediate recall; (F) delayed recall.

learning curve on the California Verbal Learning Test (correct recall of 16 words over five trials was 8, 10, 9, 8, 8). Cuing by semantic category did not aid recall, but rather increased the production of semantically related intrusions. C.A.'s immediate recall (Auditory Consonant Trigrams) was mildly impaired after 9 and 18 seconds of distraction.

Nonverbal memory functions, as assessed from her immediate and delayed reproductions of line drawings (Visual Reproduction from the WMS, Rey-Osterreith Figure), was moderately impaired (see Figure 4–3). She also displayed considerable difficulty on the Continuous Visual Memory Test, making numerous false positives and recognizing only two of the seven frequently occurring designs after a 30-minute delay.

Personality screening with the MMPI yielded an interpretive profile suggestive of significant current distress (Welsh code: 231″48′7-6950 F-LK), characterized by depression, somatic concerns, and numerous unusual experiences which may be attributed to her physical problems. People with profiles similar to C.A.'s tend to be in conflict about dependency and self-assertion. In addition, they tend to be socially nonconforming and may have feelings of social isolation and self-alienation. Overall, the personality characteristics suggested by the MMPI were consistent with C.A.'s subjective complaints and behavioral observations.

## Summary of C.A.'s Neuropsychological Evaluation

Test results indicated that C.A. was functioning in the average range of cognitive ability. Although basic language and visuoperceptual abilities were intact, she demonstrated moderate difficulties on tasks with high attention and concentration demands. Her ability to plan, organize, and integrate information was deficient, and her performance across a variety of tasks was compromised by bilateral motor slowness. She had difficulty learning repetitive or alternating motor sequences. Memory for complex, nonverbal information and learning of supraspan word lists were particularly affected. Finally, depression and somatic concerns were prominent.

## DISCUSSION OF CASE EXAMPLES

These two cases illustrate several points: (1) cognitive dysfunction in MS can range in severity from subtle to obvious; (2) there can be considerable variability among patients in the pattern of neuropsychological deficits that are identified; (3) the degree to which cognitive dysfunction interferes with a patient's life is a function of the everyday intellectual demands made of the individual; (4) the patient's self-report of cognitive dysfunction may be unreliable; and (5) personality factors may or may not be associated with cognitive disturbance. Each of these points is reviewed in the following discussion.

Consistent with knowledge derived from group studies of cognitive dysfunction, both patients performed normally on language and visuoperceptual measures, but each had difficulties on measures of intelligence, memory, and verbal fluency, sustained attention, and executive control. It is clear, however, that J.M.'s cognitive impairments are less severe than those of C.A. A range of cognitive impairment, from normal to severe dementia, has been noted in group studies of MS patients (e.g., Rao et al., 1984). In addition, the pattern of test performance for the two patients was qualitatively different. C.A. demonstrated a flat learning curve on verbal memory testing and problems in sequencing, alternating, and inhibiting motor programs, but she showed good organizational skills in copying geometric designs. J.M., on the other hand, had a normal learning curve and performed complex motor tasks without difficulty, but she was extremely disorganized in the planning and execution of copying tasks.

Both patients were college educated and had been employed earlier in their lives, but neither was working at the time of evaluation. It is not clear whether the cognitive deficits or other MS symptoms (e.g., fatigue) were the actual cause(s) of their unemployment. The neuropsychological test findings suggest that C.A., in particular, might have problems in returning to her job as a supervisor in a medical facility. Were she to seek future employment of an equally demanding nature, C.A. would need to receive comprehensive retraining of work-related activities, with emphasis on developing aids to assist her in compensating for her cognitive deficits (e.g., expanded use of logs and calendars to aid recall and organize activities).

Both patients denied having cognitive deficits that interfered with their daily activities. As noticed previously, neither patient was involved in activities that might tax her memory or problem-solving abilities. In addition, personality testing suggested that J.M. might minimize or deny problems and would be less likely to report her relatively mild cognitive deficits. In contrast, C.A. may have denied cognitive deficits because of a lack of personal insight associated with organic personality change. As noted previously, C.A. was emotionally labile, disinhibited, and showed little, if any, awareness of how she was presenting herself to others. This lack of correspondence between self-report of cognitive dysfunction and neuropsychological test performance is not uncommon in brain-damaged populations (e.g., Sunderland et al., 1983).

The cases differed in the degree of affective complaints in that C.A. presented with considerable emotional distress, while J.M. appeared to have few complaints of mood disturbance. The relationship between personality and cognitive changes is unclear in this disease: Are the cognitive deficits the side effect of a reactive depression and/or psychoactive medication usage? Does depression result as a consequence of perceived loss of cognitive abilities? Could both be the result of brain lesions that interfere with normal cognitive and affective processes? The answers to these puzzling questions await future research.

In the two cases presented, the role of the clinical neuropsychologist had been primarily to provide descriptive information to the physician about the extent and degree of neuropsychological deficits observed. Other possible functions that could have been provided include: counseling the patient regarding the effects of these deficits on work or home-related tasks, provision of referral for vocational rehabilitation assistance if symptom severity requires a change in work roles, and, finally, individual supportive psychotherapy in times of acute exacerbation of the illness. A final role, that of educating the individual patient and family about the neuropsychological consequences of MS, is a typical part of our feedback session with the patient and family. Such an education function can be very helpful in dispelling misconceptions (e.g., the patient's memory problems are viewed as a sign of laziness or obstinacy). The consulting neuropsychologist is in an excellent position to provide this clinical service.

## ACKNOWLEDGMENT

We gratefully acknowledge the assistance of Paula Dolder in the preparation of this manuscript.

## REFERENCES

Beck, A.T., Steer, S., and Garbin, M. (1988). Psychometric properties of the Beck Depression Inventory: 25 years of evaluation. *Clin. Psychol. Rev.,* **8,** 77–100.

Benton, A., and Van Allen, M. (1973). *Test of Facial Recognition. Manual. Neurosensory Center Publication No. 287.* Iowa City: University of Iowa.

Benton, A. (1974). *The Revised Visual Retention Test,* 4th ed. New York: Psychological Corporation.

Boll, T.J. (1981). The Halstead-Reitan neuropsychology battery. In: S.J. Filskov and T.J. Boll, eds., *Handbook of Clinical Neuropsychology,* pp. 577–607. New York: Wiley.

Canter, A.H. (1951). Direct and indirect measures of psychological deficit in multiple sclerosis. *J. Gen. Psychol.,* **44,** 3–50.

Casey, V.A., and Fennell, E.B. (February, 1985). Neuropsychological evidence of progressive frontal lobe dysfunction in multiple sclerosis. Paper presented at the International Neuropsychological Society Meeting, San Diego, California.

Charcot, J.M. (1877). *Lectures on the Diseases of the Nervous System Delivered at La Salpetriere.* London: New Sydenham Society.

Cutler, J.R., Aminoff, M.J., and Brant-Zawadski, M. (1986). Evaluation of patients with multiple sclerosis by evoked potentials and magnetic resonance imaging: A comparative study *Ann. Neurol.,* **20,** 645–48.

Delis, D., Kramer, J., Kaplan, E., Ober, A., and Fridlund, A. (1983). *California Verbal Learning Test.* San Antonio: Psychological Corporation.

Delis, D., Kramer, J., and Kaplan, E. (1988). *California Proverbs Test.* Unpublished manuscript.

Devins, G.M., and Seland, T.P. (1987). Emotional impact of multiple sclerosis: Recent findings and suggestions for future research. *Psychol. Bull.,* **101,** 363–75.

Educational and Industrial Testing Service. (1971). *Profile of Mood States.* San Diego: EITS.

Elpern, S.J., Gunderson, C.H., Katrah, J., and Kirsch, A.D. Cognitive and memory functioning in recently diagnosed chronic multiple sclerosis. Paper presented at the International Neuropsychological Society Meeting, Houston, February, 1984.

Elsass, P., and Zeeberg, I. (1983). Reaction time deficits in multiple sclerosis. *Acta Neurol. Scand.,* **68,** 257–61.

Goldberg, D.P. (1972). *The Detection of Psychiatric Illness by Questionnaire.* London: Oxford University Press.

Goldstein, G., and Shelly, C.H. (1974). Neuropsychological diagnosis of multiple sclerosis in a neuropsychiatric setting. *J. Nerv. Ment. Dis.,* **158,** 280–89.

Goodglass, H., and Kaplan, E. (1983). *The Assessment of Aphasia and Related Disorders,* 2nd ed. Philadelphia: Lea and Febiger.

Grant, D., and Berg, E. (1960). *Wisconsin Card Sorting Test.* San Antonio: Psychological Corporation.

Hathaway, S., and McKinley, J. (1951). *Minnesota Multiphasic Personality Inventory.* New York: Psychological Corporation.

Heaton, R.K. (1981). *A Manual for the Wisconsin Card Sorting Test.* Odessa, Florida: Psychological Assessment Resources.

Heaton, R.K., Nelson, L.M., Thompson, D.S., Burks, J.S., and Franklin, G.M. (1985). Neuropsychological findings in relapsing-remitting and chronic-progressive multiple sclerosis. *J. Consult. Clin. Psychol.,* **53,** 103–110.

Heilman, K.M., and Satz, P. (1983). *Neuropsychology of Human Emotions.* New York: Guilford.

Heilman, K.M., and Valenstein, E. (1985). *Clinical Neuropsychology,* 2nd ed. New York: Oxford.

Honer, W.G., Hurwitz, T., Li, D.K.B., Palmer, M., and Paty, D.W. (1987). Temporal lobe involvement in multiple sclerosis patients with psychiatric disorders. *Arch. Neurol.,* **44,** 187–90.

Hooper, H. (1958). *The Hooper Visual Organization Test. Manual.* Los Angeles: Western Psychological Services.

Huber, S.J., Paulson, G.W., Shuttleworth, E.C., Chakeres, D., Clapp, L.E., Pakalnis, A., Weiss, K., and Rammohan, K. (1987). Magnetic resonance imaging correlates of dementia in multiple sclerosis. *Arch. Neurol.,* **44,** 732–36.

Ivnik, R.J. (1978a). Neuropsychological stability in multiple sclerosis. *J. Consult. Clin. Psychol.,* **46,** 913–23.

Ivnik, R.J. (1978b). Neuropsychological test performance as a function of the duration of MS-related symptomatology. *J. Clin. Psychiat.,* **39,** 304–7.

Jambor, K.L. (1969). Cognitive functioning in multiple sclerosis. *Br. J. Psychiat.,* **115,** 765–775.

Kaplan, E., Goodglass, H., and Weintraub, S. (1983). *The Boston Naming Test.* Philadelphia: Lea and Febiger.

Kertesz, A. (1979). *Aphasia and Associated Disorders.* New York: Grune and Stratton.

Kurtzke, J.F. (1970). Neurologic impairment in multiple sclerosis and the Disability Status Score. *Acta Neurolog. Scand.,* **46,** 493–512.

Levin, H., Hamsher, K. de S., and Benton, A. (1975). A short form of the Test of Facial Recognition for clinical use. *J. Psychol.,* **91,** 223–28.

Lezak, M. (1983). *Neuropsychological Assessment,* 2nd ed. New York: Oxford University Press.

Litvan, I., Grafman, J., Vendrell, P., Martinez, J.M., Junque, C., Vendrell, J.M., and Barraquer-Bordas, L. (1988a). Multiple memory deficits in patients with multiple sclerosis. *Arch. Neurol.,* **45,** 607–10.

Litvan, I., Grafman, J., Vendrell, P., and Martinez, J.M. (1988b). Slowed information processing in multiple sclerosis. *Arch. Neurol.,* **45,** 281–85.

Luria, A. (1966). *Higher Cortical Functions in Man.* New York: Basic Books.

Marsh, G. (1980). Disability and intellectual function in multiple sclerosis. *J. Nerv. Ment. Dis.,* **168,** 758–62.

Matthews, C.G., Cleeland, C.S., and Hopper, C.L. (1970). Neuropsychological patterns in multiple sclerosis. *Dis. Nerv. Syst.,* **31,** 161–70.

Milner, B. (1968). Visual recognition and recall after right-temporal lobe excision in man. *Neuropsychologia,* **6,** 191–209.

Mings, E.L. (1987). *Visual-motor integration deficits in pediatric renal disease.* Doctoral dissertation, University of Florida.

Osterreith, P. (1944). Le test de copie d'une figure complexe. *Arch. Psychol.,* **30,** 206–356.

Peterson, L., and Peterson, M. (1956). Short term retention of individual verbal items. *J. Exp. Psychol.,* **58,** 193–98.

Peyser, J.M., and Poser, C.M. (1986). Neuropsychological correlates of multiple sclerosis. In: S. Filskov, and T. Boll, eds. *Handbook of Clinical Neuropsychology,* vol. 2. pp. 347–97. New York: Wiley.

Peyser, J.M., Edwards, K.R., Poser, C.M., and Filskov, S.B. (1980). Cognitive function in patients with multiple sclerosis. *Arch. Neurol.,* **37,** 377–79.

Poser, C.M., Paty, D.W., Scheinberg, L., McDonald, I., Davis, F., Ebers, G.C., Johnson, K.P., Sibley, W.A., Silverberg, D.H., and Tourtellotte, W.W. (1983). New diagnostic criteria for multiple sclerosis: Guidelines for research protocols. *Ann. Neurol.,* **13,** 227–31.

Rao, S.M. (1986). Neuropsychology of multiple sclerosis: A critical review. *J. Clin. Exp. Neuropsychol.,* **8,** 503–42.

Rao, S.M., Glatt, S., Hammeke, T.A., McQuillen, M.P., Khatri, B.O., Rhodes, A.M., and Pollard, S. (1985). Chronic-progressive multiple sclerosis: Relationship between cerebral ventricular size and neuropsychological impairment. *Arch. Neurol.,* **42,** 678–82.

Rao, S.M., Hammeke, T.A., McQuillen, M.P., Khatri, B.O., and Lloyd, D. (1984). Memory disturbance in chronic progressive multiple sclerosis. *Arch. Neurol.,* **41,** 625–31.

Rao, S.M., Hammeke, T.A., and Speech, T.J. (1987). Wisconsin card sorting test performance in relapsing-remitting and chronic-progressive multiple sclerosis. *J. Clin. Consult. Psychol.,* **55,** 263–65.

Raven, J.C. (1960). *Guide to the Standard Progressive Matrices.* London: H.K. Lewis.

Reitan, R.M., and Davison, L.A. (1974). *Clinical Neuropsychology: Current Status and Applications.* New York: Wiley.

Reitan, R. (1958). Validity of the Trail-Making Test as an indication of organic brain damage. *Percept. Motor Skills,* **8,** 271–76.

Schiffer, R.B. (1987). The spectrum of depression in multiple sclerosis. *Arch. Neurol.,* **44,** 596–99.

Schiffer, R.B., Caine, E.D., Bamford, K.A., and Levy, S. (1983). Depressive episodes in patients with multiple sclerosis. *Am. J. Psychiat.,* **140,** 1498–1500.

Speilberger, C.D., Gorsuch, R.L., and Lushene, R.E. (1970). *Manual for the Strait-Trait Anxiety Inventory.* Palo Alto, Calif.: Consulting Psychologists Press.

Spreen, O., and Benton, A. (1969). *Neurosensory Center Comprehensive Examination for Aphasia.* Victoria, B.C., Canada: Neuropsychological Laboratory, Department of Psychology, University of Victoria.

Stevens, J.C., Farlow, M.R., Edwards, M.K., and Yu, P. (1986). Magnetic resonance imaging: Clinical correlation in 64 patients with multiple sclerosis. *Arch. Neurol.,* **43,** 1145–48.

Stroop, J. (1935). Studies of interference in serial verbal reactions. *J. Exp. Psychol.,* **18,** 643–62.

Sunderland, A., Harris, J.E., and Baddeley, A.D. (1983). Do laboratory tests predict everyday memory? A neuropsychological study. *J. Verb. Learn. Verb. Behav.,* **22,** 341–57.

Thurstone, L.L., and Thurstone, T.C. (1962). *Primary Mental Abilities* (rev. ed.). Chicago: Science Research Associates.

Trahan, D.E., and Larrabee, G.J. (1984). *Continuous Visual Memory Test.* Odessa, Fla.: Psychological Assessment Resources.

Trimble, M.R., and Grant, I. (1982). Psychiatric aspects of multiple sclerosis. In: D.F. Benson and D. Blumer, eds., *Psychiatric Aspects of Neurologic Disease,* vol. 2., pp. 279–99. New York: Grune and Stratton.

Wechsler, D. (1981). *Manual for the Wechsler Adult Intelligence Scale-Revised.* New York: The Psychological Corporation.

Wechsler, D. (1987). *Wechsler Memory Scale-Revised (Manual).* New York: The Psychological Corporation.

Wechsler, D., and Stone, C.P. (1945). *Wechsler Memory Scale (Manual).* New York: The Psychological Corporation.

Yozawitz, A. (1986). Applied neuropsychology in a psychiatric center. In: Grant, I., and Adams, K., eds. *Neuropsychological Assessment of Neuropsychiatric Disorders.* pp. 121–46, New York: Oxford University Press.

# II
# Cognitive Dysfunction in Multiple Sclerosis

# Introduction

JANIS M. PEYSER

There has been a remarkable evolution in thought concerning cognitive dysfunction in multiple sclerosis (MS) since this disease was first described. At first accepted as a concomitant of MS (Charcot, 1977), cognitive deficits were given little credence or attention in the middle decades of this century (Peyser and Poser, 1986). In recent years, however, there has been an explosion of research into the neuropsychological correlates of MS, leading to the inescapable conclusion that some form of cognitive impairment is present in a significant number of patients (Rao, 1986; Peyser and Poser, 1986). A new generation of studies, many of them reviewed in this volume, is now seeking to refine our knowledge of cognitive impairment and its underpinnings, neurologic correlates, course, and clinical significance.

Some of this new research is made possible by advances in neuroimaging techniques that allow more accurate visualization of cerebral plaques, which is described by Rao in Chapter 7. With these new tools we expect to move away from the previously unproductive attempts to relate cognitive dysfunction to general disease characteristics based on signs and symptoms secondary to subtentorial lesions and to move toward explorations of the relationship of cognitive deficits to their direct anatomic substrate. Rao discusses the correlations now being made between various parameters of static cerebral and neuropsychological involvement. He also introduces us to preliminary work in cerebral metabolism and blood flow that is likely to change how we conceptualize the mechanisms of cognitive impairment in MS. These studies lay the groundwork for even more exciting future investigations of ongoing disease activity, with cognitive tasks as primary measures of lesion expression.

As more comprehensive investigations begin to delineate systematically the particular domains of cognitive function most likely to be affected in MS, it is inevitable that comparisons will be made to the other so-called subcortical dementias, as is done by Mahler and Benson in Chapter 5. While the concept of subcortical dementia remains somewhat controversial (Mayeux et al., 1983; Whitehouse, 1986; Mayeux and Stern, 1987; Rosen, 1987), Mahler and Benson present a reasoned and informative discussion of this issue as it applies to the neuropsychological literature on MS to date. The theoretical position detailed here may spur other investigators to more comparative work on MS and the other dementias as they attempt to understand more fully the nature and mechanisms of impairment in MS.

Memory loss is the most common cognitive deficit identified in MS patients, and it has received the most attention in the neuropsychological literature. In Chapter 6, Grafman and colleagues present a comprehensive review of this literature from an information-processing perspective. Based on the current state of scientific knowledge, they attempt to identify the "weak links" in the memory system that contribute to impairment in MS patients. They also present theoretical and methodological strategies for future research.

In Chapter 8, Filley and his co-authors in Colorado present the first truly prospective data on neuropsychological impairment in MS that has been controlled for disease state and type. Information gathered from their sample generally suggests little or no decline in neuropsychological function over relatively brief test-retest intervals. The natural history of cognitive function in MS represents one of our greatest research challenges, in terms of both the difficulties inherent in conducting such research and the need for such information in patient counseling. Population-based longitudinal studies that recruit subjects during the diagnostic phase are desperately needed.

Cognitive impairment has been accepted within the neuropsychological community as a common fact of illness for many patients with MS. The same cannot be said for the neurologic community at large, as Franklin and colleagues discuss in Chapter 10. Of all the potential reasons for this failure to attend to cognitive function, the sensitivity of this issue is perhaps foremost. Intellectual capacity is almost certainly the most valued of all our faculties, and thus significant threat may be attached to its potential loss. This threat may be urgently and empathically shared by the professional. But it is counterproductive to bury one's head in the sand when confronted with reported or observed cognitive deficit, employment difficulties, and financial disability issues. Parallels may be drawn to sexual dysfunction, a topic of nearly equal sensitivity from many points of view. While a neurologist or other caregiver might be unlikely to volunteer sexual dysfunction as a symptom of some frequency in MS during diagnostic counseling, he or she would be even more unlikely to foster an erroneous expectation that sexual dysfunction will never occur. And faced with a patient complaining of impotence, the physician would certainly not tell the patient that this must reflect depression or imagination. Unfortunately, we do see these false messages and responses occurring with respect to cognitive symptoms. In this volume readers will find a series of guidelines designed to help caregivers strike a reasonable balance between unnecessary alarm and realistic response in a variety of settings.

In Chapter 9, Heaton and his colleagues describe their work on brief and intermediate-length screening batteries. Such screening batteries have been proposed as useful tools to increase identification of cognitive dysfunction in the clinic or office setting and to follow large numbers of patients. They have the added advantages of increasing awareness of neuropsychological involvement by their very existence on the examination protocol and of being able to be administered by ancillary personnel in settings where a neuropsychologist is not readily available. The time and cost benefit of properly validated, sensitive screening instruments are clear, and we expect their use to proliferate. At the same time, other points need to be borne in mind. It is possible to evaluate neuropsychological functioning thoroughly and to screen simultaneously for psychiatric disturbance and functional adjustment in less than the eight hours reported by Heaton and his colleagues. To the extent that the difference between a comprehensive evaluation and a screening battery is less than several hours and several hundred dollars, many institutions will continue their present patterns of referral and testing. Most importantly, if thoughtful guidelines for use, interpretation and contingency referral are not in place, screening batteries will have as much potential for damage as no information at all.

## REFERENCES

Charcot, J.M. (1877). *Lectures on the diseases of the nervous system.* London: New Sydenham Society.

Mayeux, R., and Stern, Y. (1987). Subcortical dementia. *Arch. Neurol.,* **44,** 129–30.

Mayeux, R., Stern, Y., Rosen, J., and Benson, D.F. (1983). Is "subcortical dementia" a recognizable clinical entity? *Ann. Neurol.,* **14,** 278–283.

Peyser, J.M., and Poser, C.M. (1986). Neuropsychological correlates of multiple sclerosis. In: S.B. Filskov and T.J. Boll, eds., *Handbook of Clinical Neuropsychology,* vol. 2, pp. 364–97. New York: Wiley-Interscience.

Rao, S.M. (1986). Neuropsychology of multiple sclerosis: A critical review. *J. Clin. Exp. Neuropsychol.,* **8,** 503–42.

Rosen, J.T. (1987). Cortical vs subcortical dementia: Neuropsychological similarities. *Arch. Neurol.,* **44,** 131.

Whitehouse, P.J. (1986). The concept of subcortical and cortical dementia: Another look. *Ann Neurol.,* **19,** 1–6.

# 5

# Cognitive Dysfunction in Multiple Sclerosis: A Subcortical Dementia?

MICHAEL E. MAHLER AND D. FRANK BENSON

Charcot (1877) observed that patients with multiple sclerosis (MS) "at a certain stage of the disease" can exhibit "marked enfeeblement of the memory; conceptions are formed slowly; the intellectual and emotional faculties are blunted in their totality." Trimble and Grant (1982) pointed out that except for such early observations of dementia in some MS patients, the study of cognitive dysfunction in MS progressed little until recent years, when standardized neuropsychometric batteries were applied to MS patients. The lack of emphasis on cognitive dysfunction in MS is attributable not only to a lack of knowledge about MS, but also, in part, to misconceptions about the nature of dementia.

Dementia has long been equated with chronic, progressive, and irreversible global impairment of intellect, especially in the elderly. The prototype for this dementia syndrome is Alzheimer's disease (AD), a degenerative disease primarily affecting the cerebral cortex. Reversible and treatable causes of dementia are now known to occur (Cummings, Benson, and LoVerme, 1980; Mahler, Cummings, and Benson, 1987), however, and many of the different causes of dementia produce patterns of cognitive dysfunction that are qualitatively distinct from the symptoms and course of AD. This is especially true in diseases with predominant pathology in subcortical structures such as Huntington's disease (HD) and Parkinson's disease (PD). Although the symptoms of cognitive impairment in MS differ from those seen in AD, the cognitive deficits fulfill a broad definition of the dementia syndrome.

This chapter develops the thesis that cognitive dysfunction in MS is a subcortical dementia syndrome. First, the historical background, concepts, and clinical features of subcortical dementia are reviewed and contrasted with cortical dementia. Evidence emphasizing the features of subcortical dementia in diseases of the white matter other than MS and clinical and neuropsychological studies of cognitive dysfunction in MS demonstrating the features of subcortical dementia are presented. On this basis we then speculate about the pathophysiologic relationships between white matter disorders and subcortical dementia.

## REVIEW OF SUBCORTICAL DEMENTIA

### Historical Background

Wilson (1912) gave the first description of what has come to be known as subcortical dementia in his account of hepatolenticular degeneration. He noted decreased capacity to store and retain mental impressions, poor insight and judgment, and personality features of childishness and docility. Wilson also commented that there was no agnosia or apraxia and that memory and comprehension were affected less severely than in senile dementia. Pathologically, the brains of Wilson's patients showed gross damage in the putamen and globus pallidus, subcortical structures, but preservation of cerebral cortex. Wilson's clinical description included many of the typical features of subcortical dementia while demonstrating the locus of pathology to be in the deep gray matter, not the cortex.

The next advances occurred in the mid-1970s. Albert and colleagues (1974) studied the dementia associated with progressive supranuclear palsy (PSP), a degenerative disease affecting midbrain structures and resulting in supranuclear oculomotor difficulties and an extrapyramidal movement disorder. They noted forgetfulness, slowing of thought processes, difficulty manipulating knowledge, and mood and personality changes in PSP patients. Aphasia, apraxia, and agnosia were not present. It was suggested that a similar behavior pattern can be seen in other subcortical disorders, including PD and olivopontocerebellar atrophy (OPCA) and the term *subcortical dementia* was coined to describe the syndrome.

At nearly the same time, similar observations were made in cases of HD (McHugh and Folstein, 1973, 1975). Once again, the disordered insight, judgment, attention, problem solving, abstraction, and motivation in HD patients were contrasted with the aphasia, apraxia, alexia, agnosia, and amnesia of AD. The disease process in HD severely affects the caudate nuclei but spares cerebral cortex; once again, an association was made between a distinct dementia syndrome and subcortical pathology.

Although the distinction between cortical and subcortical dementia remains controversial (Mayeux et al., 1983; Whitehouse, 1986), recent reviews (Cummings and Benson, 1984; Cummings, 1986) clearly demarcate differences between the two types of dementia syndromes based on clinical, neuropsychological, and neuropathological evidence. Subcortical dementia has been identified in PD, HD, Wilson's disease, OPCA, PSP, and Fahr's disease (Cummings et al., 1983), as well as in thalamic degeneration (Katz et al., 1984) and infarction (Graff-Radford et al., 1984). Cummings (1986) states that this "heterogeneous group of disorders shares

a similar pattern of intellectual compromise and a common preferential involvement of subcortical gray matter structures."

The subcortical dementia picture is also seen in the dementia complex of the
acquired immunodeficiency syndrome (AIDS) (Navia et al., 1986), vascular disease
with deep white matter ischemia (Cummings and Mahler, in press), and other leu-
koencephalopathies (Cummings and Benson, 1983; Mahler et al., 1987). Since
white matter disease, too, can produce symptoms of subcortical dementia, it is reasonable to raise the question: do the cognitive deficits of MS fit the pattern of subcortical dementia?

Before proceeding to answer this question, we first explore in greater depth the
features that constitute subcortical dementia.

## What Is Subcortical Dementia?

Dementia is a clinical syndrome defined as an acquired, persistent loss of intellectual function affecting at least three of these spheres of function: (1) memory, (2)
language, (3) visuospatial skills, (4) complex cognition such as abstraction, calculation, or judgment, and (5) personality, including mood and affect (Cummings and
Benson, 1983).

Each element of this definition is important. The criterion that the intellectual
impairment be an acquired change from previously attained levels of function
eliminates from consideration mental retardation and other congenital or developmental disorders. A persistent loss enduring for more than several weeks distinguishes dementia from transient alterations of mental function that occur in acute
confusional states. When only one sphere of intellect is impaired, as in an isolated
language or memory deficit, the condition is more appropriately termed an aphasia
or amnesia. These more restricted neuropsychological conditions result from a different set of etiologies than those that must be considered when searching for the
diagnosis underlying a dementia syndrome. By not insisting that all spheres of
intellectual function be disturbed and by omitting the requirements that dementia
be chronically progressive and irreversible, the definition of dementia does not
become identical to the definition of advanced AD.

Dementia is thus defined as a clinical syndrome, not as a specific diagnosis or
a unitary disorder. Within this syndrome, various patterns of intellectual deficits
can occur, resulting from myriad etiologies. The pattern associated with any given
disorder is relatively characteristic, although not specifically pathognomonic for
that condition. There are two principal patterns of neuropsychological deficits, two
subtypes of the dementia syndrome, that can be identified as cortical and subcortical dementia (Cummings, 1986). Although each subtype fulfills the basic definition of dementia, there are clear and fundamental differences between them that
justify this demarcation.

The derivation and limitations of the terms cortical and subcortical should be
emphasized. Although cortical and subcortical are anatomic terms, they are used
only to describe clinical syndromes (dementias), not to specify pathology in full
detail. As noted, the pattern of dementia called subcortical was first described in
conditions that have predominantly subcortical pathology, primarily diseases of
the extrapyramidal system. AD, the paradigm for the cortical dementia subtype, is

known to have principally cortical pathology. Although Whitehouse (1986) suggests that AD also has subcortical pathology and many of the extrapyramidal disorders can be associated with some degree of cortical pathology, cortical and subcortical dementias are manifestly separate clinical syndromes (Cummings and Benson, 1986), and there is a correlation with the site of major pathology in the paradigmatic disorders (Cummings, 1986).

## Clinical Features of Subcortical Dementia

Subcortical dementia is characterized by a slowing of cognition, including difficulty with problem solving and visuospatial skills; a memory disturbance best described as forgetfulness; mood changes; psychomotor slowing; and motor system abnormalities (Cummings, 1986). The characteristic features of subcortical dementia are specified and contrasted with those of cortical dementia in Table 5–1.

The preservation of language function in subcortical dementia contrasts with the prominent language abnormalities (severe anomia, paraphasia, comprehension deficit) in cortical dementia. Communication in subcortical dementias, however, is often hampered by a speech disturbance, dysarthria, which is a problem that is not present in cortical dementias until very advanced, almost terminal stages.

**Table 5–1**　Features of Subcortical Dementia Contrasted with Cortical Dementia

| Features | Subcortical Dementia | Cortical Dementia |
|---|---|---|
| Prototype disorders | PD, HD, PSP | AD, Pick's disease |
| Language function | Normal or mild anomia | Empty content, anomia, paraphasia, poor comprehension |
| Memory | Forgetfulness, recall aided by clues | Amnesia, recall not aided by clues |
| Visuospatial function | Poor map reading, line orientation | Impaired figure copying; easily lost in environment; agnosias |
| Abstract reasoning | Abstraction poor, easy calculations performed; "dilapidation of cognition" | Impaired abstraction and acalculia; untestable in advancing stages |
| Psychomotor speed | Slow | Normal until very late stages |
| Personality | Apathetic, irritable | Indifferent, unconcerned, unaware; may be disinhibited |
| Mood | Depression common | Depression uncommon |
| Thought disorder | Common in some conditions, complex delusions may occur | Simple delusions common |
| Speech | Dysarthria | No dysarthria |
| Muscle tone | Abnormal | Normal until late stages |
| Posture and gait | Abnormal | Normal until late stages |
| Involuntary movements | Tremors, chorea, dystonias | None or myoclonus |

(Adapted from Cummings, 1986)

In both conditions memory is affected, but with subcortical dementia the retrieval step is more affected than is the encoding of new information. Therefore, clues and recognition tasks lead to considerably improved performance in subcortical but not in cortical dementia. Visuospatial and cognitive skills are also disturbed in subcortical dementia, but the pattern of impairment is less complete or severe than that characteristic of cortical dementia.

Mood disturbances, personality changes, and psychosis are frequent manifestations of subcortical dementia. Personality change and psychosis can also be seen in cortical dementia but are qualitatively different. The cheerful indifference and lack of awareness commonly seen in the cortical dementias is in vivid contrast to the apathetic, psychomotor-retarded, depressed state seen with subcortical dementia.

Finally, the presence of motor system abnormalities further distinguishes subcortical from cortical dementia. In disorders of the basal ganglia (PD, HD, PSP, Wilson's disease, etc.), the abnormal movements (tremors, chorea, dystonias) are often diagnostic. Less specific signs, however, such as psychomotor slowing, stooped posture, increased muscle tone, and pseudobulbar palsy are also features of subcortical dementia. Not until the terminal stages of a cortical dementia such as AD do the physical and neurologic examination become abnormal (Cummings and Benson, 1983).

Cummings (1986) reviewed the neuropathophysiology of subcortical and cortical dementias, concluding that there are differences not only in the anatomic distribution of pathology but also in the effects on neurotransmitter systems and brain metabolism. The contrast between the reduction in cortical glucose metabolism seen in AD (Benson et al., 1983; Foster et al., 1984) and decreased subcortical (caudate) metabolism seen in HD (Kuhl et al., 1982) is graphically demonstrated in Figure 5–1.

The subcortical dementias involve disturbances in fundamental functions, whereas the cortical dementias involve instrumental functions (Albert, 1978; Cummings, 1986). Fundamental functions include arousal, timing and sequencing, motor programming, motivation, and mood. These functions depend on thalamocortical, corticostriatal, and limbic-striatal projections (Nauta, 1982) that utilize dopamine and a variety of other neurotransmitters. These functions are fundamental in that they underlie the performances of many other processes. In contrast, instrumental functions include language, memory, knowledge manipulation, perceptual recognition, and praxis. Instrumental functions are relatively discrete, often with precise cortical localization or depending on specific intracortical connections. This conceptual framework supports the clinical observations that separate subcortical from cortical dementing processes, especially in the comparison between classic dementias of the basal ganglia (PD, HD) and cortical gray matter (AD).

## SUBCORTICAL DEMENTIA IN WHITE MATTER DISEASE

The white matter of the nervous system, the fibers of variable length and degree of myelination that project between neurons, can be affected by many disease processes, including ischemia, inflammation, infection, toxins, and hereditary degen-

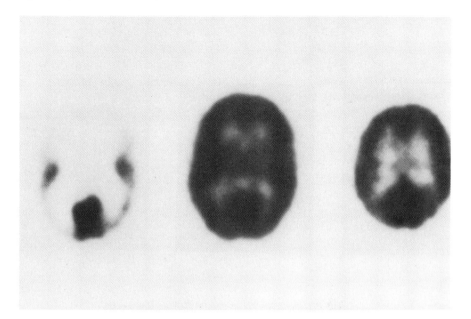

**Figure 5-1**　¹⁸FDG positron emmision tomography of a patient with AD (left), a normal control (center), and a patient with HD (right).

erations and metabolic derangements. Table 5–2 lists white matter diseases that have been associated with dementia (Cummings and Benson, 1983; Mahler et al., 1987).

When the clinical features of the dementias in these disorders have been studied, the pattern resembles that of subcortical dementia. Two conditions that have been studied intensively in recent years, Binswanger's disease and AIDS, illustrate this correlation.

## Binswanger's Disease

Subcortical arteriosclerotic encephalopathy was first described by Binswanger in 1894 and for many years was considered a rare pathological entity without specific clinical features. The neuropathology consists of diffuse ischemic demyelination of subcortical white matter, with sparing of the subcortical arcuate fibers (Olszewski, 1962). Lacunar infarctions in deep gray structures are frequent. Small artery disease, especially associated with hypertension, and cerebral hypoperfusion predispose to the development of this subcortical ischemic leukoencephalopathy (Román, 1987).

The clinical features of Binswanger's disease have been separated from those of the cortical dementias (Biemond, 1970; Caplan and Schoene, 1978; Mahler et al., 1987). The illness usually has an insidious onset between the ages of 40 and 75, with a relentless course, often punctuated by sudden strokelike events or transient ischemic attacks. The dementia is characterized by personality changes, often with depression or psychosis, and slowing of both intellectual and motor functions. Pathological laughter or weeping (pseudobulbar affect) may be observed. Focal neu-

**Table 5-2**   Dementia in Diseases with White Matter Pathology

---

*Demyelinating conditions*
  Hereditary degenerative disease
    Cerebrotendinous xanthomatosis
    Freidreich syndrome
  Idiopathic inflammatory
    Balo concentric sclerosis
    MS
  Immunologic
    Postinfectious encephalomyelopathy
    Postvaccinal encephalomyelopathy
  Infectious
    AIDS
    Progressive multifocal leukoencephalopathy
    Progressive rubella panencephalitis
    Subacute sclerosing panencephalitis
  Systemic-metabolic-nutritional
    Anoxic encephalopathy
    Central pontine myelinolysis
    Marchiafava-Bignami disease
    Vitamin $B_{12}$ deficiency
  Toxic
    Arsenic intoxication
    Carbon monoxide encephalopathy
    Ergotamine encephalopathy
    Lead encephalopathy
    Mercury intoxication
  Vascular
    Binswanger's disease (subcortical arteriosclerotic encephalopathy)

*Dysmyelinating conditions*
  Adrenoleukodystrophy
  Membranous lipodystrophy
  Metachromatic leukodystrophy

---

(Adapted from Cummings and Benson, 1983; Mahler et al., 1987)

rologic deficits such as hemianopia, hemiparesis, reflex asymmetries, and hemian-esthesia may be seen as a result of the ischemic episodes. Dysarthria, dysphagia, rigidity, bradykinesia, and difficulty walking are frequently present. The psycho-motor slowing, mood disturbance, and mixture of pyramidal and extrapyramidal motor system abnormalities fit the pattern of a subcortical dementia syndrome.

The development of sensitive neuroimaging techniques has raised Binswanger's disease from an obscure reference in neuropathology texts to a place as one of the more common causes of dementia (Román, 1987). With magnetic resonance imaging (MRI), bright signals that define discrete and sometimes confluent lesions are seen in the periventricular white matter using $T_2$-weighted sequences (Kinkel, 1985; Román, 1987). Because a similar appearance with MRI is seen, to some extent, in normal aging, AD, hydrocephalus, and other conditions (Zimmerman, 1986; George et al., 1986; Steingart et al., 1987a,b), the significance remains difficult to interpret.

The distribution and appearance of MRI lesions in MS is quite similar; the dis-crete and confluent areas of increased $T_2$ signal intensity seen in the periventricular centrum semiovale as well as in the brain stem and cerebellum are distinctive features of the disorder (Jacobs et al., 1986; Stevens et al., 1986; Huber et al., 1987).

## AIDS-Dementia Complex

With the rapidly escalating number of diagnosed cases of AIDS, much study has focused on the AIDS-dementia complex (ADC). Estimates of the frequency of cognitive dysfunction in AIDS range from 30 to 60% (Perry and Marotta, 1987). Cognitive deficits in ADC may result from the psychosocial stresses of AIDS, from opportunistic infections involving the nervous system, and from direct neurotoxicity of HIV (Shaw et al., 1985; Gabuzda et al., 1986; Gartner et al., 1986; Stoler et al., 1986).

The clinical features of ADC are variable, but the most frequent symptoms are slowing of intellect, poor concentration, forgetfulness, and mood and personality changes (Navia et al., 1986a; Benson, 1987). Perry and Marotta (1987) point out that AIDS can be "like syphilis 'the great imitator,'" meaning that its signs can mimic many neuropsychiatric disorders. Although intellectual deficits associated with cortical dysfunction (aphasia, amnesia, agnosia) may be seen (Perry and Marotta, 1987), they are rare in ADC (Benson, 1987) and severe, global dementia is a late manifestation (Navia et al., 1986a). In addition to psychomotor slowing, many ADC patients have ataxia, tremor, pyramidal tract signs, and weakness (Navia et al., 1986a).

Navia and co-workers (1986b) described the neuropathology in 70 AIDS cases, 46 of whom had ADC; fewer than 10% of the brains were normal. The brunt of the pathology involved the white matter and subcortical gray structures. The white matter had areas of pallor and rarefaction, with perivascular lymphocytic infiltrates, foamy macrophages, and multinucleated cells. There was relatively little pathology in the cortex.

The clinical pattern of cognitive deficits in AIDS closely matches the subcortical dementia syndrome (Navia et al., 1986a; Benson, 1987). Formal neuropsychological studies of patients with ADC also demonstrate findings that contrast with the pattern of patients with AD (Van Gorp et al., in submission). Perry and Marotta (1987) challenge the application of the cortical-subcortical dichotomy in ADC, noting that there is both cortical and subcortical histopathology, as well as some cortical intellectual dysfunction. The predominant histopathologic lesions affect the deep white matter, however, and the clinical and neuropsychological features of the dementia are largely those considered subcortical.

Although Binswanger's disease, ADC, and MS are quite different in terms of etiology and clinical characteristics, the distribution of cerebral pathology in the subcortical white matter is similar in the three conditions. If Binswanger's disease and ADC are accepted as models of subcortical dementia in white matter disease, the cognitive dysfunction in MS can be anticipated to follow a similar patttern.

## SUBCORTICAL DEMENTIA IN MS

Attaching the label of dementia to MS patients has been controversial. The older definitions of dementia required a chronic, irreversible, global loss of intellect; only a small number of MS patients fit these criteria. Recent neuropsychological studies reviewed by Rao (1986) and by others in this volume, however, have convincingly demonstrated that large numbers of MS patients experience decline in several areas of cognitive functioning, thereby fulfilling the definition of dementia used in this chapter. Furthermore, clinical experience reveals that many patients with MS complain of cognitive difficulties that interfere with work and occupational activities; these deficits are not merely data from tests but represent important facets of disability. The term cognitive dysfunction may be used when deficits involve only one or two areas; more extensive dysfunction deserves the term dementia.

## Neuropsychological Deficits

General intellectual function, as measured by intelligence test batteries, is adversely affected by MS (Canter, 1951; Reitan et al., 1971; Peyser et al., 1980), although some studies showed overall test scores that were not different from normals (Jambor, 1969) or actually improved over time (Fink and Houser, 1966). Correlations between either disease duration or disability level and the degree of cognitive impairment have not been observed (Marsh, 1980; Rao et al., 1985). Recent studies (Jensen et al., in press), however, do show a general relationship between disability and cognitive dysfunction.

Memory is frequently impaired in MS, and memory dysfunction was one of the more consistent neuropsychologic abnormalities found in nine separate studies cited by Rao (1986), affecting approximately half of all patients. The problem may be seen early in the disease process (Peyser et al., 1980; Grant et al., 1984; Rao et al., 1984), and difficulties on free recall tasks are much more pronounced than on recognition tasks, suggesting a defect of information retrieval, not one of encoding and storage (Rao, 1986).

Neuropsychological tests of complex cognitive functions including abstraction and conceptualization show disturbances of shifting set, concept formation, and perseveration similar to those seen in patients with frontal lobe injuries (Rao, 1986).

Aphasia has rarely been reported in MS (Olmos-Lau et al., 1977), and in general, language function is not significantly impaired in MS (Jambor, 1969; Rao, 1986), although verbal fluency may be reduced. In contrast, speech disturbances such as hypophonia, dysarthria, and scanning speech are common (Darley et al., 1975), especially in patients with brain stem and cerebellar involvement.

MS patients experience a variety of emotional changes that involve both mood (subjective emotional state) and affect (external indicators of emotional state). Depression is the most common mood change (Schiffer and Slater, 1985). Early investigators (Surridge, 1969) believed that the depression was largely a psychological reaction to the disease, but Whitlock and Siskind (1980) noted that depression occurred more frequently in MS than in other disabling disorders. MS patients with predominantly hemispheric involvement have more depression than those with equal disability primarily based on spinal involvement (Schiffer et al., 1983). Depression is more common in those MS patients without major cognitive deficits, while euphoria and irritability are more frequent in patients with widespread cerebral dysfunction (Rao, 1986). Patients experiencing exacerbation and progression of the disease are more likely to have an emotional disturbance than those whose illness is stable (Dalos et al., 1983). Inappropriate euphoria, emotional lability, or pathological laughter and weeping are terms that refer to changes in affect; they may bear no relationship to the mood state (Schiffer and Slater, 1985).

Rao (1986) discussed methodological problems that hamper the study of intellectual deficits in MS: difficulty in diagnosis, especially in the early stages; disease variability, both between individuals and over time within an individual; medication effects; emotional effects; and visual and motor impairments that interfere with test procedures. These problems impede efforts to make clinicopathological correlations between lesions seen with neuroimaging techniques (CT and MRI) and neuropsychological deficits (Huber et al., 1987). Correlation has been noted between poor memory performance and ventricular enlargement (Rao et al., 1985).

To summarize, the pattern of cognitive and affective disturbance in MS appears to be similar to that seen in other subcortical dementias. The following section describes a brief procedure for assessing subcortical dementia in patients with MS.

### Clinical Neurobehavioral Evaluation

One approach to cognitive assessment complementary to neuropsychological test batteries is the use of a brief mental status examination based on a clinical neurobehavioral evaluation. The Quick Mental Status Exam (QMSE) is a brief but broad mental status examination based on the clinical neurobehavioral exam utilized at UCLA. The QMSE probes orientation, attention and mental control, memory, cognitive and visuospatial skills, and language. The test can be administered in 20 minutes or less and is quantitative, with easy scoring of each item on the test worksheet.

When the QMSE was administered to a large number of patients with a variety of neurological and psychiatric diagnoses, including a test group of 20 MS patients and 20 matched normal controls (Mahler et al., in press), significant differences in mean total scores were found between the groups: 50% of the MS patients scored in the impaired range. The greatest difficulties were on the sequencing, memory, and complex cognition portions of the QMSE, with no difference between patients and controls on language function or orientation.

The QMSE results closely parallel the results of neuropsychological test batteries in MS patients in the proportion of patients whose scores are abnormal and the types of abnormalities seen. The pattern of QMSE dysfunction of MS patients resembles that seen in PD patients and is dissimilar to results obtained from AD patients.

### SUMMARY

Neuropsychological studies document that a high percentage of MS patients suffer cognitive dysfunction. Memory impairment is frequent and is characterized by a retrieval defect and forgetfulness rather than the defective encoding or storage of true amnesia. Concept formation, abstraction, and set shifting are disturbed, while language function and verbal intellectual skills are largely preserved. Mood and affective disturbances are common and include both depression and euphoria. Speech and other motor system abnormalities are present. This profile of neuro-psychological dysfunction in MS describes the pattern of subcortical dementia and contrasts sharply with the pattern of cortical dementia exemplified by AD.

## Mechanism of Subcortical Dementia in White Matter Disease

Binswanger's disease is of ischemic origin, ADC results from a viral infection, and MS is an idiopathic inflammatory condition with a presumed immunologic basis. Despite the different etiologies and clinical courses, similarities exist in the nature of the dementia that accompanies these conditions. The common location of lesions in each of these diseases is in the deep cerebral white matter, particularly in the periventricular area and the centrum semiovale.

Subcortical structures mediate fundamental functions. When these structures are directly affected by pathological processes, as in PD, PSP, or HD, subcortical dementia results from the effects on arousal, activation, attention, sequencing, motivation, and mood. The thalamus, striatum, and other important subcortical structures do not function in isolation, however, and have important reciprocal links with cortex, especially the frontal cortex, and with the limbic system. Discon-nection of pathways linking subcortical structures with the frontal and limbic cortex appears to be the mechanism producing subcortical dementia in white matter diseases, including MS.

## ACKNOWLEDGMENT

Support is acknowledged from an NIA Academic Award AG00260 and from the Veterans Administration.

## REFERENCES

Albert, M.L. (1978). Subcortical dementia. In R. Katzman, R.D. Terry, and K.L. Bick, eds., *Alzheimer's Disease: Senile Dementia and Related Disorders.* New York: Raven Press.

Albert, M.L., Feldman, R.G., and Willis, A.L. (1974). The 'subcortical dementia' of progres-sive supranuclear palsy. *J. Neurol. Neurosurg., Psychiat., 37,* 121–30.

Benson, D.F. (1987). Guest editorial—the spectrum of dementia: A comparison of the clin-ical features of AIDS/dementia and dementia of the Alzheimer type. *Alzheimer's Dis. Associated Disorders, 1,* 217–20.

Benson, D.F., Kuhl, D.E., Hawkins, R.A., Phelps, M.E., Cummings, J.L., and Tsai, S.Y. (1983). The fluorodeoxyglucose $^{18}$F scan in Alzheimer's disease and multi-infarct dementia. *Arch. Neurol., 40,* 711–14.

Biemond, A. (1970). On Binswanger's subcortical arteriosclerotic encephalopathy and the possibility of its clinical recognition. *Psychiatr. Neurol. Neurochir., 73,* 413–17.

Canter, A.H. (1951). Direct and indirect measures of psychological deficit in multiple scle-rosis. *J. Gen. Psychol., 44,* 3–50.

Caplan, L.R., and Schoene, W.C. (1978). Clinical features of subcortical arteriosclerotic encephalopathy (Binswanger disease). *Neurology, 28,* 1206–15.

Charcot, J.M. (1877). *Lectures on the Diseases of the Nervous System Delivered at La Salpetriere.* London: New Sydenham Society, pp. 194–95.

Cummings, J.L. (1986). Subcortical dementia: neuropsychology, neuropsychiatry, and pathophysiology. *Br. Rev. Psychiat., 149*, 682–97.

Cummings, J.L., and Benson, D.F. (1983). *Dementia: A Clinical Approach.* Boston: Butterworths.

Cummings, J.L., and Benson, D.F. (1984). Subcortical dementia: Review of an emerging concept. *Arch. Neurol., 41*, 874–79.

Cummings, J.L., and Benson, D.F. (1986). Dementia of the Alzheimer type: an inventory of diagnostic clinical features. *J. Am. Geriatr. Soc., 34*, 12–19.

Cummings, J.L., Benson, D.F., and LoVerme, S., Jr. (1980). Reversible dementia. *J.A.M.A., 243*, 2434–39.

Cummings, J.L., Gosenfeld, L., Houlihan, J., McCaffrey, T. (1983). Neuropsychiatric manifestations of idiopathic calcification of the basal ganglia: a case report and review. *Biol. Psychiat., 18*, 591–601.

Cummings, J.L., and Mahler, M.E. (in press). Vascular dementia. In: R.A. Bornstein and G.G. Brown, eds., *Neurobehavioral Aspects of Cerebrovascular Disease.* New York: Oxford University Press.

Dalos, N.P., Rabins, P.V., Brooks, B.R., and O'Donnell, P. (1983). Disease activity and emotional state in multiple sclerosis. *Ann. Neurol., 13*, 573–77.

Darley, F.L., Aronson, A.E., and Brown, J.R. (1975). *Motor Speech Disorders.* Philadelphia: Saunders.

Fink, S.L., and Houser, H.B. (1966). An investigation of physical and intellectual changes in multiple sclerosis. *Arch. Phys. Med. Rehab., 47*, 56–61.

Foster, N.L., Chase, T.N., Mansi, L., Brooks, R., Fedio, P., Patronas, N.T., and Di Chiro, G. (1984). Cortical abnormalities in Alzheimer's disease. *Ann. Neurol., 16*, 649–54.

Gabuzda, D.H., Ho, D.D., de la Monte, S.M., Hirsch, M.S., Rota, T.R., Sobel, R.A. (1986). Immunohistochemical identification of HTLV-III antigen in brains of patients with AIDS. *Ann. Neurol., 20*, 289–95.

Gartner, S., Markovits, P., Markovitz, D.M., Betts, R.F., Popovic, M. (1986). Virus isolation from and identification of HTLV-III/LAV-producing cells in brain tissue from a patient with AIDS. *J.A.M.A., 256*, 2365–71.

George, A.E., de Leon, M.J., Kalnin, A., Rosner, L., Goodgold, A., and Chase, N. (1986). Leukoencephalopathy in normal and pathologic aging: II. MRI of brain lucencies. *Am. J. Neuroradiol., 7*, 567–70.

Graff-Radford, N.R., Eslinger, P.J., Damasio, A.R., and Yamada, T. (1984). Nonhemorrhagic infarction of the thalamus: behavioral, anatomic, and physiologic correlates. *Neurology, 34*, 14–23.

Grant, I., McDonald, W.I., Trimble, M.R., Smith E., and Reed, R. (1984). Deficient learning and memory in early and middle phases of multiple sclerosis. *J. Neurol., Neurosur., Psychiat., 47*, 250–55.

Huber, S.J., Paulson, G.W., Shuttleworth, E.C., Chakeres, D., Clapp, L.E., Pakalnis, A., Weiss, K., and Rammohan, K. (1987). Magnetic resonance imaging correlates of dementia in multiple sclerosis. *Arch. Neurol., 44*, 732–36.

Jacobs, L., Kinkel, W.R., Polachini, I., and Kinkel, R.P. (1986). Correlations of nuclear magnetic resonance imaging, computerized tomography, and clinical profiles in multiple sclerosis. *Neurology, 36*, 27–34.

Jambor, K.L. (1969). Cognitive functioning in multiple sclerosis. *Br. J. Psychiat., 115*, 765–75.

Jensen, K., and Grant, I. eds (in press). *Mental Disorders, Cognitive Deficits and Their Treatment in Multiple Sclerosis,* London: J. Libbey.

Katz, A., Naseem, A., Horoupian, D.S., Rothner, A.D., and Davies, P. (1984). Familial multisystem atrophy with possible thalamic dementia. *Neurology*, **34**, 1213–17.

Kinkel, W.R., Jacobs, L., Polachini, I., Bates, V., and Heffner, R.R., Jr. (1985). Subcortical arteriosclerotic encephalopathy (Binswanger's disease): computed tomographic, nuclear magnetic resonance, and clinical correlations. *Arch. Neurol.*, **42**, 951–59.

Kuhl, D.E., Phelps, M.E., Markham, C.H., Metter, E.J., Riege, W.H., and Winter, J. (1982). Cerebral metabolism and atrophy in Huntington's disease determined by $^{18}$FDG and computed tomographic scan. *Ann. Neurol.*, **12**, 425–34.

Mahler, M.E., Cummings, J.L., and Benson, D.F. (1987). Treatable dementias. *West. J. Med.*, **146**, 705–12.

Mahler, M.E., Cummings, J.L., and Tomiyasu, U. (1987). Atypical dementia syndrome in an elderly man. *J. Am. Geriat. Soc.*, **35**, 1116–26.

Mahler, M.E., Davis, R.J., Spiegel, J., and Benson, D.F. (in press). Screening multiple sclerosis patients for cognitive impairments. In: K. Jensen, and I. Grant, eds., *Mental Disorders, Cognitive Deficits and Their Treatment in Multiple Sclerosis,* London: J. Libbey.

Marsh, G. Disability and intellectual function in multiple sclerosis. (1980). *J. Nerv. Ment. Dis.*, **168**, 758–62.

Mayeux, R., Stern, Y., Rosen, J., and Benson, D.F. (1983). Is 'subcortical dementia' a recognizeable clinical entity? *Ann. Neurol.*, **14**, 278–83.

McHugh, P.R., and Folstein, M.F. (1973). Recent advances in dementia. Address to the American Academy of Neurology (unpublished).

McHugh, P.R., and Folstein, M.F. (1975). Psychiatric syndromes of Huntington's chorea: a clinical and phenomenologic study. In: D.F. Benson and D. Blumer, eds., *Psychiatric Aspects of Neurologic Disease,* pp. 267–85. New York: Grune and Stratton.

Nauta, W.J.H. (1982). Limbic innervation of the striatum. In: A.J. Friedhoff and T.N. Chase, eds., *Gilles de la Tourette Syndrome.* New York: Raven Press.

Navia, B.A., Jordan, B.D., and Price, R.W. (1986). The AIDS dementia complex: I. clinical features. *Ann. Neurol.*, **19**, 517–24.

Navia, B.A., Cho, E-S., Petito, C.K., and Price, R.W. (1986). The AIDS dementia complex: II. neuropathology, *Ann. Neurol.*, **19**, 525–35.

Olmos-Lau, N., Ginsberg, M.D., and Geller, J.B. (1977). Aphasia in multiple sclerosis. *Neurology*, **27**, 623–26.

Olszewski, J. (1962). Subcortical arteriosclerotic encephalopathy: review of the literature on the so-called Binswanger's disease and presentation of two cases. *World Neurol.*, **3**, 359–75.

Perry, S., and Marotta, R.F. (1987). AIDS dementia: a review of the literature. *Alzheimer Disease and Associated Disorders,* **1**, 221–35.

Peyser, J.M., Edwards, K.R., Poser, C.M., and Filskov, S.B. (1980). Cognitive function in patients with multiple sclerosis. *Arch. Neurol.*, **37**, 577–79.

Rao, S.M. (1986). Neuropsychology of multiple sclerosis: a critical review. *J. Clin. Exp. Neuropsychol.*, **8**, 502–42.

Rao, S.M., Glatt, S., Hammeke, T.A., McQuillen, M.P., Khatri, B.O., Rhodes, A.M., and Pollard, S. (1985). Chronic progressive multiple sclerosis: Relationship between cerebral ventricular size and neuropsychological impairment. *Arch. Neurol.*, **42**, 678–82.

Rao, S.M., Hammeke, T.A., McQuillen, M.P., Khatri, B.O., Lloyd, D. (1984). Memory disturbance in chronic progressive multiple sclerosis. *Arch. Neurol.*, **41**, 625–31.

Reitan, R.M., Reed, J.C., and Dyken, M. (1971). Cognitive, psychomotor, and motor correlates of multiple sclerosis. *J. Nerv. Ment. Dis.*, **153**, 218–24.

Román, G.C. (1987). Senile dementia of the Binswanger type: a vascular form of dementia in the elderly. *J.A.M.A.*, **258**, 1782–88.

Schiffer, R.B., Caine, E.D., Bamford, K.A., and Levy, S. (1983). Depressive episodes in patients with multiple sclerosis. *Am. J. Psychiat.,* **140,** 1498–1500.

Schiffer, R.B., and Slater, R.J. (1985). Neuropsychiatric features of multiple sclerosis: recognition and management. *Semin. Neurol.,* **5,** 127–33.

Shaw, G.M., Harper, M.E., Hahn, B.H., Epstein, L.G., Gajdusek, D.G., Price, R.W., Navia, B.A., Petito, C.K., O'Hara, C.J., Groopman, J.E., Cho, E-S., Oleske, J.M., Wong-Staal, F., and Gallo, R.C. (1985). HTLV-III infection in brains of children and adults with AIDS encephalopathy. *Science,* **227,** 177–82.

Steingart, A., Hachinski, V.C., Lau, C., Fox, A.J., Diaz, F., Cape, R., Lee, D., Inzitari, D., and Merskey, H. (1987a). Cognitive and neurologic findings in subjects with diffuse white matter lucencies on computed tomographic scan (leukoaraiosis). *Arch. Neurol.,* **44,** 32–35.

Steingart, A., Hachinski, V.C., Lau, C., Fox, A.J., Fox, H., Lee, D., Inzitari, D., and Merskey, H. (1987b). Cognitive and neurologic findings in demented patients with diffuse white matter lucencies on computed tomographic scan (leukoaraiosis). *Arch. Neurol.,* **44,** 36–39.

Stevens, J.C., Farlow, M.R., Edwards, M.K., and Yu, P. (1986). Magnetic resonance imaging: clinical correlation in 64 patients with multiple sclerosis. *Arch. Neurol.,* **43,** 1145–48.

Stoler, M.H., Eskin, T.A., Benn, S., Angerer, R.C., Angerer, I.M. (1986). Human T-cell lymphotropic virus type III infection of the central nervous system: a preliminary in situ analysis. *J.A.M.A.,* **256,** 2360–64.

Surridge, D. (1969). An investigation into some aspects of multiple sclerosis. *Br. J. Psychiat.,* **114,** 749–64.

Trimble, M.R., and Grant, I. (1982). Psychiatric aspects of multiple sclerosis. In D.F. Benson and D. Blumer, eds., *Psychiatric Aspects of Neurologic Disease,* vol. 2, pp. 279–99. New York: Grune and Stratton.

Van Gorp, W.G., Mitrushina, M., Cummings, J.L., Satz, P., and Modesitt, J. (1989). AIDS encephalopathy, Alzheimer's disease, and normal aging: a comparison study. *Neuropsychiat., Neuropsychol., and Beh. Neurol.,* **2,** 5–20.

Whitehouse, P.J. (1986). The concept of subcortical and cortical dementia: another look. *Ann. Neurol.,* **19,** 1–6.

Whitlock, F.A., and Siskind, M.M. (1980). Depression as a major symptom of multiple sclerosis. *J. Neurol., Neurosurg., and Psychiat.,* **43,** 861–65.

Wilson, S.A.K. (1912). Progressive lenticular degeneration: a familial nervous disease associated with cirrhosis of the liver. *Brain,* **34,** 295–509.

Zimmerman, R.D., Fleming, C.A., Lee, B.C.P., Saint-Louis, L.A., and Deck, M.D.F. (1986). Periventricular hyperintensity as seen by magnetic resonance: prevalance and significance. *Am. J. Neuroradiol.,* **7,** 13–20.

# 6

# Disorders of Memory

JORDAN GRAFMAN, STEPHEN M. RAO, AND
IRENE LITVAN

Memory impairment is the most common form of cognitive dysfunction reported by multiple sclerosis (MS) patients. It has also been the most widely studied cognitive disability in the scientific literature. Neuropsychological investigations indicate that 40–60% of MS patients perform below expectations on learning and memory tests when compared with control groups (Beatty et al., 1988; Fischer, 1988; Rao et al., 1984; Staples and Lincoln, 1979). These studies also demonstrate that not all aspects of memory are uniformly disrupted by this demyelinating disease. In the following review of the memory literature, we have taken the traditional information-processing approach used in cognitive psychology as the framework for integrating the results of empirical studies.

According to this view of memory (Waugh and Norman, 1965), information flows "linearly" from sensory input to a limited-capacity store, referred to as primary (short-term) memory (see Figure 6–1). Information held in primary memory is lost to conscious awareness if not immediately rehearsed. Secondary (long-term) memory represents a larger-capacity, more permanent store of acquired information that has been consolidated from primary memory. Both recent and remote personal information and historical events are considered part of secondary memory. Memory failure in MS, therefore, may result from a breakdown of either or both of these representational stores and their linked processes.

In this chapter we examine the experimental findings that relate to each representational store. In addition, we discuss the role of attentional and motivational factors in memory dysfunction, the relationship of memory impairment to various illness variables (i.e., degree of disability, disease duration, medication use), and

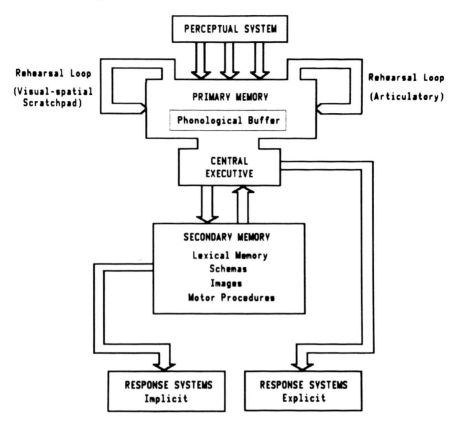

**Figure 6-1** This figure represents a simplified model of some of the information-processing stages required for encoding, storage, and retrieval of information. Many of these stages are described in the chapter in the context of our effort to identify the cause of the memory problems experienced by many MS patients.

the resemblance (or lack thereof) between the memory disorder in MS and that observed in dementing and amnesic conditions. Finally, we make suggestions for future research.

## PRIMARY MEMORY

We define primary memory as the information-processing system dedicated to the temporary storage of information. This system is hypothesized to include postperceptual storage of information, rehearsal mechanisms required to reactivate information for greater processing, and consolidation processes. Each part of this memory system has a limited capacity and constraints on the speed of processing. This system can be assessed by using experimental techniques that measure the amount of information that can be held briefly in short-term store (e.g., digit span), the rate of scanning information held in short-term store (e.g., Sternberg Memory Scanning Paradigm), the effects of subsequent processing of information on accessibility of information held in short-term store (e.g., the Brown-Peterson Paradigm), and the effects of a parallel task load on temporary storage and rehearsal mechanisms in short-term store.

If one or more components of this system were impaired relative to intact secondary memory, then MS patients would have trouble in learning new information but would show little forgetting of information once encoded.

The digit span test is a simple task that estimates the capacity of primary memory. Jambor (1969) found no significant differences on digit span between patients with MS, muscular dystrophy, and psychiatric disorders. This finding of a relatively intact digit span in MS patients has been confirmed by later studies (Heaton et al., 1985; Litvan et al., 1988a,b; Rao et al., 1984; Rao, et al., in press; Staples and Lincoln, 1979).

Immediate free recall of a supraspan word list is consistently impaired in patients with MS (Beatty et al., 1988; Caine et al., 1986; Rao et al., 1984; van den Burg et al., 1987), although it is not clear whether the problem lies with primary or secondary memory. In normal subjects, the first and last items of a list have a higher probability of being recalled. This well-documented finding is known as the serial position effect (Baddeley, 1976); the enhanced recall of words in the beginning and end of a list are commonly referred to as the primacy and recency effects. Theoretical and experimental evidence suggests that the relative contributions of primary and secondary memory to list recall are represented by the recency and primacy effects, respectively (Baddeley, 1976). Caine et al. (1986) and Rao et al. (in press) found no MS–control group differences for the recency effect, while Litvan et al. (1988a,b) reported that MS patients have a tendency toward diminished recall in the recency portion of the learning curve, but this tendency did not reach statistical significance.

Although there is general agreement that MS patients perform as matched controls do on standard digit span tasks and in retaining the last few items on a word list learning task, there have been contradictory results in studies using the Sternberg paradigm, a task that assesses the rate of scanning information held in primary memory. The information scanned in this paradigm is within the number of digits learned in digit span tasks where MS patients perform normally. Litvan et al. (1988a) reported no difference in the reaction time slope to verify whether a single probe digit was a member of the target set (no matter whether the target set was two, four, or six digits) between MS patients and matched normal controls. Rao et al. (1989b), however, found a significant difference in slope between MS patients and controls, suggesting impaired scanning of information independent of reaction-time speed. In this study there was a small but significant relationship between the degree of physical disability and the $y$-intercept (a pure measure of motor response time), but not with slope. No such relationship was found in the Litvan et al. (1988a) study. Differences in age, education, medication usage, and degree of disability may have accounted for the different results in these studies.

The Brown-Peterson task has been used as a measure of consolidation of information in primary memory as well as an index of interference in primary memory activation of stimulus information. In this task, immediately following presentation of stimulus information (usually three words or consonants) interference in the form of counting aloud or reading is begun for various durations (e.g., 0, 3, 6, 12, 18, and 36 seconds), after which recall of the three words or consonants is required. Grant et al. (1984) found that MS patients were impaired on the Brown-Peterson task following interference, and they considered this finding reflective of a defect in short-term storage. This finding was replicated by Beatty et al. (1988), although they did not adequately describe their methods in the paper. In contrast, both Litvan et al. (1988b) and Rao et al. (in press) found no impairment in MS patients on the Brown-Peterson distractor task. Rao et al. (in press) have criticized Grant et al.'s (1984) method of collapsing data on this task, making comparisons of *rate of decay* (which is the critical variable on this task) impossible. Other criticisms of the Grant et al. (1984) paper were voiced by Litvan et al. (1988b). The strongest evidence indicates a normal rate of forgetting by MS patients on the Brown-Peterson task.

Recently, Litvan et al. (1988b) adapted the working memory model of Baddeley (1986) to evaluate learning in MS patients. They hypothesized that despite a normal digit span, MS patients were restricted in the amount of information that could be held in a buffer during encoding. They evaluated this hypothesis by administering letters and words of different syllabic length and phonologic similarity with and without simultaneous articulatory suppression and then asking patients to recall the items. They found that MS patients were significantly impaired compared with controls when five-syllabic words were presented in both the suppression and nonsuppression control conditions. This finding suggested that patients with MS have an impairment to the articulatory loop but have an intact phonologic buffer. While not ruling out other memory deficits, Litvan et al. (1988b) claimed that MS patients' performance on this task was correlated with their performance on secondary memory measures. Unfortunately, because the results for the five-syllabic word control condition was weaker than for the suppression condition (the opposite effect should have occurred for strong confirmation of the articulatory loop deficit hypothesis), the Litvan et al. (1988b) study should be considered promising but tentative.

## Conclusion

It appears that MS patients have a normal digit span, recency retrieval, and decay from primary store. There is some evidence that their scanning of information in primary memory is affected by the number of items held in primary memory. Finally, the findings of Litvan et al. (1988b) provide support for a deficit in working memory (i.e., the articulatory rehearsal loop) that could account for at least some secondary memory deficits, and predict that encoding information to a "deeper" level would result in normal secondary memory performance, a prediction that has been confirmed by Carroll et al. (1984).

## SECONDARY MEMORY

The preponderance of memory studies involving MS patients have evaluated the role of secondary memory impairment. Tasks that assess secondary memory typically require the patient to recall or recognize units of information that exceed the capacity of primary memory (i.e., at least eight or nine units). The importance of the distinction between span and supraspan stimulus presentations is illustrated in one study (Rao et al., in press) where MS patients were found to perform normally on a digit span task but were impaired relative to controls when asked to recall a digit sequence that was two digits longer than their maximal forward digit span.

The most commonly employed secondary memory task in the MS literature has been the immediate recall of a paragraph-length story. In all studies that have used this technique, MS patients have recalled significantly fewer details of the story than controls (Caine et al., 1986; Grant et al., 1984; Rao et al., 1984; Rao et al., in press; Staples and Lincoln, 1979). In a subset of these studies patients were also asked to recall the same stories after a delay of, typically, 30–60 minutes. Relative to controls, MS patients are impaired if the variable examined is the number of informational bits recalled (Caine et al., 1986; Rao et al., in press; Rao et al., 1984; Staples and Lincoln, 1979). In those studies in which the amount of information recalled after the delay is represented as a percentage of immediate recall, however, the evidence is equivocal: some studies indicate that MS patients perform normally (Rao, et al., in press; van den Burg et al., 1987), while others show impairment (Fischer, 1988). Thus it is unclear from this procedure whether MS patients exhibit any abnormalities in their rate of forgetting from secondary memory.

Some studies have examined the primacy effect in the free recall of a supraspan word list (see above). Using the Tulving and Colotla's (1970) scoring procedure for classifying words recalled from primary or secondary memory, Rao et al (in press) found that MS patients were impaired in recalling words from the beginning of the word list (primacy effect), suggesting a specific impairment in secondary memory. While a similar pattern of results have been observed by Caine et al. (1986), Litvan et al. (1988b) found no MS–control group differences for the primacy effect.

Other studies have examined the rate of word list learning on multitrial stimulus presentations. In general, while the absolute amount of words recalled by MS patients over a series of trials is inferior to that of controls, the slope of the learning curves has been found to be similar to those of controls (Rao et al., 1984; van den Burg et al., 1987) or only minimally reduced (Beatty and Gange, 1977; Litvan et al., 1988b). These findings suggest that while MS patients' diminished retrieval capacity places an upper limit on the number of words recalled on a given trial, their capacity for learning with repeated stimulus presentations is relatively preserved. It is also noteworthy that MS patients do not make an abnormal number of intrusive or perseverative errors on free-recall tasks (Beatty and Gange, 1977; Rao et al, in press).

The Selective Reminding Test is a list-learning task that differentiates words recalled from primary or secondary memory (Buschke and Fuld, 1974). Rao et al. (in press) found that MS patients were less likely to recall words from long-term storage than a control group. No group differences were observed in the number of words recalled from short-term storage, however. Furthermore, MS patients exhibited less consistent recall of those words that had already entered into long-term storage, suggesting a problem with memory retrieval.

All these studies have examined verbal memory. Virtually identical results have been found in studies that have used nonverbal stimuli in their memory tasks. Specifically, MS patients are less effective than controls at reproducing geometric designs (Caine et al., 1986; Fischer, 1988; Grant et al., 1984), checkerboard patterns (i.e., 7/24 test) (Rao et al., 1984; Vowels, 1979), or locations of cities on a fictitious map (Beatty et al., 1988). As in the studies using multitrial verbal learning tasks, MS patients recalled less overall information, but they had normal or near normal learning curves for nonverbal stimuli (Rao et al., 1984; Beatty et al., 1988). Delayed recall of nonverbal information, as reflected by percentage of retention from initial learning, also appears to be normal (Caine et al., 1986; Heaton et al., 1985), although impaired performance was found by Fischer (1988).

All the secondary memory tasks discussed thus far have relied on a free-recall paradigm. Recognition memory tests are useful for examining the relative contributions of encoding and storage versus retrieval failure to secondary memory impairment. It is assumed that if a patient is unable to recall an item of information spontaneously, but can successfully discriminate this item in a list combining old and new information, then the item must have entered into long-term storage. Hence the patient's deficits occur primarily in gaining access to information in long-term store. The results of recognition memory testing in MS patients suggest that recognition memory is normal (Carroll, Gates, and Roldan, 1984; Rao et al., in press) or less impaired than recall (Caine et al., 1986; Rao et al., 1984; van den Burg et al., 1987).

The results of recognition memory testing suggest that the secondary memory deficits of most MS patients result from retrieval failure (Caine et al., 1986; Rao, 1986). This conclusion is also supported by studies that have administered letter and category fluency tasks to MS patients. Performance on such tasks is felt to be indicative of the patient's ability to search semantic memory (Butters et al., 1986; Martin and Fedio, 1983). In all studies that have assessed fluency in MS patients, significant impairment has been found (Beatty et al., 1988; Caine et al., 1986; Rao et al., in press; van den Burg et al., 1987).

All the memory tasks used in these studies were designed to measure the patient's conscious and explicit recollection of factual material. Recent studies have suggested that there is an alternate memory system in which learning is expressed implicitly. On implicit memory tasks, such as motor skill acquisition (e.g., pursuit rotor task) or priming (e.g., stem-completion task), patients with global amnesia have been found to perform normally (Corkin, 1968; Shimamura et al., 1987). An interesting double dissociation has been noted in two dementing conditions: patients with Huntington's disease (HD) exhibit deficits in motor skill learning (Heindel, Butters, and Salmon, 1988) but have normal priming (Shimamura et al., 1987), while patients with Alzheimer's disease (AD) have the opposite pattern of deficits, abnormal priming (Salmon et al., 1988) and intact motor skill learning (Heindel et al., 1988). Beatty et al. (in press) administered both types of implicit learning tasks to MS patients and found them to perform comparable to controls.

Only one study has examined remote memory in MS patients (Beatty et al., 1988). Beatty et al. administered the Famous Faces test to patients with chronic-progressive MS. For this test the patient must identify famous faces from the 1940s through the 1980s. MS patients, particularly those with signs of global dementia (Mini-Mental State $<$ 28), were impaired relative to controls. The MS patients were equally impaired for each decade (so-called flat gradient).

## Conclusion

Results of secondary memory testing suggest that MS patients are impaired on verbal and nonverbal, supraspan, and free-recall memory tasks. Much less impairment is observed on recognition testing, which suggests primary problems with retrieval. The retrieval hypothesis is supported by the consistent finding that MS patients are impaired on fluency tasks. Acquisition on multitrial learning tasks is reduced on early trials, but the rate of learning is normal thereafter. Information held in secondary memory appears to be resistant to decay after a delay. The retrieval deficits appear to affect both recent and remote events. Finally, while MS patients are impaired on explicit memory tasks, implicit memory tasks are performed normally.

## OVERALL SUMMARY OF MEMORY RESEARCH

Some general conclusions can be reached regarding the evidence of memory deficits in patients with MS. The evidence suggests that memory processes at the level of both *primary* and *secondary* memory are impaired in many MS patients. Retrieval deficits have been found with both semantic and episodic *secondary* memory tasks. Interestingly, tasks that measure implicit memory and recognition memory show normal or near normal performance in MS patients. Therefore, instead of all aspects of retrieval, mainly processes that allow retrieved information to reach consciousness are impaired. MS patients perform similarly to controls on percentage of information forgotten from immediate to delayed recall. Any retrieval deficit explanation would have to explain the relative consistency in performance at delayed retrieval (given immediate recall) by MS patients. MS and control learning slopes are also similar, although MS patients recall proportionately fewer items across trials. Both maintenance rehearsal and scanning of information in *primary* memory also appear to be impaired in MS patients. Maintenance rehearsal is especially impaired when the information to be encoded places a relatively greater phonological load on processing or when encoding of target information must be accomplished despite a simultaneous information-processing load, however simple (e.g., repeating numbers or counting down from 100). There is some evidence that this impairment at the level of *primary* memory maintenance rehearsal capacity is related to the amount of information that can be immediately freely recalled on a standard *secondary* memory task (e.g., story recall). A graphic summary of the information processing components that are believed to be defective in MS is presented in Figure 6–2.

## ROLE OF ATTENTION PROCESSES IN MEMORY DYSFUNCTION

Attention, for the purposes of this chapter, can be segregated into focal and sustained processes. Focused attention refers to the process of the search for, and localization of, target stimuli. Sustained attention, sometimes used interchangeably with

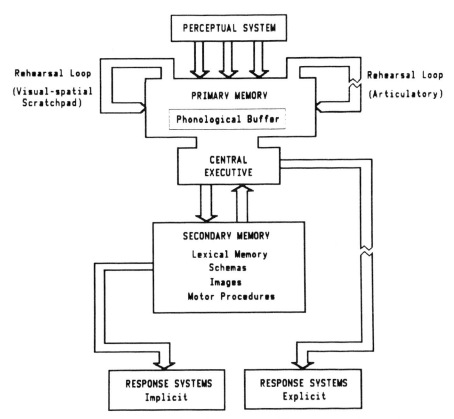

**Figure 6-2** On the basis of our review, the strongest evidence suggests that two information-processing routes are affected in MS. The first route corresponds to an articulatory rehearsal loop and affects encoding capacity. The second route corresponds to a retrieval pathway in the response system concerned with explicit recall of both episodic and semantic information.

the term vigilance, refers to the monitoring of target stimuli over an extended duration of time. So-called preattentive processes have not been examined in MS patients and so are not discussed in this chapter.

There has only been one study of sustained attention. Rao (1988) administered a series of auditory tones that varied by duration (600 versus 800 milliseconds). The long tone (the *signal*) was randomly presented 20% of the time. Stimuli were presented once every 2 seconds. Subjects were required to press a telegraph key whenever the signal tone occurred. The task lasted for 12 minutes; errors of omission and commission were reported for four consecutive 3-minute blocks. Both the MS patients and the controls made an equal number of commission errors during the first block of trials; however, while the controls steadily decreased their commission errors during blocks 2–4, the MS patients made slightly more errors, a statistically significant interaction effect. No group differences were observed on errors of omission.

Van den Burg et al. (1987) administered a task that most closely approximates a test of focused attention to MS patients and controls. They required subjects to attend to a target array while keeping their hand on a button. In one condition, subjects were required to lift their hand off the button and press a target button that was illuminated. In another condition, distracting lights in another row of buttons were flashed at the same time as a target light. Subjects had to both search for the target button and ignore the distractor button in this second condition. Decision times were determined by measuring the time it took the subject to lift his or her finger off the button following target button illumination onset. Movement times were recorded as the duration of time between finger lift and target button press. As expected, there were differences that were independent of conditions in movement times between MS and controls. Decision times also showed a difference between MS patients and controls which increased in the distractor condition. Van den Burg et al. point out, however, that decision times are also affected by movement initiation, so that their results should be viewed with caution.

We next report on tasks that have been traditionally described as attentional tasks in the clinical literature but that clearly have more complex processing requirements than the reaction time tasks used by van den Burg et al. (1987). One such task is the Paced Auditory Serial Addition Test (PASAT). Devised by Gronwall and Wrightson (1974), this test requires that the patient add 60 pairs of randomized single digits so that each is added to the digit immediately preceding it. Litvan et al. (1988a) found that MS patients performed significantly worse than controls at the faster presentation rates (1.6. and 1.2 second per digit), but were intact at slower rates (2.4 and 2.0 second per digit). They interpreted this result as reflecting the limited ability of MS patients to process rapidly presented information rather than a deficit in computational ability, memory, or resource allocation. Rao (1988) administered a slightly different version of the PASAT and found that MS patients were equally impaired with both fast *and slow* rates of presentation (2 and 3 seconds per digit, respectively). While these two studies agree that PASAT test performance is impaired in MS patients, it is unclear whether the disturbance is dependent on rate of stimulus presentation.

Van der Burg et al. (1987) used the Trail Making Test as a measure of attention in their study. The Trail Making Test consists of two conditions: Part A requires the patient to draw lines to connect consecutively numbered circles on a single sheet of paper, while for Part B the same number of consecutively numbered and lettered circles are connected by alternating between the sequences. Time to completion is the primary dependent variable. Van den Burg et al. found significant differences between MS patients and controls for Parts A and B. These differences were eliminated in a covariance analysis in which a motor manipulation task served as the covariate. Complexity in cognitive processing (i.e., the difference in performance between Parts A and B) was not examined in their covariance analysis, however. Heaton et al. (1985), on the other hand, found that chronic-progressive, but not relapsing-remitting, MS patients performed significantly more poorly when performance on Trails A was subtracted from performance on Trails B.

To summarize, there is some evidence to suggest that MS patients have both focal and sustained attentional deficits. Unfortunately, the relationship between these deficits and performance on primary and secondary memory tasks has not been examined.

## ROLE OF DEPRESSION IN MEMORY DYSFUNCTION

Studies of depressed individuals have noted improvement in memory test performance after patients are treated with antidepressants or other therapies, although other studies have not found differences between depressed and normal individuals on memory tests (for a review, see Niederehe, 1986). Weingartner and his colleagues (1986) administered two types of memory tasks to depressed patients: those requiring mental effort and those involving automatic processing. Depressed patients were found to be impaired on the former and normal on the latter, prompting these researchers to propose a "central motivational deficit" to account for impaired memory performance in depressed patients.

Patients with MS are known to exhibit a higher rate of depression than other patient groups with equal degree, or greater, of physical disability (Joffe et al., 1987; Schiffer et al., 1983; Whitlock and Siskind, 1980). These clinical observations raise the question as to what extent the memory problems in MS can be attributed to depression. Rao et al. (1984) found that MS patients with mild memory disorders were more likely to report depression on the MMPI than patients with normal memory or patients with moderate to severe memory disturbance. In a subsequent study (Rao et al., in press), depression was assessed with the Zung Depression Scale; scores on this self-report scale did not correlate with any of the indices derived from an extensive battery of memory tests. Fischer (1988) administered the Beck Depression Scale and the revised version of the Wechsler Memory Scale. While the MS group reported more depression than the control group, no relationship was found between severity of memory disturbance and self-reported depression. Finally, Beatty et al. (1988) found differences between depressed (Beck Depression Scale > 9) and nondepressed MS patients on a subset of memory measures; if the depressed patients were excluded from the analysis, however, the MS patients still performed defectively relative to controls on memory testing.

The modest relationship, if any, between measures of depression and memory performance in these studies could be related to the use of self-report depression scales. Patients with mild memory problems may have adequate personal insight to report their mood state accurately, while patients with more severe memory problems (and more global dementia) are incapable of reporting depression accurately. Two studies have examined the relationship between depression, as diagnosed from a psychiatric interview, and memory performance. Jambor (1969) found that nondepressed MS patients actually scored lower on memory test scores than depressed patients. Lyon-Caen et al. (1986) also found no relationship between the presence of depression (DSM-III criteria) and memory impairment.

Magnetic resonance imaging (MRI) studies indicate that memory disturbance cannot entirely be caused by depression. These studies (Franklin et al., 1988; Rao et al., 1989a; Chapter 7, this volume) have found robust correlations beween measures of memory performance and the total area of lesion involvement on MRI scans. Instead of the usual explanation that depression produces memory dysfunction, two alternative explanations may be offered. In the first, depression results as a normal emotional reaction to lost cognitive abilities, particularly in the mildly memory impaired MS patient with intact personal insight. For the second, both depression and memory disturbance result as a direct consequence of demyelinating lesions within the limbic system. Indeed one of us (Rao) has found significant correlations between total lesion involvement on MRI and measures of depression (self-report and relative ratings) in MS patients (unpublished data). Similar clinicopathological correlations have been noted by Honer et al. (1987).

## RELATIONSHIP TO ILLNESS VARIABLES

In most research studies the degree of disability is quantified using either the 10-point Kurtzke Disability Status Scale (DSS) (Kurtzke, 1955) or the revised 20-point Expanded Kurtzke DSS (Kurtzke, 1983). This scale is heavily weighted toward disabilities associated with ambulation. As a result, patients whose MS lesions are confined primarily to the spinal cord can experience severe physical disability but have minimal, if any, cognitive impairment. It is not surprising, therefore, that most studies have not found this scale or similar scales to correlate with the severity of memory disturbance (Beatty et al., 1988; Fischer, 1988; Heaton et al., 1985; Lyon-Caen et al., 1986; Rao et al., 1984, 1989b, in press; Vowels, 1979), although some exceptions have been noted (Litvan et al., 1988b; van den Burg et al., 1987).

All studies of memory disturbance in MS published thus far have relied on cross-sectional research designs. Surprisingly, these studies have not found relationships between length of symptom duration and degree of memory dysfunction (Grant et al., 1984; Heaton et al., 1985; Lyon-Caen et al., 1986; Rao et al., 1984, 1989b, in press; van den Burg et al., 1987; Vowels, 1979). Longitudinal studies are clearly needed to address this issue.

Some studies have noted a relationship between disease course (relapsing-remitting versus chronic-progressive) and memory disturbance (Heaton et al., 1985). In general, patients with a chronic-progressive course perform more poorly on memory testing. It should also be noted that these patients frequently are older and have had symptoms longer than relapsing-remitting patients.

Several studies have examined the possible role of psychoactive medications as an explanation for memory loss in MS. Rao et al. (1984) found that MS patients with mild memory disturbance were more likely to be taking medications than patients without memory disturbance or patients with moderate/severe disturbance. Grant et al. (1984) found no relationship between steroid use and memory performance. Likewise, Heaton et al. (1985) and Rao et al. (in press) found no differences between medicated and nonmedicated MS patients on a variety of memory measures. Overall, these findings suggest that medication use is not a major contributor to memory loss in MS patients.

## RELATIONSHIP TO OTHER NEUROLOGIC DISORDERS

How do the memory problems in MS compare with other neurologic disorders that are known to impair memory functions? From a quantitative standpoint, it is clear that MS patients *as a group* do not exhibit the same degree of memory loss as patients with progressive dementia (AD and HD) or with stable amnesia (Korsak-off's syndrome). This conclusion is illustrated in Figure 6–3 using subscale data provided in the manual of the revised Wechsler Memory Scale (Wechsler, 1987). Caine et al. (1986) also concluded that their MS patients' overall degree of memory dysfunction was less severe than that of patients with HD.

The conclusion that MS patients have less severe memory dysfunction relative to dementing and amnesic patients is somewhat misleading. Whereas memory loss is a defining problem in dementing and amnesic conditions and is therefore observed to some extent in all patients, considerable interpatient variability is observed in MS. Neuropsychological studies indicate that approximately 40–60% of MS patients exhibit little, if any, memory disturbance (Beatty et al., 1988; Fischer, 1988; Rao et al., 1984; Staples and Lincoln, 1979). When the performance of these intact individuals is averaged with that of patients with disordered memory, it gives the mistaken impression that all MS patients exhibit mild memory loss.

The study by Caine et al. (1986) is the only one to compare directly the perfor-mance of MS patients with another memory disordered group (i.e., HD). MS patients were found to perform poorly on recall tasks but normally on recognition tasks, while HD patients performed poorly on both tasks. They concluded that HD patients exhibit deficits with storage, encoding, and retrieval, while MS patients have problems solely with retrieval mechanisms.

Although no direct comparisons have been reported, it would appear that the pattern of memory problems in MS patients are *qualitatively* different from those of patients with presumed AD. In this group, deficits in primary memory (i.e., digit span, short-term forgetting) are prominent, particularly in the middle to late stages of the illness (Kaszniak et al., 1986). Likewise, MS patients appear unlike the dien-cephalic amnesics, who have normal performance on fluency tasks, but impaired recognition testing due to faulty encoding strategies (Kaszniak et al., 1986). MS patients are also unlike temporal lobe amnesics, who exhibit a rapid and abnormal rate of forgetting from secondary memory, which undoubtedly contributes to their impaired recognition test performance (Squire, 1982).

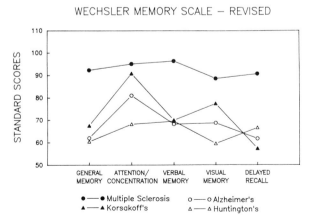

**Figure 6–3**  Subscale scores derived from the revised Wechsler Memory Scale for MS, Korsak-off's, Alzheimer's, and Huntington's patients (adapted from Wechsler, 1987).

From a review of the memory literature, Rao et al. (in press) proposed that the qualitative features of the memory loss in MS most closely resemble that found in HD. While Caine et al. found recognition deficits in HD patients, this result has not been observed consistently (Butters et al., 1986). Furthermore, HD patients, unlike amnesic patients and similar to MS patients, are impaired on fluency tasks (Butters et al., 1986). Thus the basic deficits in retrieval may be similar in MS and HD, despite the fact that the absolute degree of impairment is clearly worse in the latter group.

## FUTURE DIRECTIONS

Although we have been able to specify some memory processes that appear reliably impaired in MS patients, much remains to be learned about the course and the characterization of the memory deficits. To distinguish whether the memory deficits noted in MS have unique features or can be found in patients with other CNS disorders, a better categorization of study patients is required. For example, dividing the patients by their disease course (e.g., chronic-progressive or relapsing-remitting), duration, MRI lesion severity, and stage of mental decline (e.g., severity of general dementia) would be a required first step. The memory performance of MS patients could be then described within the category of disease stage in which they fall. This categorization, particularly in the context of longitudinal studies, would enable investigators to note how memory deficits manifested themselves over time. For example, it is probable that the pattern of memory deficits in the early stages of the disorder may be different than the pattern seen with increasing MS severity. Location of the MS plaques in the brain may clearly predict the appearance of specific memory deficits. This approach to classifying patients is used with other CNS disorders (e.g., AD or head injury) and is appropriate for MS patients.

Experimental designs of memory tasks that better control for encoding strategies and that manipulate processing capacity are needed. For example, if a retrieval deficit is considered as a possible mechanism for the observed memory deficit(s) in MS patients, how can retrieval be manipulated to ascertain what component of retrieval is affected? Cued retrieval, implicit retrieval, error analysis, associate retrieval, controlled retrieval, all can be used under varying encoding procedures (controlling for motor ability) to obtain a more accurate identification of the involved component processes in the memory deficit displayed by MS patients. The use of neuroimaging and event-related potential methodologies may enhance the explanatory power of the results of such cognitive experiments.

To this point, we have not discussed possible treatments for the memory disorders of MS patients. While the scientific literature contains several illustrations of successful applications of cognitive rehabilitation procedures for memory loss in stroke and head injury populations (Gasparrini and Satz, 1979; Grafman, 1984), no study has addressed the efficacy of these procedures with MS patients (although see Chapters 14 and 15, this volume). Likewise, only one study (Leo and Rao, 1988) has evaluated the effects of medication as a treatment of memory in MS patients. Leo and Rao (1988) found significant improvement on the Selective Reminding Test in three of four memory-impaired MS patients while receiving intravenous physostigmine, an acetylcholinesterase inhibitor, in a double-blind, crossover study. Replication of this study using oral physostigmine in a larger patient population is currently underway. Clearly, further work is needed to develop clinically effective treatments for memory loss in MS patients.

There is ample documentation that many MS patients suffer from memory impairment. This chapter has been able to identify some possible memory processes where the impairment may be located. Greater precision in describing and treating the impaired memory process in conjunction with improved patient staging is one direction that memory research with MS patients needs to take during the last decade of the twentieth century.

## ACKNOWLEDGMENTS

The National Institute of Neurological Disorders and Stroke and the Medical Neurology Branch provided the facilities and support for J.G. to prepare this chapter. S.M.R. was supported in part by a Research Career Development Award (K04 NS01055) and a Research Grant (R01 NS22128) from the National Institute of Neurological Disorders and Stroke.

The opinions and assertions contained herein are the private views of the authors and are not to be construed as official or necessarily reflecting views of the National Institutes of Health, the United States Public Health Service, the Department of Health and Human Services or the Uniformed Services University of the Health Sciences.

## REFERENCES

Baddeley, A.D. (1976). *The Psychology of Memory.* New York: Basic Books.

Baddeley, A.D. (1986). *Working Memory.* Oxford: Clarendon Press.

Beatty, P.A. and Gange, J.J. (1977). Neuropsychological aspects of multiple sclerosis. *J. Nerv. Ment. Dis.,* **164,** 42–50.

Beatty, W.W., Goodkin, D.E., Monson, N., and Beatty, P.A. (in press). Implicit learning in patients with chronic progressive multiple sclerosis. *Int. J. Clin. Neuropsychol.*

Beatty, W.W., Goodkin, D.E., Monson, N., Beatty, P.A., and Hertsgaard, D. (1988). Anterograde and retrograde amnesia in patients with chronic progressive multiple sclerosis. *Arch. Neurol.,* **45,** 611–19.

Buschke, H., and Fuld, P.A. (1974). Evaluating storage, retention, and retrieval in disordered memory and learning. *Neurology,* **24,** 1019–25.

Butters, N., Martone, M., White, B., Granholm, E., and Wolfe, J. (1986). Clinical validators: Comparisons of demented and amnesic patients. In: L.W. Poon, ed., *Clinical Memory Assessment of Older Adults,* pp. 337–52. Washington, D.C.: American Psychological Association.

Caine, E.D., Bamford, K.A., Schiffer, R.B., Shoulson, I., and Levy, S. (1986). A controlled neuropsychological comparison of Huntington's disease and multiple sclerosis. *Arch. Neurol.,* **43,** 249–54.

Carroll, M., Gates, R., and Roldan, F. (1984). Memory impairment in multiple sclerosis. *Neuropsychologia,* **22,** 297–302.

Corkin, S. (1968). Acquisition of a motor skill after bilateral medial temporal-lobe excision. *Neuropsychologia,* **6,** 255–64.

Fischer, J.S. (1988). Using the Wechsler Memory Scale-Revised to detect and characterize memory deficits in multiple sclerosis. *Clin. Neuropsychol.* **2,** 149–72.

Franklin, G.M., Heaton, R.K., Nelson, L.M., Filley, C.M., and Seibert, C. (1988). Correlation of neuropsychological and MRI findings in chronic/progressive multiple sclerosis. *Neurology,* **38,** 1826–29.

Gasparrini, B., and Satz, P. (1979). A treatment for memory problems in left hemisphere CVA patients. *J. Clin. Psychol.,* **1,** 137–50.

Grafman, J. (1984). Memory assessment and remediation in brain-injured patients: From theory to practice. In: B.A. Edelstein and E.T. Couture, eds., *Behavioral Assessment and Rehabilitation of the Traumatically Brain-Damaged,* pp. 151–89. New York: Plenum.

Grant, I., McDonald, W.I., Trimble, M.R., Smith E., and Reed, R. (1984). Deficient learning and memory in early and middle phases of multiple sclerosis. *J. Neurol. Neurosurg. Psychiat.,* **47,** 250–55.

Gronwall, D., and Wrightson, P. (1974). Recovery after minor head injury. *Lancet,* **2,** 1452.

Heaton, R.K., Nelson, L.M., Thompson, D.S., Burks, J.S., and Franklin, G.M. (1985). Neuropsychological findings in relapsing-remitting and chronic-progressive multiple sclerosis. *J. Consult. Clin. Psychol.,* **53,** 103–10.

Heindel, W.C., Butters, N., and Salmon, D.P. (1988). Impaired learning of a motor skill in patients with Huntington's disease. *Beh. Neurosci.,* **102,** 141–47.

Honer, W.G., Hurwitz, T., Li, D.K.B., Palmer, M., and Paty, D.W. (1987). Temporal lobe involvement in multiple sclerosis patients with psychiatric disorders. *Arch. Neurol.,* **44,** 187–90.

Jambor, K.L. (1969). Cognitive functioning in multiple sclerosis. *Br. J. Psychiat.,* **115,** 765–75.

Joffe, R.T., Lippert, G.P., Gray, T.A., Sawa, G., and Horvath, Z. (1987). Mood disorder and multiple sclerosis. *Arch. Neurol.,* **44,** 376–78.

Kaszniak, A.W., Poon, L.W., and Riege, W. (1986). Assessing memory deficits: An information-processing approach. In: L.W. Poon, ed., *Clinical Memory Assessment of Older Adults,* pp. 168–88. Washington, D.C.: American Psychological Association.

Kurtzke, J.F. (1955). A new scale for evaluating disability in multiple sclerosis. *Neurology,* **5,** 580–83.

Kurtzke, J.F. (1983). Rating neurologic impairment in multiple sclerosis: An expanded disability status scale (EDSS). *Neurology,* **33,** 1444–52.

Leo, G.J., and Rao, S.M. (1988). Effects of intravenous physostigmine and lecithin on memory loss in multiple sclerosis: Report of a pilot study. *J. Neurol. Rehab.,* **2,** 123–29.

Litvan, I., Grafman, J., Vendrell, P., and Martinez, J.M. (1988a). Slowed information processing in multiple sclerosis. *Arch. Neurol.,* **45,** 281–85.

Litvan, I., Grafman, J., Vendrell, P., Martinez, J.M., Junque, C., Vendrell, J.M., and Barraquer-Bordas, J.L. (1988b). Multiple memory deficits in patients with multiple sclerosis: Exploring the working memory system. *Arch. Neurol.,* **45,** 607–10.

Lyon-Caen, O., Jouvent, R., Hauser, S., Chaunu, M.-P., Benoit, N., Widlocher, D., and Lhermitte, F. (1986). Cognitive function in recent-onset demyelinating diseases. *Arch. Neurol.,* **43,** 1138–41.

Martin, A., and Fedio, P. (1983). Word production and comprehension in Alzheimer's disease: The breakdown of semantic knowledge. *Brain Lang.,* **19,** 124–41.

Niederehe, G. (1986). Depression and memory impairment in the aged. In: L.W. Poon, ed., *Handbook for Clinical Memory Assessment of Older Adults,* pp. 226–37. Washington, D.C.: American Psychological Association.

Rao, S.M. (1986). Neuropsychology of multiple sclerosis: A critical review. *J. Clin. Exp. Neuropsychol.,* **8,** 503–42.

Rao, S.M., Hammeke, T.A., McQuillen, M.P., Khatri, B.O., and Lloyd, D. (1984). Memory disturbance in chronic progressive multiple sclerosis. *Arch. Neurol.,* **41,** 625–31.

Rao, S.M. (1988). Issues in the assessment of information processing speed in subcortical dementia. *J. Clin. Exp. Neuropsychol.,* **10,** 54.

Rao, S.M., Leo, G.J., Haughton, V.M., St. Aubin-Faubert, P., and Bernardin, L. (1989a). Correlation of magnetic resonance imaging with neuropsychological testing in multiple sclerosis. *Neurology,* **39,** 161–66.

Rao, S.M., Leo, G.J., and St. Aubin-Faubert, P. (in press). On the nature of memory disturbance in multiple sclerosis. *J. Clin. Exp. Neuropsychol.*

Rao, S.M., St. Aubin-Faubert, P., and Leo, G.J. (1989b). Information processing speed in patients with multiple sclerosis. *J. Clin. Exp. Neuropsychol.,* **11,** 471–77.

Salmon, D.P., Shimamura, A.P., Butters, N., and Smith, S. (1988). Lexical and semantic priming deficits in patients with Alzheimer's disease. *J. Clin. Exp. Neuropsychol.,* **10,** 477–94.

Schiffer, R.B., Caine, E.D., Bamford, K.A., and Levy, S. (1983). Depressive episodes in patients with multiple sclerosis. *Am. J. Psychiat.,* **140,** 1498–1500.

Shimamura, A.P., Salmon, D.P., Squire, L.R., and Butters, N. (1987). Memory dysfunction and word priming in dementia and amnesia. *Beh. Neurosci.,* **101,** 347–51.

Squire, L.R. (1982). The neuropsychology of human memory. *Ann. Rev. Neurosci.,* **5,** 241–73.

Staples, D., and Lincoln, N.B. (1979). Intellectual impairment in multiple sclerosis and its relation to functional abilities. *Rheumatol. Rehab.,* **18,** 153–60.

Tulving, E., and Colotla, V.A. (1970). Free recall of trilingual lists. *Cognitive Psychol.,* **1,** 86–98.

van den Burg, W., van Zomeren, A.H., Minderhoud, J.M., Prange, A.J.A. and Meijer, N.S.A. (1987). Cognitive impairment in patients with multiple sclerosis and mild physical disability. *Arch. Neurol.,* **44,** 494–501.

Vowels, L.M. (1979). Memory impairment in multiple sclerosis. In: M. Molloy, G.V. Stanley, and K.W. Walsh, eds., *Brain Impairment: Proceedings of the 1978 Brain Impairment Workshop,* pp. 10–22. Melbourne: University of Melbourne.

Waugh, N.C., and Norman, D.A. (1965). Primary memory. *Psychol. Rev.,* **72,** 89–104.

Wechsler, D. (1987). *Wechsler Memory Scale-Revised.* New York: Psychological Corporation.

Weingartner, H. (1986). Automatic and effort-demanding cognitive processes in depression. In: L.W. Poon, ed., *Handbook for Clinical Memory Assessment of Older Adults* (pp. 218–25). Washington, D.C.: American Psychological Association.

Whitlock, F.A., and Siskind, M.M. (1980). Depression as a major symptom of multiple sclerosis. *J. Neurol. Neurosurg. Psychiat.* **43,** 861–65.

# 7

# Neuroimaging Correlates
# of Cognitive Dysfunction

STEPHEN M. RAO

Autopsy studies have demonstrated that the cerebrum is widely and commonly involved in multiple sclerosis (MS) patients (Adams, 1977; Brownell and Hughes, 1962; Powell and Lampert, 1983). Characteristically, lesions involve periventricular white matter, although they may also appear in the gray-white matter junction and occasionally extend into gray matter (Brownell and Hughes, 1962). Recent advances in brain imaging technology make it possible for the clinician to visualize MS-related pathology during life (see Chapter 3). Such information has the potential of delineating important clinicopathological relationships, particularly with regard to the study of cognitive dysfunction in MS. In this chapter the results of investigations that attempt to relate cognitive test findings with pathological data derived from computed tomography (CT), magnetic resonance imaging (MRI), and positron emission tomography (PET) are reviewed. Methodological problems are also discussed, along with directions for future research.

## COMPUTED TOMOGRAPHY

The standard unenhanced CT scan is relatively insensitive to demyelination in the cerebrum of MS patients. For example, Haughton et al. (1979) obtained high-resolution CT images from the cadaver brains of two MS patients. Three radiologists independently measured the number and size of plaques from CT images and corresponding brain slices. Although nearly 70 discrete lesions were observed at autopsy, only 4 lesions were observed on CT. The authors offered two possible explanations for this discrepancy: (1) the resolving power of even the most recent generation of CT scanners is incapable of visualizing lesions smaller than 0.7 cm; and (2) subacute or chronic demyelinated lesions may be difficult to observe because they are isodense with surrounding "normal" brain tissue. Enhanced CT provides the possibility of detecting some acute lesions; these lesions appear on CT because of leakage of contrast medium resulting from breakdown of the blood-brain barrier, which occurs primarily in the acute stages of lesion development (see Chapter 2).

More recently, the relative insensitivity of CT to demyelination has been highlighted in studies that compare CT with MRI. These studies have consistently shown an approximately 20:1 ratio between the number of lesions observed on MRI when compared with CT, respectively (Jacobs et al., 1986; Lukes et al., 1983; Reese et al., 1986; Young et al., 1981). The differences in sensitivity between CT and MRI are somewhat diminished if CT scans are performed with a double dose of contrast agent with delayed scanning (Jackson et al., 1985; Reese et al., 1986). Nevertheless, CT performed in this way is still not as effective as MRI in identifying lesions (Jackson et al., 1985; Reese et al., 1986).

Despite its limitations in detecting MS lesions, CT provides an accurate index of ventricular size. Table 7–1 provides the number of MS patients diagnosed as having age-inappropriate cerebral atrophy on CT from several published series. Overall, ventricular dilatation is observed in approximately 40% of MS patients. While the exact mechanism causing ventricular enlargement is unknown, it is assumed to occur as a consequence of diffuse periventricular demyelination (Brownell and Hughes, 1962). Cerebral atrophy, therefore, can serve as an indirect and probably late marker of cerebral disease activity in MS.

Three studies have correlated cerebral atrophy from CT with cognitive testing. Brooks et al. (1984) administered the Wechsler Adult Intelligence Scale (WAIS), standardized reading tests, and CT scans to 12 MS patients. Cognitive dysfunction was defined as a significant discrepancy between IQ and reading-test scores. The former measure served as an indicator of acquired cognitive deterioration, while the latter was used as a predictor of premorbid ability level. Eight patients were rated as having cerebral atrophy on CT scans. Seven of these eight patients exhib-

**Table 7–1** Percentage of MS Patients with Atrophy on CT Scan in Previously Reported Series[a]

| Study | N | % with Atrophy |
|---|---|---|
| Hershey et al. (1979) | 66 | 20 |
| Radue and Kendall (1978) | 49 | 35 |
| Reisner and Maida (1980) | 43 | 37 |
| Jacobs and Kinkel (1976) | 34 | 38 |
| Cala et al. (1978) | 100 | 44 |
| Gyldenstad (1976) | 110 | 46 |
| de Weerd (1979) | 23 | 57 |
| Rao et al. (1985) | 47 | 60 |
| Total | 472 | 41 |

[a]In order of increasing incidence.
(Reproduced with permission from Rao et al., 1985.)

ited cognitive dysfunction, while none of the four patients without atrophy showed signs of cognitive decline.

Rabins et al. (1986) examined 37 MS patients with CT and the Mini-Mental State (MMS) cognitive screening examination. In addition, patients were also rated for "euphoric mood state." A venticular-brain ratio (VBR) was computed by dividing a linear measure of the lateral ventricles at the greatest width by the intracranial width at the same level. Rabins et al. found that patients with large ventricles were also more likely to be impaired cognitively and to be rated as euphoric. A significant negative correlation was observed between VBR and MMS score ($r = -.33$).

We obtained subjective ratings and linear measurements of ventricular size from CT scans of 47 chronic-progressive MS patients (Rao et al., 1985). The cognitive measures included: the verbal subtests of the revised WAIS (WAIS-R), the complete Wechsler Memory Scale, and two experimental measures of verbal and visuospatial learning and memory. CT scans were classified as having either no, mild, or moderate/severe cerebral atrophy. The CT rater was provided only with the patient's age, which was used to make appropriate adjustments in the atrophy ratings; 19 patients (40%) were judged to have no ventricular enlargement, 19 (40%) had mildly enlarged ventricles, and 9 (20%) had moderate-to-severe ventricular dilatation. Statistically significant ($p < .05$) group differences were observed on the WAIS-R Comprehension subtest and on 10 of 13 measures of learning and memory; no group differences were seen on three measures of orientation and attention span, skills that are rarely affected in MS (Rao, 1986). Post hoc analyses revealed significant differences between the no atrophy and moderate/severe atrophy groups. These group differences were particularly noteworthy on measures of verbal and visuospatial learning (see Figure 7–1).

Ventricular size was also measured from illuminated roentgenographic transparencies using the linear procedures described by Huckman et al. (1975). These measurements included: (1) the length of the distance between the most lateral portion of each of the frontal horns of the lateral ventricles ("bifrontal" span), (2) the width of the lateral ventricles in the region of the caudate nuclei, that being the width of the two lateral ventricles just anterior to the third ventricle ("bicaudate"), and (3) the maximum width of the third ventricle ("third"). A ventricular-cranial

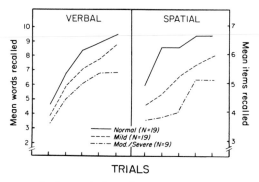

TRIALS

**Figure 7–1**  Learning curves for free verbal recall test (left) and 7/24 spatial recall test (right) for three subgroups of patients with MS having normal ventricular size, mild dilatation, and moderate to severe ventricular enlargement. (Reproduced with permission from Rao et al., 1985.)

ratio was computed by dividing each measure by its internal transverse cranial diameter recorded at the same level. The third ventricle measure correlated significantly, albeit modestly, with 16 of 19 cognitive measures ($r = -.25$ to $-.41$); the bifrontal and bicaudate indices, by comparison, were relatively poor predictors of memory/cognitive dysfunction.

These findings suggested the possibility that relatively focal areas of demyelination involving structures surrounding the third ventricle may play a significant role in the development of memory/cognitive disturbance in MS. Alternatively, we conjectured that the third ventricle measure may have been the best predictor of cognitive decline because of an artifact in the linear measurement procedure. The third ventricle is easier to visualize in the CT axial plane than the larger and more tortuous lateral ventricles. As a result, the third ventricle may have been a better indicator of cognitive dysfunction because it was more reliably measured than the lateral ventricles.

To address these two competing hypotheses, we (Rao and Glatt, unpublished manuscript) reanalyzed the scans of 41 of our original 47 patients using the General Electric 9800 CT scanner's computer software routines to obtain more precise measurements of ventricular size (CT computer data could not be located for 6 patients). These measurements were accomplished by placing the region of interest cursor within the ventricles and measuring all contiguous regions with densities between $-10$ and 23 CT density units in square centimeters. This number was multiplied by slice thickness (1 cm) to yield a ventricular volume per slice. Because ventricular size may be influenced by the size of the cranium, intracranial volume was analyzed by placement of the ROI cursor within the cranial cavity and measuring contiguous areas with densities between $-10$ and 150 CT units. VBRs were computed by dividing ventricular by intracranial volumes. VBRs were calculated for the third and lateral ventricules separately and in combination (total).

Table 7–2 compares correlations between cognitive measures and three methods of quantifying ventricular dilatation from CT scans. The blind, subjective ratings and VBR measurements correlated better with cognitive measures than the linear measurements did. With the slightly smaller sample size in the reanalysis, the superior correlations between cognitive and linear third ventricle measurements were no longer evident, suggesting that our original finding (Rao et al., 1985) was a chance observation. This conclusion is supported by the VBR measurements in which no significant differences were found between the third and lateral ventricles in predicting cognitive dysfunction.

The primary conclusion that may be drawn from the CT studies is that size of the ventricular spaces is a gross indicator of cognitive decline in MS. Nevertheless, cerebral atrophy is at best an indirect and late index of cerebral demyelination. As a result of CT's inability to provide useful information regarding the location and size of MS lesions, correlations with cognitive testing are small. This may occur because recently diagnosed patients with extensive cerebral plaque involvement and cognitive disturbance may not show ventricular dilatation on CT. Thus more accurate information regarding cerebral pathology may be essential to a better understanding of cognitive disturbance in MS. These studies also suggest that the methods used to quantify brain imaging may significantly affect clinicopathological correlations.

**Table 7–2**  Significant Partial Correlations ($p<.05$) Between Three Measures of CT Atrophy and Measures of Verbal Intelligence and Memory Controlling for the Effects of Age and Education ($N=41$)

| Neuropsychological Test | Subjective | Linear | | | Volumetric | | |
|---|---|---|---|---|---|---|---|
| | | Bifrontal | Bicaudate | Third | Total | Lateral | Third |
| *Verbal intelligence* | | | | | | | |
| WAIS-R Verbal IQ | −.32 | | | −.27 | −.37 | −.37 | −.30 |
| Comprehension | −.38 | | | | −.31 | −.31 | |
| Similarities | −.30 | −.34 | −.32 | −.34 | −.30 | −.30 | |
| *Wechsler Memory Scale* | | | | | | | |
| Memory quotient | −49 | −.29 | −.30 | | −.47 | −.47 | −.44 |
| Mental Control | −.35 | | | | −.30 | −.30 | −.30 |
| Digit Span | −.35 | −.27 | −.28 | | −.46 | −.46 | −.45 |
| Logical Memory | −.44 | −.31 | −.33 | −.31 | −.39 | −.39 | −.38 |
| Visual Reproduction | −.38 | | | | −.27 | | −.33 |
| Associate Learning | −.47 | | | | −.43 | −.43 | −.44 |
| *Free Verbal Recall Test* | | | | | | | |
| List A (total recall) | −.41 | | | | −.32 | −.32 | −.36 |
| List B | | | | | | | −.30 |
| List A recall | −.41 | | | | −.44 | −.44 | −.42 |
| List A delayed | −.46 | | | | −.41 | −.41 | −.37 |
| *Spatial Recall Test* | | | | | | | |
| Design A (total recall) | −.41 | | | | −.28 | −.28 | −.29 |
| Design B | −.35 | | | | −.44 | −.44 | −.41 |

## MAGNETIC RESONANCE IMAGING

The recent introduction of magnetic resonance imaging (MRI) has emphasized the significant involvement of the cerebrum in MS patients. So sensitive is MRI to MS pathology that several studies have suggested that this imaging technique is the most useful laboratory measure in the initial diagnosis of MS when compared with CT scans, evoked potentials, and spinal fluid analysis (Gebarski et al., 1985; Kirshner et al., 1985). In addition, the shape, location, and distribution of lesions on MRI closely resemble those observed in MS patients at autopsy (see Chapter 3).

Despite the high degree of sensitivity of MRI, the procedure does have some limitations. First, like CT, it cannot resolve small demyelinating lesions because of limitations in current imaging technology. Second, the standard MRI procedures are incapable of differentiating the chronicity of MS lesions. Third, MRI does not appear to differentiate plaque from surrounding edema and inflammation. Finally, the high-intensity signals observed in the periventricular white matter on MRI may not be specific to MS. Several studies have observed such lesions, referred to as leuko-araiosis (thinning of the white matter; Hachinski, Potter, and Merskey, 1987) or unidentified bright objects, in otherwise healthy individuals (Bradley et al., 1984; George et al., 1986; Gerard and Weisberg, 1986; Naheedy et al., 1985; Zimmerman et al., 1986). While multiple etiologies may ultimately explain these lesions (Drayer, 1988; Kirkpatrick and Hayman, 1987), in a small percentage of cases leuko-araiosis may represent unsuspected MS (Gilbert and Sadler, 1983; MacKay and Hirano, 1967). The neuropsychological significance of leuko-araiosis is as yet unclear (Brant-Zawadzki et al., 1985; Rao et al., 1989b; Steingart et al., 1987).

Two recent studies (Franklin et al., 1988; Huber et al., 1987) have attempted to correlate MRI findings with neuropsychological testing in patients with MS. In the first, 60 patients with chronic-progressive MS underwent MRI scanning (unspecified scanner and magnet strength) with spin echo (SE) pulse sequences of $T_R = 2000$ ms and $T_E = 60–80$ ms. A neuroradiologist recorded the number, size (using a three-point scale), and location (left versus right hemisphere) of lesions. Weighted lesion scores were developed based on the number and size of lesions. These values were summed to obtain an overall brain lesion score and separate summary scores for the left and right hemispheres. The overall brain lesion summary score correlated significantly ($r = .35$) with a summary score derived from a brief (30–45 minute) cognitive screening battery. Franklin et al. were unable to find specific relationships between laterality lesion scores and component abilities measured by their test battery, noting that the cerebral lesions in their MS population appeared to be diffuse.

Huber et al. (1987) examined 30 definite MS patients with MRI (GE Signa system, 1.5-T magnet strength). Axial scans with a 5-mm slice thickness were obtained using two SE pulse sequences: proton density ($T_R = 2500$ ms and $T_E = 20–25$ ms) and relative $T_2$ ($T_R = 2500$ ms and $T_E = 75–100$ ms) weighted images; $T_1$-weighted partial saturation parameters ($T_R = 600$ ms and $T_E = 20$ ms) were used for obtaining images in the sagittal plane. The MRI scans were quantified by four methods: (1) a total score that reflected the sum of five-point ratings applied on the basis of the size of each lesion, (2) a five-point rating of cerebral atrophy, (3) a five-point rating of corpus callosum atrophy based on midsagittal images, and (4) a five-point rating of periventricular plaque severity.

All subjects were administered a brief (30-minute) battery of neurospychological tests, including the MMS and measures of language, memory, apraxia, visuospatial ability, and depression (Zung Self-Rated Depression Scale). On the basis of this testing protocol, 9 patients (28%) were classified as demented, 11 (34%) were moderately impaired, and 12 (38%) were minimally impaired. No significant group differences were observed on three of the four MRI indices: total lesion score, cerebral atrophy, and severity of periventricular involvement. On the corpus callosum atrophy ratings, "demented" patients had significantly higher ratings of atrophy than the moderate and minimal cognitive impairment groups. Huber et al. concluded that atrophy of the corpus callosum is a meaningful indicator of dementia in MS, whereas the number and size of lesions and the degree of generalized atrophy are of relatively little importance.

These two studies found significant correlations between MRI variables and cognitive testing, but the strength of the correlations was weak. Three methodological factors may have influenced their ability to find meaningful relationships. First, both studies relied on rating scales to measure the size of lesions from MRI scans. Rating scales, by definition, are subjective and prone to human error. In addition, rating scales provide a more restricted range of data values than quantitative systems that measure lesions in area units; this restricted range may seriously limit the size of obtained correlations. Second, both studies used brief cognitive screening examinations. It is well known that MS does not produce a uniform decline of all cognitive skills (Peyser and Poser, 1986; Rao, 1986); consequently, a brief examination may miss the salient cognitive deficiencies of MS patients. A more comprehensive neuropsychological examination may be more successful in measuring those cognitive functions that are influenced by MS-related cerebral pathology. Finally, cognitive test performance is affected by education and age (Prigatano and Parsons, 1976). Thus relatively uneducated or older patients may be classified as impaired on testing when they are functioning close to their premorbid level. Conversely, highly educated or younger patients may have experienced declines in cognitive performance that were undetected because their performance remained in the average range. Neither study attempted to control for these potential confounds either experimentally or statistically.

We recently completed a study of 53 patients with definite or probable MS (see Table 7–3 for patient characteristics) (Rao et al., 1989a). All patients underwent MRI using the identical scanner, magnet strength, slice thickness, and pulse sequences as in the Huber et al. (1987) study. Outlines of lesions and cerebral structures were traced on the MRI scanner computer console (see Figure 7–2); software routines were used to compute the area (in square centimeters) subtended by each tracing. The following cerebral structures were measured: size of the corpus callosum (SCC) from the midsagittal slice, the third and lateral ventricles from axial slices, and the entire area of the brain for each axial slice in which the third and/ or lateral ventricles could be visualized. Total lesion area (TLA) was computed by adding the measurements of lesion size. VBR was computed by dividing the sum of the ventricular measurements by the sum of the brain area measurements. All patients were administered a five-hour battery of neuropsychological tests (see Table 7–4) over the course of two days. The neuropsychological test battery consisted of measures of verbal intelligence, memory, abstract/conceptual reasoning,

**Table 7–3**   Clinical Characteristics of the MS Sample (N = 53)

| | | |
|---|---|---|
| Sex, males/females | 13/40 | |
| Age in years, mean | 43.9 | (range, 27–61) |
| Education in years, mean | 13.6 | (range, 8–20) |
| Occupation (6-pt. scale), mean | 4.1 | (range, 2–6) |
| Estimated premorbid IQ, mean[a] | 106.1 | (range, 89–118) |
| Length of symptoms in years, mean | 12.2 | (range, 1–33) |
| Years since diagnosis, mean | 7.8 | (range, 1–28) |
| Kurtzke EDSS, mean | 3.8 | (range, 0–8) |
| Diagnostic category: | | |
|    Clinically definite | 37 | (70%) |
|    Laboratory definite | 10 | (19%) |
|    Clinically probable | 6 | (11%) |
| Clinical course: | | |
|    Relapsing-remitting | 21 | (40%) |
|    Chronic-progressive | 10 | (19%) |
|    Chronic-stable | 21 | (39%) |
|    Benign | 1 | (2%) |
| MMS (max. = 30), mean | 28.8 | (range, 12–30) |

[a]Estimated from demographic variables using regression formula derived from WAIS-R standardization sample (Barona, Reynolds, and Chastain, 1984).
(Reproduced with permission from Rao et al., 1989a.)

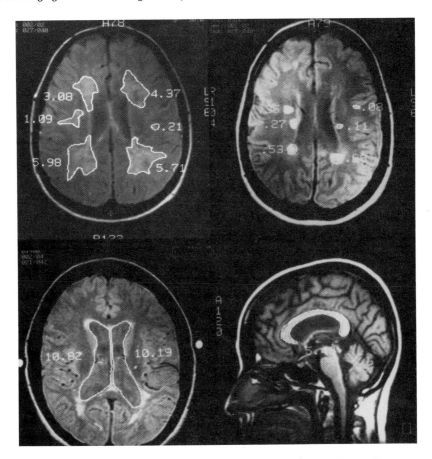

**Figure 7-2**   The two top scans illustrate the outlining and measurement of lesions (in square cen-timeters) for two patients. Note that while the number of lesions is the same for both patients (six), a sizable difference exists in the TLA (20.4 vs. 2.0 cm²). The lower left scan demonstrates the outlining and measurement of the lateral ventricular spaces (used to compute VBRs), while the lower right scan shows the measurement of the corpus callosum from the midsagittal scan. (Repro-duced with permission from Rao et al., 1989a.)

attention/concentration, language, and visuospatial skills. MRI was obtained at the end of the second examination day.

SCC was obtained for 45 of 53 patients in which precise midline saggital cuts were obtained. The mean TLA was 21.7 cm² (range: 0–95), SCC was 4.49 cm² (range: 1.01–7.08), and VBR was 0.044 (range: 0.006–0.133). TLA correlated positively with VBR (.61), while SCC correlated negatively with VBR (−.48) and TLA (−.46). Age correlated with VBR (.61), but did not correlate significantly with TLA or SCC.

Table 7–4 presents the results of stepwise multiple regression analyses for each of the cognitive variables; age and education were forced into the regression equation on the first step to minimize the effects of premorbid ability level on cognitive test performance. Only those MRI variables making a significant ($p < .05$) contribution to the prediction of cognitive test performance were listed. Of 34 cognitive

**Table 7–4**   Results of Stepwise Multiple Regression Analyses

| Cognitive Test | MRI Variable | Partial |
|---|---|---|
| *Verbal intelligence* | | |
| WAIS-R verbal IQ | SCC | .37 |
| Information | — | |
| Vocabulary | TLA | −.31 |
| Comprehension | SCC | .38 |
| Similarities | — | |
| Arithmetic | SCC | .39 |
| *Memory* | | |
| Selective Reminding Test: | | |
| Long-term storage | TLA | −.40 |
| Consistent long-term retrieval | TLA | −.38 |
| 7/24 Spatial Recall Test: | | |
| Total recall | TLA | −.31 |
| Delayed recall | TLA | −.35 |
| Story Recall Test: | | |
| Immediate recall | TLA | −.41 |
| 1-hour delayed recall | TLA | −.43 |
| 24-hour delayed recall | TLA | −.48 |
| President's Test: | | |
| Total score | — | |
| Brown-Peterson Interference Test: | | |
| 0–18 sec. delay | — | |
| *Abstract/conceptual reasoning:* | | |
| Wisconsin Card Sorting Test: | | |
| Categories completed | TLA | −.49 |
| Perseverative errors | TLA | .44 |
| Booklet Category Test: | | |
| Total errors | SCC | −.48 |
| | TLA | .34 |
| Raven Progressive Matrices: | | |
| Number correct | TLA | −.54 |
| Stroop Interference Test: | | |
| Color/word—word condition (sec) | TLA | .38 |
| *Attention/concentration* | | |
| Digit span: | | |
| Forward | — | |
| Backward | — | |
| Reaction Time: | | |
| Complex—simple RT (msec) | — | |
| Sternberg High Speed Scanning Test: | | |
| Scan rate (msec per digit) | SCC | −.48 |
| Y-intercept (msec) | — | |
| Paced Auditory Serial Addition Test: | | |
| Percent correct—easy | — | |
| Percent correct—hard | SCC | .40 |
| *Language* | | |
| Abbreviated Boston Naming Test: | | |
| Total correct | TLA | −.35 |
| Controlled Oral Word Association Test: | | |
| Total words generated | SCC | .39 |

**Table 7–4**  Results of Stepwise Multiple Regression Analyses

| Cognitive Test | MRI Variable | Partial |
|---|---|---|
| Category Word Generation: | | |
|   Total words generated | TLA | −.38 |
| *Visuospatial skills* | | |
| Hooper Visual Organization Test: | | |
|   T-Score | TLA | .49 |
| Judgment of Line Orientation Test: | | |
|   Number correct | SCC | .47 |
| Facial Recognition Test: | | |
|   Number correct | TLA | −.34 |
| Visual Form Discrimination Test: | | |
|   Number correct | TLA | −.35 |

Note: Partial, significant ($p < .05$) partial correlations between cognitive and MRI variables correcting for age, education, and previously entered MR variables;—, no MRI variable significantly predicted cognitive variable.

(Reproduced with permission from Rao et al., 1989a.)

variables assessed in this study, 25 (74%) were significantly ($p < .05$) predicted by at least one MRI variable. Of these 25 cognitive variables, 18 were predicted by TLA and 8 were predicted by SCC; one cognitive test, the Booklet Category Test, was predicted by two MRI variables, SCC and TLA. VBR, as predicted in the CT section of this chapter, did not *independently* predict any of the cognitive variables.

The partial correlation coefficients (labeled Partial in Table 7–4) represent the magnitude of the relationship between the cognitive and MRI variables after the effects of age and education are statistically removed. The sign of the coefficient indicates whether the relationship was positive or negative. The partial correlations ranged from −.31 (Vocabulary subtest of the WAIS-R with TLA) to −.54 (Raven Progressive Matrices and TLA).

TLA was the best predictor of performance on measures of recent memory and abstract/conceptual reasoning, skills that are most often impaired in MS patients (Peyser and Poser, 1986; Rao, 1986). Various tests of linguistic processes and visuo-spatial problem-solving skills were also predicted by both TLA and SCC. These skills are not systematically assessed in controlled neuropsychological studies of MS patients. These findings suggest that cerebral demyelination may affect a wider range of cognitive functions than had previously been suspected.

SCC was the best predictor of information-processing speed (scan rate on the Sternberg test), sustained and rapid problem solving (hard form of the Paced Auditory Serial Addition Test), and mental arithmetic (Arithmetic subtest of the WAIS-R). This finding suggests the possibility that intact performance on such tasks depends on precisely timed interhemispheric communication, which may be disrupted by demyelinated callosal fiber tracts.

MRI variables did not predict cognitive performance on measures of general (remote) information (Information subtest of the WAIS-R), verbal abstraction skills (Similarities subtest), immediate memory (Brown-Peterson test), remote memory (President's test), sustained and slow problem solving (easy form of the

**Table 7–5**   Results of Cluster Analysis

| Variable | Intact ($N = 34$) | Impaired ($N = 19$) |
|---|---|---|
| Sex, males/females | 10/24 | 3/16 |
| Age in years, mean (s.d.) | 43.7 (7.7) | 44.2 (10.0) |
| Education in years | 13.9 (2.3) | 13.0 (2.4) |
| Occupation (6-pt. scale) | 4.3 (1.3) | 3.8 (1.7) |
| Estimated premorbid verbal IQ | 107.8 (5.8) | 104.7 (8.4) |
| Tested verbal IQ | 105.6 (11.6) | 91.8 (11.5)[a] |
| MMS | 29.5 (0.9) | 27.6 (4.2)[b] |
| Currently employed, number (%) | 15 (44%) | 3 (16%)[b] |
| Length of symptoms, years | 12.0 (7.8) | 12.6 (7.1) |
| Years since diagnosis | 7.6 (7.1) | 8.1 (5.8) |
| Kurtzke Expanded DDS | 3.4 (2.2) | 4.6 (1.9) |
| Diagnostic category | | |
|   Clinically definite | 25 | 12 |
|   Laboratory definite | 5 | 5 |
|   Clinically probable | 4 | 2 |
| Clinical course | | |
|   Relapsing-remitting | 16 | 5 |
|   Chronic-progressive | 6 | 4 |
|   Chronic-stable | 11 | 10 |
|   Benign | 1 | 0 |
| MR variables | | |
|   TLA | 12.2 (13.4) | 38.5 (29.2)[a] |
|   VBR | 0.037 (0.020) | 0.057 (0.033)[c] |
|   SCC[d] | 4.9 (1.0) | 3.6 (1.3)[c] |

[a]$p < .001$.
[b]$p < .05$.
[c]$p < .01$.
[d]Intact: $N = 30$; Impaired: $N = 15$.
(Reproduced with permission from Rao et al., 1989a.)

Paced Auditory Serial Addition Test), and speed of fine upper extremity motor response (Reaction Time, $Y$-intercept on the Sternberg test). Overlearned verbal skills, short-term memory, and remote memory functions are relatively well preserved in patients with MS (Rao, 1986; Rao et al., in press), while fine motor speed can be influenced by extra-cerebral lesions (Rao et al., 1989).

The data were also analyzed to examine differences between patients with and without cognitive dysfunction on MRI and demographic variables. Table 7–5 presents the results of a two-group solution to a cluster analysis performed on 10 representative cognitive measures. The cluster analysis was based on the residual scores derived from regression equations, in which each cognitive variable was regressed with age and education. This was done to eliminate premorbid differences in cognitive ability statistically. Nineteen patients (36%) performed below expectations on neuropsychological testing (impaired group; mean cluster center = −.691), while thirty-four patients (64%) performed at or slightly above expectations (intact group; mean cluster center = +.358).

As expected, no significant group differences were observed on demographic variables and on an estimate of *premorbid* verbal IQ derived from demographic variables (Barona et al., 1984). In contrast, a highly significant group difference was observed on *current* WAIS-R verbal IQ (t = 4.13, *d.f.* = 51, *p* < .0001). The two groups also differed on the MMS (*t* = 2.55, *d.f.* = 51, *p* < .02), although the mean values for both groups were in the nondemented range (Folstein, Folstein, and McHugh, 1975). While the two groups did not differ in duration of symptoms, disease course, or overall physical disability [Kurtzke Expanded Disability Status Score (EDSS)], patients in the cognitively impaired group were less likely to be employed than patients in the cognitively intact group (16% versus 44%, respectively; $\chi^2$ = 4.36, *d.f.* = 1, *p* < .04). This employment statistic could not be explained by other disease factors, such as physical disability, length of illness, or disease course. Thus the significance of identifying cognitive dysfunction is highlighted by the observation that MS patients with cognitive impairment are less likely to be employed than patients without cognitive impairment.

Means and standard deviations for the three MRI variables in the impaired and unimpaired groups are also listed in Table 7–5. The impaired group had significantly greater TLA (*p* < .001) and VBR (*p* < .01) and a smaller SCC (*p* < .01) than the intact group. MRI values for individual subjects in each group are presented in Figure 7–3. Of the three MRI variables, TLA has the least amount of group overlap. Ten of twelve (83%) patients with a TLA greater than 30 $cm^2$ were cognitively impaired, while nine of forty-one (22%) patients with TLA less than 30 $cm^2$ were impaired. Thus results of the cluster analysis suggest that if the total lesion area exceeds a critical value (using our quantitation method, 30 $cm^2$), there is a high probability that the patient will have cognitive impairment.

Finally, a study by Honer et al. (1987) requires brief mention. These investigators compared the MRIs of eight MS patients having severe psychiatric disturbance with eight demographically matched MS patients without history of psychiatric illness. TLA and VBR were similar for both groups; however, the psychiatric group had significantly more temporal lobe involvement than the control group.

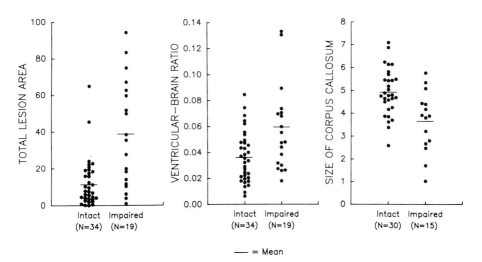

**Figure 7–3**  TLA, VBR, and SCC for cognitively intact and impaired MS patients. (Reproduced with permission from Rao et al., 1989a.)

To conclude, MRI is a more precise indicator of cognitive dysfunction in MS than CT. While virtually all definite MS patients have abnormal MRI, the overall amount of brain involvement varies considerably among patients. The correlational studies suggest that the overall lesion load is proportional to the amount of cognitive dysfunction. In addition, our finding that atrophy of the corpus callosum is correlated with sustained attentional deficits and Honer et al.'s finding that temporal lobe lesions are associated with psychiatric disturbance suggest the possibility that relatively focal MS lesions may have impact on specific neurobehavioral functions.

## POSITRON EMISSION TOMOGRAPHY

Three studies have examined the possible relationship between degree of cognitive dysfunction and altered cerebral physiology as imaged by positron emission tomography (PET) (Brooks et al., 1984; Herscovitch et al., 1984; Sheremata et al., 1984). Brooks et al. (1984) measured regional cerebral oxygen utilization, oxygen extraction, blood flow, and blood volume in 15 MS patients in remission. Patients were administered intelligence and reading tests; 13 patients also underwent CT scanning. Compared with a normal control group ($N = 13$), cerebral oxygen utilization and blood flow were found to be reduced in both the white and peripheral gray matter of the MS patients. This effect was most dramatic in those patients with ventricular dilatation on CT scan and in patients with a significant drop in intelligence relative to a premorbid prediction of cognitive ability (i.e., based on reading test scores). They concluded that reduced blood flow in MS is diffuse and caused by a loss of cerebral brain tissue rather than cerebral ischemia.

Sheremata et al. (1984) tested the hypothesis that MS patients were more likely to experience hypometabolism in the frontal lobes on PET imaging. They based their hypothesis on previous neuropsychological studies that have demonstrated a high rate of failure of MS patients on "frontal lobe" cognitive tests (e.g., Wisconsin Card Sorting Test, Verbal Fluency, Category Test). Scanning was performed on three MS patients and three normal controls while they performed a word-learning task. Mean metabolic rates were lower in the frontal lobes of the MS patients than in the controls, but the group difference was even larger for the temporal lobes. Metabolic rates for the parietal and occipital lobes were not presented. Sheremata et al. concluded that although their original hypothesis was not supported, the overall findings indicated generalized cortical hypometabolism in MS, possibly due to deafferentation.

We would also note that the larger difference in temporal than frontal lobe metabolic rate in the Sheremata et al. study may have resulted from the activation task administered during PET scanning. Their learning task would be predicted to engage activity of the temporal lobes in light of the role of the hippocampus in memory consolidation (Squire, 1986). Hypometabolism of the temporal lobes, therefore, might not be surprising, given the high incidence of memory impairment in patients with MS (Peyser and Poser, 1986; Rao, 1986).

Finally, Herscovitch et al. (1984) used PET to study myelin distribution and regional cerebral blood flow in a 24-year-old clinically definite MS patient, who developed a left hemiparesis and hemisensory deficit during an acute exacerbation. CT demonstrated a hypodense lesion of the right central white matter, which was supported by a diminished radiotracer accumulation in the same region on the myelin image. Regional cerebral blood flow was noted to be decreased in the right frontoparietal cortex superficial to the white matter lesion. A subsequent PET scan noted improvement in cortical blood flow corresponding with resolution of the patient's left-sided deficits. They hypothesized that the reductions in regional cortical blood flow were associated with conduction block in white matter pathways. It should be noted that the patient described by Herscovitch et al. may not be representative of other cognitively impaired MS patients, in that focal cortical symptoms (i.e., aphasia, apraxia, lateralized sensorimotor deficits due to cerebral lesions) are relatively rare in MS (Rao, 1986) and likely occur only in association with large, acute lesions extending into gray matter structures.

Overall, PET scan studies have conveyed a single, important message: cerebral hypometabolism may extend well beyond the white matter lesions visualized on structural brain imaging (CT, MRI). This may be particularly true for acute lesions. Consequently, researchers attempting to relate specific cognitive functions to subcortical brain sites may also need to consider the neurobehavioral effects of white matter lesions on distant cortical structures.


## CONCLUSIONS AND CONSIDERATIONS FOR FUTURE RESEARCH

The studies described in this chapter suggest that brain imaging can shed light on the anatomic abnormalities associated with cognitive dysfunction in MS. No longer can it be said that cerebral lesions in MS are clinically "silent." Furthermore, these studies lay to rest arguments that poor cognitive test performance in MS patients is attributed to extraneous factors, such as depression, anxiety, psychoactive medication usage, or fatigue.

The identification of MS patients with cognitive dysfunction is important, since evidence is accumulating that such impairment may have as devastating an impact on the psychosocial and vocational adjustment of patients as physical disability (Lincoln, 1981; Rao et al., 1989a). While MRI has become the diagnostic procedure of choice for forming the diagnosis of MS, studies reviewed in this chapter suggest that severity of lesions on MRI can be used to generate hypotheses about possible cognitive dysfunction in a given patient. Such information, coupled with anamnestic information from the patient and family members, could be used in determining whether a patient should receive a comprehensive neuropsychological evaluation. In contrast, the degree of physical disability, at least as measured by the Kurtzke scale, is a poor indicator of cognitive disturbance (Heaton et al., 1985; Lyon-Caen et al., 1986; Marsh, 1980; Peyser et al., 1980; Rao et al., 1984; van den Burg et al., 1987), despite the widely held belief that cognitive dysfunction occurs only in severely disabled patients (McKhann, 1982).

Continuing advances in imaging techniques should greatly enhance our ability to make clinicopathological correlations. Early work with contrast agents in MRI (i.e., gadolinium) (Gonzalez-Scarano et al., 1987; Grossman et al., 1986) suggests the possibility that acute lesions can be discriminated from chronic. Neuropsychological studies of diverse brain-damaged patient groups have shown differing patterns of cognitive deficits as a function of lesion chronicity (Fitzhugh, Fitzhugh and Reitan, 1962). Chronicity may also influence patterns of cognitive impairment in MS.

Recent work by Paty and colleagues (see Chapter 3), in which patients underwent MRI on a once or twice per month basis for 6 months, suggests that MS lesions are anything but static. Lesions appear and expand over a 4–6-week period, followed by a reduction in size and almost complete disappearance over a 6–10-week period. A given MRI scan may contain lesions that are in different stages of development. Paty has noted that most of these new cerebral lesions are asymptomatic, at least with regard to the neurologic examination. Prospective neuropsychological studies using repeatable batteries administered on a once per month basis may address the question of the significance of changing lesion patterns.

As shown in our reviews of the CT and MRI literature, the method used to quantify lesions can make a difference in the ability to predict cognitive performance. Studies that relied on subjective rating scales generally obtained weaker correlations with cognitive testing than those studies that used computer software to measure lesion size. In addition, subjective ratings are incapable of recording changes in lesion size and location over time (see Chapter 3). Recording the number of lesions should be also avoided, since patients with equivalent numbers of lesions may have significantly different brain lesion lodes (see Figure 7–2).

The studies reviewed in this chapter did not find on brain imaging a relationship between length of illness and severity of lesion involvement. This finding is counterintuitive, since it is assumed that cognitive functions deteriorate as the disease advances. In a disease that produces considerable interpatient variability in symptom presentation, cognitive deterioration may be masked by cross-sectional research designs. Cognitive functions may slowly deteriorate in some MS patients, while in others there is relative stability between exacerbations. Prospective longitudinal research is needed, therefore, to examine the natural history of cognitive dysfunction in MS, with brain-imaging tools serving as the marker of cerebral disease progression.


## ACKNOWLEDGMENTS

The author gratefully acknowledges the invaluable assistance of Gary J. Leo, D. O., Sander Glatt, M. D., Victor Haughton, M. D., Linda Bernardin, and Patricia St. Aubin-Faubert. Support is also acknowledged from a Research Career Development Award (K04 NS01055) and a Research Grant (R01 NS22128) from NINDS. The assistance of the Multiple Sclerosis Society of Milwaukee is gratefully appreciated.


## REFERENCES

Adams, C.W.M. (1977). Pathology of multiple sclerosis: Progression of the lesion. *Br. Med. Bull.*, **33**, 15–19.

Barona, A., Reynolds, C.R., and Chastain, R. (1984). A demographically based index of premorbid intelligence for the WAIS-R. *J. Consult. Clin. Psychol., 52,* 885–87.

Bradley, W.G., Waluch, V., Brant-Zawadzki, M., Yadley, R.A., and Wycoff, R.R. (1984). Patchy, periventricular white matter lesions in the elderly: A common observation during NMR imaging. *Noninvasive Med. Imaging,* **1,** 35–41.

Brant-Zawadzki, M., Fein, G., Van Dyke, C., Kiernan, R., Davenport, L., and de Groot, J. (1985). MR imaging of the aging brain: Patchy white-matter lesions and dementia. *AJNR,* **6,** 675–82.

Brooks, D.J., Leenders, K.L., Head, G., Marshall, J., Legg, N.J., and Jones, T. (1984). Studies on regional cerebral oxygen utilization and cognitive function in multiple sclerosis. *J. Neurol. Neurosurg. Psychiat.* **47,** 1182–91.

Brownell, B., and Hughes, J.F. (1962). The distribution of plaques in the cerebrum in multiple sclerosis. *J. Neurol. Neurosurg. Psychiat.* **25,** 315–20.

Cala, L.A., Mastaglia, F.L., and Black, J.L. (1978). Comptuerized tomography of brain and optic nerve in multiple sclerosis: Observations in 100 patients, including serial studies in 16. *J. Neurol. Sci.,* **36,** 411–26.

de Weerd, A.W. (1979). Computerized tomography in multiple sclerosis. *Clin. Neurol. Neurosurg.,* **80,** 258–63.

Drayer, B.P. (1988). Imaging of the aging brain. Part I. Normal findings. *Radiology,* **166,** 785–96.

Fitzhugh, K.B., Fitzhugh, L.C., and Reitan, R.M. (1962). Wechsler-Bellevue comparisons in groups with "chronic" and "current" lateralized and diffuse brain lesions. *J. Consult. Psychol.,* **26,** 306–10.

Folstein, M.F., Folstein, S.E., and McHugh, P.R. (1975). Mini-Mental State: A practical method for grading the cognitive state of patients for the clinician. *J. Psychiat. Res.* **12,** 189–98.

Franklin, G.M., Heaton, R.K., Nelson, L.M., Filley, C.M., and Seibert, C. (1988). Correlation of neuropsychology and MRI findings in chronic/progressive multiple sclerosis. *Neurology,* **38,** 1826–29.

Gebarski, S.S., Gabrielsen, T.O., Gilman, S., Knake, J.E., Latack, J.T., and Aisen, A.M. (1985). The initial diagnosis of multiple sclerosis: Clinical impact of magnetic resonance imaging. *Ann. Neurol.,* **17,** 469–74.

George, A.E., de Leon, M.J., Kalnin, A., Rosner, L., Goodgold, A., and Chase, N. (1986). Leukoencephalopathy in normal and pathologic aging: 2. MRI of brain lucencies. *AJNR,* **7,** 567–70.

Gerard, G., and Weisberg, L.A. (1986). MRI periventricular lesions in adults. *Neurology,* **36,** 998–1001.

Gilbert, J.J., and Sadler, M. (1983). Unsuspected multiple sclerosis. *Arch. Neurol.,* **40,** 533–36.

Gonzalez-Scarano, F., Grossman, R.I., Galetta, S., Atlas, S.W., and Silberberg, D.H. (1987). Multiple sclerosis disease activity correlates with gadolinium-enhanced magnetic resonance imaging. *Ann. Neurol.,* **21,** 300–6.

Grossman, R.I., Gonzalez-Scarano, F., Atlas, S.W., Galetta, S., and Silberberg, D.H. (1986). Multiple sclerosis: Gadolinium enhancement in MR imaging. *Radiology,* **161,** 721–25.

Gyldensted, C. (1976). Computer tomography of the cerebrum in multiple sclerosis. *Neuroradiology,* **12,** 33–42.

Hachinski, V.C., Potter, P., and Merskey, H. (1987). Leuko-araiosis. *Arch. Neurol.,* **44,** 21–3.

Haughton, V.M., Ho, K.-C., Williams, A.L., and Eldevik, P. (1979). CT detection of demyelinated plaques in multiple sclerosis. *Am. J. Roentgen.,* **132,** 213–15.

Heaton, R.K., Nelson, L.M., Thompson, D.S., Burks, J.S., and Franklin, G.M. (1985). Neuropsychological findings in relapsing-remitting and chronic-progressive multiple sclerosis. *J. Consult. Clin. Psychol.,* **53,** 103–10.

Herscovitch, P., Trotter, J.L., Lemann, W., and Raichle, M.E. (1984). Positron emission tomography (PET) in active MS: Demonstration of demyelination and diaschisis. *Neurology,* **34(Suppl. 1),** 78.

Hershey, L.A., Gado, M.H., and Trotter, J.L. (1979). Computerized tomography in the diagnostic evaluation of multiple sclerosis. *Ann. Neurol.,* **5,** 32–9.

Honer, W.G., Hurwitz, T., Li, D.K.B., Palmer, M., and Paty, D.W. (1987). Temporal lobe involvement in multiple sclerosis patients with psychiatric disorders. *Arch. Neurol.,* **44,** 187–90.

Huber, S.J., Paulson, G.W., Shuttleworth, E.C., Chakeres, D., Clapp, L.E., Pakalnis, A., Weiss, K., and Rammohan, K. (1987). Magnetic resonance imaging correlates of dementia in multiple sclerosis. *Arch. Neurol.,* **44,** 732–36.

Huckman, M.S., Fox, J.H., and Topel, J. (1975). The validity of criteria for the evaluation of cerebral atrophy by computed tomography. *Radiology,* **116,** 85–92.

Jackson, J.A., Leake, D.R., Schneiders, N.J., Rolak, L.A., Kelley, G.R., Ford, J.J., Appel, S.H., and Bryan, R.N. (1985). Magnetic resonance imaging in multiple sclerosis: Results in 32 cases. *AJNR,* **6,** 171–76.

Jacobs, L., and Kinkel, W.R. (1976). Computerized axial tomography in multiple sclerosis. *Neurology,* **26,** 390–91.

Jacobs, L., Kinkel, W.R., Polachini, I., and Kindel, R.P. (1986). Correlations of nuclear magnetic resonance imaging, computerized tomography, and clinical profiles in multiple sclerosis. *Neurology,* **36,** 27–34.

Kirkpatrick, J.B., and Hayman, L.A. (1987). White-matter lesions in MR imaging of clinically healthy brains of elderly subjects: Possible pathologic basis. *Radiology,* **162,** 509–11.

Kirshner, H.S., Tsai, S.I., Runge, V.M., and Price, A.C. (1985). Magnetic resonance imaging and other techniques in the diagnosis of multiple sclerosis. *Arch. Neurol.,* **42,** 859–63.

Lincoln, N.B. (1981). Discrepancies between capabilities and performance of activities of daily living in multiple sclerosis patients. *Int. Rehabil. Med.,* **3,** 84–8.

Lukes, S.A., Crooks, L.E., Aminoff, M.J., Kaufman, L., Panitch, H.S., Mills, C., and Norman, D. (1983). Nuclear magnetic resonance imaging in multiple sclerosis. *Ann. Neurol.,* **13,** 592–601.

Lyon-Caen, O., Jouvent, R., Hauser, S., Chaunu, M.-P., Benoit, N., Widlocher, D., and Lhermitte, F. (1986). Cognitive function in recent-onset demyelinating diseases. *Arch. Neurol.,* **43,** 1138–41.

MacKay, R.P., and Hirano, A. (1967). Forms of benign multiple sclerosis: Report of two "clinically silent" cases discovered at autopsy. *Arch. Neurol.,* **17,** 588–600.

Marsh, G. (1980). Disability and intellectual function in multiple sclerosis. *J. Nerv. Ment. Dis.,* **168,** 758–62.

McKhann, G.M. (1982). Multiple sclerosis. *Ann. Rev. Neurosci.,* **5,** 219–39.

Naheedy, M.H., Gupta, S.R., Young, J.C., Ghobrial, M., Rubino, F.A., Ross, E.R., and Hindo, W. (1985). Periventricular white matter changes and subcortical dementia: Clinical, neuropsychological, radiological and pathological correlation. *AJNR,* **6,** 468.

Peyser, J.M., Edwards, K.R., Poser, C.M., and Filskov, S.B. (1980). Cognitive function in patients with multiple sclerosis. *Arch. Neurol.,* **37,** 577–79.

Peyser, J.M., and Poser, C.M. (1986). Neuropsychological correlates of multiple sclerosis. In S.B. Filskov, and T.J. Boll, eds., *Handbook of Clinical Neuropsychology, vol. 2,* pp. 364–97. New York: Wiley.

Powell, H.C., and Lampert, P.W. (1983). Pathology of multiple sclerosis. *Neurologic Clinics,* **1,** 631–44.

Prigatano, G.P., and Parsons, O.A. (1976). Relationship of age and education to Halstead Test performance in different patient populations. *J. Consult. Clin. Psychol.,* **44,** 527–33.

Rabins, P.V., Brooks, B.R., O'Donnell, P., Pearlson, G.D., Moberg, P., Jubelt, B., Coyle, P., Dalos, N., and Folstein, M.F. (1986). Structural brain correlates of emotional disorder in multiple sclerosis. *Brain,* **109,** 585–97.

Radue, E.W., and Kendall, B.E. (1978). Iodide and xenon enhancement of computed tomography (CT) in multiple sclerosis (MS). *Neuroradiology,* **15,** 153–58.

Rao, S.M., Glatt, S., Hammeke, T.A., McQuillen, M.P., Khatri, B.O., Rhodes, A.M., and Pollard, S. (1985). Chronic progressive multiple sclerosis: Relationship between cerebral ventricular size and neuropsychological impairment. *Arch. Neurol.,* **42,** 678–82.

Rao, S.M., Hammeke, T.A., McQuillen, M.P., Khatri, B.O., and Lloyd, D. (1984). Memory disturbance in chronic progressive multiple sclerosis. *Arch. Neurol.,* **41,** 625–31.

Rao, S.M. (1986). Neurospychology of multiple sclerosis: A critical review. *J. Clin. Exp. Neuropsychol.,* **8,** 503–42.

Rao, S.M., Leo, G.J., Haughton, V.M., St. Aubin-Faubert, P., and Bernardin, L. (1989a). Correlation of magnetic resonance imaging with neuropsychological testing in multiple sclerosis. *Neurology,* **39,** 161–66.

Rao, S.M., Leo, G.J., and St. Aubin-Faubert, P. (in press). On the nature of memory disturbance in multiple sclerosis. *J. Clin. Exp. Neuropsychol.*

Rao, S.M., Mittenberg, W., Bernardin, L., Haughton, V., and Leo, G.J. (1989b). Neuropsychological test findings in subjects with leukoaraiosis. *Arch. Neurol.,* **46,** 40–4.

Rao, S.M., St. Aubin-Faubert, P., and Leo, G.J. (1989). Information processing speed in patients with multiple sclerosis. *J. Clin. Exp. Neuropsychol.,* **11,** 471–77.

Reese, L., Carr, T.J., Nicholson, R.L., and Lepp, E.K. (1986). Magnetic resonance imaging for detecting lesions of multiple sclerosis: Comparison with computed tomography and clinical assessment. *Can. Med. Assoc. J.,* **135,** 639–43.

Reisner, T., and Maida, E. (1980). Computerized tomography in multiple sclerosis. *Arch. Neurol.,* **37,** 475–77.

Sheremata, W.A., Sevush, S., Knight, D., and Ziajka, P. (1984). Altered cerebral metabolism in MS. *Neurology,* **34 (Suppl. 1),** 118.

Squire, L.R. (1986). Mechanisms of memory. *Science,* **232,** 1612–19.

Steingart, A., Hachinski, V.C., Lau, C., Fox, A.J., Diaz, F., Cape, R., Lee, D., Inzitari, D., and Merskey, H. (1987). Cognitive and neurologic findings in subjects with diffuse white matter lucencies on computed tomographic scan (leuko-araiosis). *Arch. Neurol.,* **44,** 32–5.

van den Burg, W., van Zomeren, A.H., Minderhoud, J.M., Prange, A.J.A., and Meijer, N.S.A. (1987). Cognitive impairment in patients with multiple sclerosis and mild physical disability. *Arch. Neurol.,* **44,** 494–501.

Young, I.R., Hall, A.S., Pallis, C.A., Legg, N.J., Bydder, G.M., and Steiner, R.E. (1981). Nuclear magnetic resonance imaging of the brain in multiple sclerosis. *Lancet,* **2,** 1063–66.

Zimmerman, R.D., Fleming, C.A., Lee, B.C.P., Saint-Louis, L.A., and Deck, M.D.F. (1986). Periventricular hyperintensity as seen by magnetic resonance: Prevalence and significance. *AJR,* **146,** 433–50.

# 8

# Effects of Disease Course on Neuropsychological Functioning

CHRISTOPHER M. FILLEY, ROBERT K. HEATON,
LAETITIA L. THOMPSON, LORENE M. NELSON, AND
GARY M. FRANKLIN

Multiple sclerosis (MS) is a chronic disease of the central nervous system that typically begins in young adulthood. Because it usually afflicts patients for extended periods of time, knowledge of the natural history of the disease is of great importance. Although progress has been made in classifying the disease into various types that have prognostic significance, these classifications are founded primarily on motor, sensory, and other elemental neurologic criteria. In terms of cognitive functioning, the natural history of MS remains virtually unknown.

Prospective follow-up studies are difficult to conduct in any disease because of such factors as patient relocation, differing means of assessment, varying test-retest intervals, and cost. These problems are compounded further in MS, a disease that is often difficult to diagnose and frequently unpredictable in its course. Cognitive function in MS is still more elusive, as deficits may be apparent only on detailed neuropsychological examination (Heaton et al., 1985). Nevertheless, data on the longitudinal course of cognitive status are needed if the full impact of MS on an individual patient is to be appreciated.

In this chapter we report neuropsychological findings on 46 MS patients who had comprehensive testing at two different times in their disease course. These results provide some preliminary information on the natural history of cognitive disturbances in MS, but before describing these studies, we first review the literature pertaining to changes in cognitive function over time in MS.

## REVIEW OF THE LITERATURE

A steady accumulation of information over the past few decades has led to a growing appreciation of cognitive dysfunction in many MS patients (Peyser and Becker, 1984). Many investigators have demonstrated such dysfunction by comparing MS patients with normal controls or control groups of patients with other illnesses (Rao, 1986). Others have used a case study format to highlight cognitive dysfunction that can occur early in the disease course, even preceding other neurologic disturbances (Young et al., 1976). Such investigations point out the existence of cognitive dysfunction but leave unanswered the question of natural history.

A landmark study of the longitudinal course of cognitive function in MS was done by Canter (1951). Using the Army General Classification Test, he was able to obtain pre- and postmorbid data on 23 men who entered the military and then developed symptoms of MS; after four years, these patients showed a drop of 13.5 IQ points (Canter, 1951). In addition, he performed a longitudinal study of 47 MS patients and 38 normal controls over six months with the Wechsler-Bellevue Intelligence Scale; the MS group dropped a mean of 3.7 points on the verbal IQ and 7.8 points on the performance IQ, while the normals gained 4.1 and 7.8 points on the verbal and performance IQs, respectively. Although the patients in these studies appear to comprise a representative sample, details of diagnostic procedure were not provided, and the patients' clinical status at the time of retesting was unclear. Nevertheless, these data suggest that cognitive deterioration may be an early feature of MS and that it may occur in less than one year.

Other investigators have found conflicting data. Fink and Houser (1966) administered the Wechsler Adult Intelligence Scale (WAIS) verbal subtests to 44 MS patients on two occasions separated by one year. The mean verbal IQ rose from 106 to 110, suggesting the possibility that intellectual decline may not be common in MS (Fink and Houser, 1966). It should be noted, however, that verbal IQ is not a measure that is sensitive to cognitive impairment in MS (Heaton et al., 1985).

The clinical variability of cognitive status in MS has been demonstrated by Young et al. (1976), who found that one patient had a WAIS full scale IQ decline of 21 points over one year, whereas another had no neuropsychological change over eight years. More needs to be learned of the factors that can account for such variability.

Ivnik (1978a) presented data on neuropsychological impairment in MS as a function of duration of illness. Using an extensive neuropsychological battery, he found little difference between MS patients with disease durations of 0–5, 6–10, and greater than 10 years. No attempt was made to distinguish between clinical types of MS. These findings indicated that length of illness does not necessarily portend intellectual impairment.

In another study the same investigator (Ivnik, 1978b) concluded that increased neuropsychological impairment in MS patients who were tested after a three-year interval was more likely due to sensorimotor dysfunction than to cognitive disturbance. The control group in this study, which showed slight improvement over approximately the same time period, was made up of a diverse group of neurologic and neurosurgical patients (Ivnik, 1978b).

In summary, although the literature is somewhat contradictory, there is good evidence that mild intellectual deterioration is encountered in some MS patients, even early in the disease. It should be noted that these studies used different diagnostic criteria and widely varying neuropsychological techniques. Furthermore, none attempted to subdivide patients into categories with potentially meaningful implications. For example, Heaton et al. (1985) found a much higher prevalence of cognitive impairment in patients who had a chronic-progressive disease course as compared to those with a relapsing-remitting course. Given the great variability of cognitive status in MS, it is evident that some method of attempting to predict cognitive course is desirable.

## THE PRESENT STUDY

We prospectively followed a group of 46 MS patients for an average of 18.8 months and repeated a neuropsychological test battery to address two questions. First, over this test-retest interval, what was the prevalence of *worsening* neuropsychological deficits in patients who have a relapsing-remitting versus chronic-progressive disease course? Second, for relapsing-remitting MS patients, how pronounced an effect did a diagnosed exacerbation of neurologic symptoms have on results of comprehensive neuropsychological testing?

The patients were members of a consecutive series of 100 MS patients who had participated in a previous study (Heaton et al., 1985), and had been administered their baseline neuropsychological evaluations while clinically stable. A total of 46 patients were available for repeat testing. Of these, 36 had relapsing-remitting MS, defined as having a clinical course characterized by acute exacerbations that are separated in time by periods of relative disease stability (Heaton et al., 1985). Of these 36 cases, 18 were retested during a documented relapse, and the other 18 during a period of remission; in the exacerbating relapsing-remitting MS group, retesting always took place during the patient's first relapse after baseline testing, whereas in the stable relapsing-remitting MS group, no clinically detectable relapse had occurred between baseline and follow-up. The remaining 10 patients had chronic-progressive MS, defined as having a clinical course characterized by steady progression of neurologic defects without periods of significant remission (Heaton et al., 1985).

Mean test-retest intervals for the three groups were as follow: 23 months (range 8–38) for the stable relapsing-remitting MS group, 15 months (range 7–33) for the exacerbating relapsing-remitting MS group, and 18 months (range 17–19) for the chronic-progressive MS group. Analysis of variance (ANOVA) revealed a significant difference in test-retest interval among the groups ($F(2, 43) = 8.06, p < .01$). Post hoc analysis using Scheffe's procedure showed that the test-retest interval for the stable relapsing-remitting MS group was significantly longer than for the exacerbating relapsing-remitting MS group ($p < .01$). Conceivably, this longer test-retest interval for the stable relapsing-remitting MS group would slightly lessen their "practice effect" on some tests, making it more difficult to demonstrate any neuropsychological advantage for them over the exacerbating relapsing-remitting MS group.

All patients had clinically definite MS according to the diagnostic criteria proposed by Schumacher et al. (1965). Other details of patient selection may be found in Heaton et al. (1985). An MS exacerbation was defined as the development of any new neurologic sign(s) and/or symptom(s) or significant worsening of existing symptoms lasting at least 24 hours (Schumacher et al., 1965). The examining neurologist was careful to exclude transient fluctuations in neurologic status that could be related to other factors such as a viral illness.

The stable relapsing-remitting MS group had 16 women (89%), a mean age of 38 years, and a mean of 13.7 years of education. The exacerbating relapsing-remitting MS group also had 16 women (89%), with a mean age of 32 years and mean educational level of 13.4 years. The chronic-progressive MS group had 6 women (60%), a mean age of 42, and a mean of 12.9 years of education. No group differences were found for sex or education, but there was an age difference ($F(2, 43) = 6.56$, $p < .01$), with the chronic-progressive MS group significantly older than the exacerbating relapsing-remitting MS group.

Patients were administered an expanded Halstead-Reitan Battery (HRB), as described in Heaton et al. (1985). As in the previous study, test measures were grouped according to whether they reflect cognitive functioning (Table 8–1), cognitive plus sensorimotor functioning (Table 8–2), or only sensorimotor functioning (Table 8–3). Summary measures from the WAIS and HRB were considered separately (Table 8–4), because they cut across these categories.

The primary method of analyzing the neuropsychological data in this study relied on "blind" clinical ratings, described below. Previous research has demonstrated the reliability and validity of this approach, both for neurodiagnostic purposes and for detecting relatively subtle changes in patients' functioning (Heaton et al., 1981; Grant et al., 1982; Heaton et al., 1983). In the present study the clinical rating approach had two major advantages. The first was that it provided for considerable data reduction. This was desirable because of the large number of variables in the expanded HRB, which raised concerns about error rate in the experiment. In addition, however, there was a more important reason for our focusing on clinical ratings of the neuropsychological data: in detecting "spotty" changes in neuropsychological functioning, the clinician potentially has a considerable advantage over univariate or multivariate comparisons of group data. This is because MS can cause discrete changes in abilities that differ from patient to patient, reflecting differences in discrete loci of central nervous system (CNS) involvement. If the abilities affected are inconsistent across patients within a group, the changes will be poorly reflected by group mean scores; that is, on any given test measure, the good scores of the patients who do not have that ability affected (or changed from baseline) tend to "wash out" or overshadow the poor scores of the (possibly very few) individuals who are impaired on that measure. On the other hand, the clinician analyzes the test data of individuals, rather than groups, and can therefore give full weight to a major change in any of a number of abilities being considered.

Clinical ratings of the degree of change between evaluations were carried out using direct comparison of the two data sets for each patient. These ratings were conducted by two experienced neuropsychologists who were blinded to the patient's diagnostic group, and a five-point scale was used to rate the change in performance: 1 = significantly improved, 2 = slightly improved, 3 = no change,

4 = slightly worse, 5 = significantly worse. Ratings were performed independently by the clinicians, and $\chi^2$ analyses comparing the two raters revealed highly significant associations among the four rating categories: cognitive rating, $\chi^2(9) = 37.68$, $p < .0001$; cognitive-sensorimotor rating, $\chi^2(9) = 23.25$, $p < .006$; sensorimotor rating, $\chi^2(9) = 66.55$, $p < .0001$. In a few cases in which disagreements were found, a consensus rating was reached for each patient in each category. In keeping with the organization of data in the previous study (Heaton et al., 1985), clinical ratings were generated for cognitive function, cognitive/sensorimotor function, sensorimotor function, and overall "global" performance. Tables 8–1 to 8–4 list the data that were used by the raters in judging the change, if any, seen in the respective areas of neuropsychological evaluation. $T1$ signifies the initial evaluation, and $T2$ the second testing. Asterisks indicate the occasional tests that one or two subjects were unable to complete.

Statistical analyses of the raw test data were performed using repeated measures ANOVAs to compare the three groups at $T1$ and $T2$. A multivariate analysis of variance was not performed because of the inadequate subject-to-variable ratio. When significant main effects or interaction effects were detected, post hoc analyses on difference scores ($T1 - T2$) for the three groups were performed using Scheffe's procedure.

The expectation, based on the findings of the Heaton et al. (1985) study, was that baseline group differences would tend to favor the relapsing-remitting MS groups over the chronic-progressive MS group. Significant main effects for test administration could go in either direction: improvement could occur on the basis of practice effects on the second administration, whereas worse performance on follow-up could reflect gradual deterioration in functioning (chronic-progressive MS group) or the effects of an acute MS exacerbation (exacerbating relapsing-remitting MS group). Finally, significant group by time interaction effects would indicate group differences in the amount of change over the test-retest interval. Preliminary expectations were that the chronic-progressive MS group and exacerbating relapsing-remitting MS group would be more likely to show deterioration in functioning at follow-up than would the stable relapsing-remitting MS group.

Clinical ratings were analyzed using the $\chi^2$ statistic. Although the full range of clinical ratings were considered, of greatest interest was whether the groups differed with respect to the proportion of patients who were classified as "worse" at the time of follow-up. Again, the expectation was that the stable relapsing-remitting MS group would show no significant change, whereas some deterioration would occur in the chronic-progressive MS group and in the exacerbating relapsing-remitting MS group.

Table 8–1 presents data for cognitive function and includes measures that involve only a minor sensorimotor component. ANOVAs revealed main effects for diagnostic group on only 3 of the 13 measures: Category Test errors [$F(2,43) = 3.21$, $p = .05$], Trails $B - A$ [$F(2,43) = 8.04$, $p = .001$], and Aphasia errors [$F(2,43) = 8.26$, $p = .001$]. For Trails $B - A$ and Aphasia errors, as expected, the chronic-progressive MS group performed more poorly than the two relapsing-remitting MS groups ($p < .01$). Post hoc comparisons of Category Test errors across the three groups revealed no significant difference. With regard to main effects for time, several were of interest: WAIS Comprehension [$F(1,42) = 8.81$, $p$

**Table 8-1** Cognitive Measures

| | Stable Relapsing-Remitting MS (*n* = 18) | | Exacerbating Relapsing-Remitting MS (*n* = 18) | | Chronic-Progressive MS (*n* = 10) | |
|---|---|---|---|---|---|---|
| | *T*1 | *T*2 | *T*1 | *T*2 | *T*1 | *T*2 |
| *WAIS* | | | | | | |
| Information[a] | 12.50 | 12.89 | 11.56 | 11.59* | 12.50 | 12.70 |
| | (1.69) | (1.32) | (2.23) | (2.40) | (3.47) | (3.33) |
| Comprehension[a] | 13.06 | 11.94 | 11.39 | 11.41* | 13.10 | 11.20 |
| | (1.89) | (1.86) | (1.65) | (2.18) | (4.07) | (2.30) |
| Arithmetic[a] | 11.17 | 12.28 | 10.61 | 11.41* | 10.90 | 11.20 |
| | (1.95) | (2.70) | (2.89) | (3.00) | (3.93) | (3.68) |
| Similarities[a] | 12.50 | 12.06 | 12.39 | 12.18* | 11.30 | 12.30 |
| | (1.10) | (.73) | (1.33) | (1.13) | (2.79) | (1.57) |
| Digit Span[a] | 11.72 | 11.28 | 11.17 | 10.76* | 10.90 | 10.00 |
| | (1.78) | (1.84) | (3.42) | (3.56) | (3.18) | (2.31) |
| Vocabulary[a] | 12.44 | 12.61 | 11.78 | 12.06* | 11.90 | 12.20 |
| | (1.69) | (1.58) | (2.76) | (2.14) | (2.73) | (2.53) |
| Category Test (errors)[b] | 33.50 | 27.50 | 36.17 | 29.00 | 58.20 | 44.80 |
| | (20.70) | (19.44) | (27.93) | (22.90) | (21.06) | (23.19) |
| Wisconsin Card Sorting Test (perseverative responses)[b] | 14.44 | 9.56 | 17.67 | 16.78 | 29.40 | 22.00 |
| | (15.50) | (9.48) | (12.32) | (15.99) | (28.58) | (22.01) |
| Trails B-A[b] | 29.67 | 31.00 | 36.67 | 31.41* | 57.90 | 70.70 |
| | (13.95) | (14.57) | (19.07) | (19.23) | (38.25) | (50.25) |
| Aphasia Screening Test Errors[b] | 2.00 | 4.17 | 3.61 | 3.56 | 7.10 | 10.10 |
| | (2.45) | (2.23) | (4.03) | (4.20) | (5.28) | (6.31) |
| Verbal Learning[b] | 1.56 | 1.78 | 1.72 | 1.67 | 1.70 | 1.90 |
| | (.62) | (.65) | (.83) | (1.03) | (.67) | (1.29) |
| Verbal Memory (% loss)[b] | 15.53 | 19.26 | 12.51 | 18.27 | 17.03 | 27.14 |
| | (12.60) | (21.08) | (9.65) | (12.51) | (9.88) | (17.51) |
| Figure Memory (% loss)[b] | 13.62* | 13.97 | 8.88 | 11.84 | 12.53 | 16.08 |
| | (12.44) | (15.33) | (12.66) | (14.00) | (12.28) | (9.15) |

All data in parentheses are standard deviations.
[a]higher score indicates better performance.
[b]higher score indicates worse performance.
**n* = 17

< .01], WAIS Digit Span [$F(1,42) = 4.33$, $p < .05$], Aphasia errors [$F(1,43) = 11.48$, $p < .01$], and Verbal Memory (% loss) [$F(1,43) = 6.63$, $p < .05$]. On each of these tests the overall trend was for performance to be poorer at the second testing. For three of the cognitive measures, the time main effect suggested that scores were better on the second testing: WAIS Arithmetic [$F(1,42) = 4.4$, $p < .05$], Category Test errors [$F(1,43) = 28.86$, $p < .001$], and Wisconsin Card Sorting [$F(1,43) = 6.19$, $p < .05$]. The latter two tests are known to be particularly susceptible to practice effects on repeated administrations.

The more interesting finding of an interaction between group and time was found for only two of the measures: WAIS Similarities [$F(2,42) = 3.89$, $p < .05$]

and Aphasia errors [$F$ (2,43) = 3.43, $p < .05$]. Post hoc analyses using Scheffe's procedure revealed that for Similarities, the chronic-progressive MS group was significantly different only from the stable relapsing-remitting MS group, in that the chronic-progressive MS group *improved* slightly between $T1$ and $T2$ while the stable relapsing-remitting MS group did not ($p < .05$). Post hoc comparisons of Aphasia errors revealed no significant differences among the groups. In sum, none of the

**Table 8-2**  Cognitive/Sensorimotor Measures

| | Stable Relapsing-Remitting MS ($n$ = 18) | | Exacerbating Relapsing-Remitting MS ($n$ = 18) | | Chronic Progressive MS ($n$ = 10) | |
|---|---|---|---|---|---|---|
| | $T1$ | $T2$ | $T1$ | $T2$ | $T1$ | $T2$ |
| *WAIS* | | | | | | |
| Digit Symbol[a] | 10.78 | 13.00 | 10.56 | 11.88* | 7.70 | 7.89** |
| | (1.99) | (3.07) | (2.73) | (3.94) | (2.06) | (2.89) |
| Picture Completion[a] | 11.11 | 11.61 | 10.94 | 11.24* | 10.10 | 10.20 |
| | (1.37) | (1.54) | (2.24) | (2.02) | (1.20) | (1.62) |
| Block Design[a] | 11.94 | 12.28 | 11.50 | 11.24* | 8.30 | 9.40 |
| | (2.88) | (2.89) | (3.00) | (2.51) | (1.83) | (2.72) |
| Picture Arrangement[a] | 10.94 | 10.78 | 9.72 | 9.82* | 9.20 | 8.70 |
| | (2.51) | (2.18) | (2.42) | (3.23) | (1.61) | (2.21) |
| Object Assembly[a] | 10.39 | 11.39 | 10.39 | 10.94* | 9.00 | 8.90 |
| | (2.06) | (2.81) | (2.70) | (2.84) | (2.36) | (2.38) |
| *TPT* | | | | | | |
| Time/Block[b] | .812 | .677 | .592 | .700 | 2.125 | 2.639 |
| | (.818) | (.578) | (.301) | (.560) | (1.734) | (2.329) |
| Memory[a] | 7.83 | 7.78 | 7.78 | 7.50 | 5.20 | 5.80 |
| | (1.29) | (1.26) | (1.26) | (1.58) | (2.86) | (3.05) |
| Location[a] | 3.56 | 3.56 | 4.00 | 4.39 | 2.00 | 2.10 |
| | (1.79) | (2.43) | (2.87) | (3.03) | (2.21) | (2.28) |
| Trails B[b] | 58.11 | 55.83 | 68.33 | 57.94* | 94.30 | 108.00 |
| | (15.53) | (17.12) | (25.02) | (24.83) | (43.99) | (60.46) |
| Spatial Relations[b] | 2.83 | 2.78 | 2.61 | 3.11 | 3.10 | 3.40 |
| | (1.15) | (.65) | (.92) | (.90) | (.99) | (.97) |
| Figure Learning[b] | 1.67 | 1.33 | 1.39 | 1.11 | 1.90 | 1.50 |
| | (.97) | (.69) | (.61) | (.32) | (.74) | (.71) |
| Thurstone Word Fluency[a] | 53.22 | 59.00 | 45.50 | 53.89 | 40.10 | 43.20 |
| | (15.11) | (14.40) | (17.26) | (23.06) | (12.39) | (10.77) |
| Seashore Rhythm[a] | 26.39 | 26.33 | 26.39 | 26.72 | 26.10 | 26.10 |
| | (2.73) | (2.50) | (2.83) | (2.61) | (2.60) | (2.69) |
| Tonal Memory[a] | 22.44 | 23.00 | 22.61 | 24.28 | 16.50 | 20.10 |
| | (6.34 | (6.06) | (4.57) | (4.56) | (7.85) | (7.22) |
| Speech Perception (errors)[b] | 5.00 | 3.50 | 4.72 | 4.06 | 7.30 | 7.90 |
| | (3.34) | (1.79) | (2.93) | (2.34) | (7.96) | (9.92) |

All data in parentheses are standard deviations.

[a]higher score indicates better performance.

[b]higher score indicates worse performance.

*$n$ = 17.

**$n$ = 9.

cognitive measures indicated that a significant decline between $T1$ and $T2$ had occurred in either the exacerbating relapsing-remitting MS group or the chronic-progressive MS group.

Table 8–2 presents means and standard deviations for measures having substantial cognitive and sensorimotor components. Main effects for diagnostic group were found for 5 of the 15 measures, indicating that the chronic-progressive MS group performed more poorly than the relapsing-remitting MS groups: WAIS Digit Symbol [$F(2,41) = 6.93, p < .01$], WAIS Block Design [$F(2,42) = 5.49, p < .01$], Tactual Performance Test (TPT) Time/Block [$F(2,43) = 10.21, p < .001$], TPT Memory [$F(2,43) = 6.83, p < .01$], and Trails B [$F(2,42) = 8.80, p < .001$]. For all these measures except WAIS Block Design, the chronic-progressive MS group obtained poorer scores than both relapsing-remitting MS groups; for Block Design, chronic-progressive MS patients did worse than the stable relapsing-remitting MS group only. A significant difference between $T1$ and $T2$ was also found on five measures, indicating better performance (probably due to practice effects) at $T2$: WAIS Digit Symbol [$F(1,41) = 14.13, p < .001$], TPT Time/Block [$F(1,43) = 4.29, p < .05$], Figure Learning (Trials) [$F(1,43) = .946, p < .01$], Thurstone Word Fluency [$F(1,43) = 17.20, p < .001$], and Tonal Memory [$F(1,43) = 12.18, p < .001$].

On only two measures did we find a significant interaction: WAIS Digit Symbol [$F(2,41) = 3.62, p < .05$] and TPT Time/Block [$F(2,43) = 5.17, p < .05$]. Using Scheffe's procedure, the only significant findings were that the chronic-progressive MS group performed worse over time than the stable relapsing-remitting MS group ($p < .05$). The exacerbating relapsing-remitting MS group did not differ from either the chronic-progressive MS group or the stable relapsing-remitting MS group.

Table 8–3 shows means and standard deviations for measures that are primarily sensorimotor in nature. Main effects for diagnostic group were found for three of the five measures. In two instances, the chronic-progressive MS group performed

**Table 8–3**  Sensorimotor Measures

| | Stable Relapsing-Remitting MS (n = 18) | | Exacerbating Relapsing-Remitting MS (n = 18) | | Chronic-Progressive MS (n = 10) | |
|---|---|---|---|---|---|---|
| | T1 | T2 | T1 | T2 | T1 | T2 |
| Sensory-perceptual errors[b] | 4.00 (4.70) | 5.14 (6.48) | 5.33 (5.81) | 8.44 (7.10) | 8.60 (5.25) | 12.75 (10.13) |
| Finger Tapping[a] | 83.73 (10.91) | 89.68 (13.04) | 91.07 (11.95) | 97.23* (13.24) | 67.73 (17.86) | 68.95 (15.14) |
| Grip Strength[a] | 55.23 (17.37) | 56.47 (16.91) | 61.74 (20.92) | 59.19* (18.83) | 50.50 (21.11) | 51.80 (15.28) |
| Grooved Pegboard[b] | 171.94 (57.07) | 162.00 (42.08) | 159.17 (38.31) | 164.47* (52.95) | 339.80 (153.54) | 357.30 (141.28) |

All data in parentheses are standard deviations.

[a]higher score indicates better performance.

[b]higher score indicates worse performance.

*$n = 17$.

more poorly than both relapsing-remitting MS groups: Finger Tapping [$F$ (2,42) = 13.08, $p < .001$] and Grooved Pegboard [$F$ (2,42) = 21.20, $p < .001$]. A main effect for Perceptual Errors was also found [$F$ (2,43) = 3.57, $p < .05$], but post hoc analysis revealed only that the chronic-progressive MS group made more errors than the stable relapsing-remitting MS group ($p < .05$). Main effects for differences between $T1$ and $T2$ were found for Perceptual errors [$F$ (1,43) = 8.91, $p < .01$] and Static Steadiness [$F$ (1,43) = 6.12, $p < .05$] with scores being worse at $T2$, and Finger Tapping [$F$ (1,42) = 12.08, $p < .001$], on which scores were better at $T2$.

Only one significant interaction between group and time was found, on Static Steadiness [$F$ (2,43) = 4.66, $p < .05$]. Post hoc analysis revealed that the chronic-progressive MS group declined significantly more than did either relapsing-remitting MS group.

Four summary scores are presented in Table 8–4. ANOVAs revealed a group main effect for three of the four: WAIS PIQ [$F$ (2,42) = 6.52, $p < .01$], Halstead Impairment Index (HII) [$F$ (2,41) = 3.96, $p < .05$], and Average Impairment Rating (AIR) [$F$ (2,41) = 11.38, $p < .001$]. On the WAIS PIQ, chronic-progressive MS patients performed more poorly than stable relapsing-remitting MS patients; on the HII and AIR, chronic-progressive MS patients were more impaired than each of the relapsing-remitting MS groups. Post hoc analysis showed that on the HII, chronic-progressive MS patients performed worse than the exacerbating relapsing-remitting MS group, whereas the chronic-progressive group did worse than either relapsing-remitting group on the AIR. In addition, WAIS PIQ and HII measures showed a main effect for time, with scores better at $T2$ than at $T1$ [$F$ (1,42) = 17.82, $p < .001$] and [$F$ (1,41) = 7.00, $p < .05$, respectively]. None of the summary scores, however, showed an interaction between group and time. Therefore, when analyzing summary scores that combine discrete units of data according to tradi-

**Table 8–4** Summary Scores

|  | Stable Relapsing-Remitting MS ($n = 18$) | | Exacerbating Relapsing-Remitting MS ($n = 18$) | | Chronic-Progressive MS ($n=10$) | |
|---|---|---|---|---|---|---|
|  | $T1$ | $T2$ | $T1$ | $T2$ | $T1$ | $T2$ |
| WAIS Verbal IQ[a] | 113.78 | 114.33 | 108.22 | 108.65* | 111.30 | 110.40 |
|  | (6.31) | (6.12) | (9.63) | (10.45) | (14.91) | (12.08) |
| WAIS Performance IQ[a] | 112.28 | 118.94 | 106.11 | 109.06* | 100.10 | 101.80 |
|  | (7.71) | (10.50) | (11.27) | (13.23) | (9.65) | (12.89) |
| Halstead Impairment Index[b] | .417 | .333 | .361 | .338** | .680 | .570 |
|  | (.268) | (.243) | (.283) | (.307) | (.235) | (.275) |
| Average Impairment Rating[b] | 1.073 | .991 | 1.061 | 1.00* | 1.988 | 1.899*** |
|  | (.459) | (.400) | (.478) | (.472) | (.615) | (.743) |

All data in parentheses are standard deviations.
[a]higher score indicates better performance.
[b]higher score indicates worse performance.
*$n = 17$.
**$n = 16$.
***$n = 9$.

**Table 8–5** Global Clinical Ratings of Performance Between *T*1 and *T*2

| Group | Significantly improved | Slightly improved | No change | Slightly worse | Significantly worse |
|---|---|---|---|---|---|
| Stable relapsing-remitting MS | 0 | 2 (11.1%) | 13 (72.2%) | 2 (11.1%) | 1 (5.6%) |
| Exacerbating relapsing-remitting MS | 0 | 0 | 7 (38.9%) | 10 (55.6%) | 1 (5.6%) |
| Chronic-progressive MS | 0 | 0 | 3 (30%) | 5 (50%) | 2 (20%) |

tional guidelines, we found no evidence of a differential course for specific diagnostic groups of MS patients over the test-retest interval.

Clinical ratings were used to provide an independent assessment of change in performance over time which would complement the raw data analyses; $\chi^2$ analysis disclosed no significant differences between the groups for any of the three specific ratings (cognitive, cognitive-sensorimotor, sensorimotor), but did reveal a significant result for the global rating [$\chi^2(6) = 13.41$, $p < .05$]. This result supports the prior hypothesis that the stable relapsing-remitting MS group would fare better than the other groups (see Table 8–5). If categories 1 and 2 are collapsed into a single rating (better), and categories 4 and 5 into another single rating (worse), 11.1% of stable relapsing-remitting MS patients were better at *T*2, whereas 72.2% were unchanged, and only 16.7% were worse. In the exacerbating relapsing-remitting MS group, on the other hand, none were better, 38.9% were the same, and 61.2% were worse. Faring still worse was the chronic-progressive MS group, in which none was better, 30% were unchanged, and 70% were worse. It is thus apparent that when experienced clinicians made a global judgment regarding change over time for individual subjects, differences among groups were found that did not appear when discrete units of data were examined.

## DISCUSSION

The finding that the chronic-progressive MS group showed greater neuropsychological impairment than did both relapsing-remitting MS groups was predictable from the Heaton et al. (1985) study. These same subjects participated in both studies, although only the baseline data were analyzed before.

The focus of the present study was on group change over the one–two year test-retest interval. In considering the change data, it should be noted that practice effects on some measures undoubtedly biased the study against finding evidence of progressive deficits; that is, in the absence of real change in the patients, some improvement in their performance might occur as a consequence of their previous exposure to the same test items and materials. Indeed, across all groups, significant improvements were noted on two of the four summary measures (WAIS, PIQ, and HII) and on four individual test measures.

Nevertheless, even if we allow for some bias due to practice effects, the finding that significant worsening of performance at follow-up was noted on only 6 of the

36 test measures is hardly impressive. In general, the group data on individual test measures did not show substantial deterioration in the neuropsychological functioning of MS patients over a one–two year period.

The group data on individual test measures also provided minimal support for the hypothesized differences among patient groups in progression of neuropsychological impairment. Only 3 of the 36 measures indicated significantly greater increases in impairment for the chronic-progressive MS group, in relation to one or both of the relapsing-remitting MS groups. Moreover, the exacerbating relapsing-remitting MS group failed to show significantly greater deterioration than the stable relapsing-remitting MS group did on any of the test measures.

As noted, clinical ratings were expected to be more sensitive to any "spotty" changes in functioning that might be manifested by individual patients within our three groups. The results in Table 8–5 clearly support this expectation and further indicate that the group differences in change rating are in the hypothesized direction. Our raters found the individuals in the stable relapsing-remitting MS group to be least changed over the test-retest interval, whereas the chronic-progressive MS group showed the most consistent (albeit quite mild) deterioration in their functioning. The exacerbating relapsing-remitting MS group resembled the chronic-progressive MS group, suggesting that relapse in MS may cause neuropsychological changes that are, temporarily at least, similar to those of progressive demyelinating disease. Because only the global ratings disclosed these differences, it seems likely that the disease progression or relapse affected the three categories of ability inconsistently, from patient to patient, again depending on the locus of new demyelination.

Since relapses in MS are defined by elemental (i.e., noncognitive) neurologic criteria, it may not be surprising that cognitive changes do not accompany clinical relapses with regularity. Our study does not address the issue of whether MS relapses can be *defined* as events involving cognitive deterioration, although we suspect such relapses are a part of the natural history of MS. It seems plausible to us that cognitive relapses may be as common as other types, depending on where demyelination occurs. Moreover, greater clinical sensitivity to the possibility of isolated cognitive changes during exacerbation might permit better documentation of this phenomenon using formal neuropsychological testing (see Chapter 9 in this volume).

Our finding of either mild or absent neuropsychological deterioration in 42 (91%) of our 46 patients suggests a more favorable prognosis than has been implied by some previous studies (e.g., Canter, 1951). Nevertheless, this optimism should be tempered by the fact that our test-retest intervals were rather brief. Evaluation at much longer intervals would be likely to reveal more significant changes in neuropsychological function, since MS is a chronic disease whose effects may require many years or decades to become apparent. Another factor to be considered is our relatively small sample size, and future studies with larger samples are certainly desirable. Finally, the absence of a control group in our study raises the possibility that the observed neuropsychological stability of MS may be due to practice effects. These are all legitimate issues that can be meaningfully addressed in further research.

Despite these limitations, however, our clinical rating data provide preliminary evidence that the natural history of cognitive impairment in MS may depend in part on the severity of illness and, by implication, on the degree and location of demyelination. Another useful approach would involve magnetic resonance imaging (MRI) in conjunction with neuropsychological evaluation, since there is now evidence that cognitive impairment correlates with the burden of cerebral white matter involvement (Franklin, et al., 1988). If cognitive stability or progression over time in MS were correlated with MRI data that had been collected simultaneously, important new information could be obtained.

## ACKNOWLEDGMENT

We are grateful to Nanci S. Avitable, M.S., for her assistance with statistical analyses.

## REFERENCES

Canter, A.H. (1951). Direct and indirect measures of psychological deficit in multiple sclerosis. *J. Gen. Psychol.,* **44,** 3–50.

Fink, S.L., and Houser, H.B. (1966). An investigation of physical and intellectual changes in multiple sclerosis. *Arch. Phys. Med. Rehab.,* **47,** 56–61.

Franklin, G.M., Heaton, R.K., Nelson, L.M., Filley, C.M., and Seibert, C. (1988). Correlation of neuropsychological and magnetic resonance imaging findings in chronic/progressive multiple sclerosis. *Neurology,* **38,** 1826–29.

Grant, I. (1986). Neuropsychological and psychiatric disturbances in multiple sclerosis. In W.I. McDonald, and D.H. Silberberg, eds., *Multiple Sclerosis.* London: Butterworths, pp. 134–152.

Grant, I., Heaton, R.K., McSweeny, A.J., Adams, K.M., and Timms, R.M. (1982). Neuropsychological findings in hypoxemic chronic obstructive pulmonary disease. *Arch. Int. Med.,* **142,** 1470–76.

Heaton, R., Grant, I., Anthony, W.Z., and Lehman, R.A.W. (1981). A comparison of clinical and automated interpretation of the Halstead-Reitan Battery. *J. Clin. Neuropsychol.,* **3,** 121–41.

Heaton, R.K., McSweeny, A.J., Grant, I., Adams, K.M., and Petty, T.L. (1983). Psychological effects of continuous and nocturnal oxygen therapy in hypoxemic chronic obstructuve pulmonary disease. *Arch. Int. Med.,* **143,** 1941–47.

Heaton, R.K., Nelson, L.M., Thompson, D.S., Burks, J.S., and Franklin, G. M. (1985). Neuropsychological findings in relapsing-remitting and chronic-progressive multiple sclerosis, *J. Consult. Clin. Psychol.* **53,** 103–10.

Ivnik, R.J. (1978a). Neuropsychological test performance as a function of the duration of MS-related symptomatology. *J. Clin. Psychiat.,* **39,** 304–7, 311–12.

Ivnik, R.J. (1978b). Neuropsychological stability in multiple sclerosis. *J. Consult. Clin. Psychol.,* **46,** 913–23.

Peyser, J.M., and Becker, B. (1984). Neuropsychological evaluation in patients with multiple sclerosis. In C.M. Poser, D.W. Paty, L. Scheinberg, W.I. McDonald, and G.C. Ebers, eds., *The Diagnosis of Multiple Sclerosis.* New York: Thieme-Stratton, pp. 143–158.

Rao, S.M. (1986). Neuropsychology of multiple sclerosis: a critical review. *J. Clin. Exp. Neuropsychol.,* **8,** 503–42.

Schumacher, G.A., Beebe, G., Kibler, R.F., Kurland, L.T., Kurtzke, J.F., McDowell, J.F., Nagler, F., Sibley, W.A., Tourtellotte, W.W., and Wilman, T.L. (1965). Problems of experimental trials of therapy in multiple sclerosis: report by the panel on the evaluation of experimental trials of therapy in multiple sclerosis. *Ann. N.Y. Acad. Sci.,* **122,** 552–68.

Young, A.C., Saunders, J., and Ponsford, J.R. (1976). Mental change as an early feature of multiple sclerosis. *J. Neurol. Neurosurg. Psychiat.,* **39,** 1008–13.

# 9

# Brief and Intermediate-Length Screening of Neuropsychological Impairment in Multiple Sclerosis

ROBERT K. HEATON, LAETITIA L. THOMPSON,
LORENE M. NELSON, CHRISTOPHER M. FILLEY, AND
GARY M. FRANKLIN

Until fairly recently, significant cognitive impairment has been considered rare in patients who have multiple sclerosis (MS). Now, however, several studies using comprehensive neuropsychological test batteries have shown that MS groups perform worse than control groups do on a variety of cognitive as well as sensorimotor tasks. A recent study of 100 consecutive outpatients with clinically definite MS has found significant cognitive impairment in 57% (Heaton et al., 1985). In an extensive review of the neuropsychological literature on MS, Rao (1986) concluded that the pattern of cognitive deficits associated with this disease represents a prototype subcortical dementia. This pattern of mental deficits is consistent with the widely disseminated lesions frequently found in the cerebral white matter of MS patients who have advanced disease. It should also be noted that, especially early in the course of MS and in relatively benign cases, one may see only one or two discrete mental deficits (e.g., poor verbal or nonverbal memory) that represent a part of the overall pattern described by Rao.

The cognitive deficits of MS patients tend to be relatively mild when compared with those found in other dementing illnesses such as Alzheimer's or Huntington's diseases. Nevertheless, even mild cognitive impairment can have significant negative effects on vocational functioning and other aspects of daily living (Heaton and Pendleton, 1981). Moreover, such impairment frequently goes undetected by treating neurologists because of the insensitivity of clinical mental status examinations and the fact that more readily detected sensorimotor disability is not helpful in predicting cognitive disability (Rao, 1986).

Perhaps ideally, the neuropsychological status of all MS patients who have known or suspected cerebral involvement would be assessed using a comprehensive (six–eight hour) test battery. Such batteries are sensitive to even subtle impairment, and they yield detailed information about a wide range of abilities that are important for both neurological diagnosis and everyday functioning. On the other hand, comprehensive neuropsychological testing is expensive and very time-consuming, and it is not available in all clinical settings.

In many clinical and research situations, it would be helpful to have a relatively brief, standardized assessment approach that is intermediate between the insensitive bedside mental status exams and the day-long test batteries. In this chapter we compare the results of three such approaches in groups of 40 MS patients and 90 demographically matched controls. The first two cognitive screening procedures included in our comparison take only 5–10 minutes to administer and essentially are standardized and slightly expanded versions of bedside mental status exams: the Mini-Mental State (MMS) (Folstein et al., 1975) and the Cognitive Capacity Screening Examination (CCSE) (Jacobs et al., 1977). Both of these screening tests were developed to help detect diffuse organic mental syndromes (e.g., dementias) on medical and psychiatric services. Although various elementary cognitive abilities are tapped by different items in these exams, no individual abilities are assessed in sufficient detail to warrant separate scoring. For each screening exam only a single score, reflecting global cognitive status, is generated. Although the MMS and CCSE are helpful in detecting and grading gross neurocognitive impairment, these exams have been criticized as lacking sensitivity to milder cognitive deficits (Nelson et al., 1986).

The third screening procedure to be considered here is called the Neuropsychological Screening Battery (NSB). This is a collection of 18 brief, standardized tests that generate both summary scores and individual test scores reflecting the adequacy of a variety of individual abilities. Although much longer than the MMS and CCSE (i.e., it takes 30–45 minutes to administer), the NSB is more comprehensive and includes subtests that might be sensitive to a broader spectrum of neurocognitive impairment. In a previous study of 60 chronic-progressive MS patients, their NSB summary scores correlated significantly with independent ratings of their cerebral lesions as demonstrated by magnetic resonance imaging (MRI) (Franklin et al., 1988). Also, the NSB can be administered by various clinical personnel after relatively brief training, and it is much briefer and less expensive than a comprehensive neuropsychological examination.

We were interested in exploring the usefulness of these three approaches to screen for cognitive impairment as well as general (cognitive and sensorimotor) neuropsychological impairment in MS. For two reasons, MS represents a particularly difficult challenge for such screening instruments. First, unlike other illnesses that cause dementia, this disease is not always associated with significant cerebral involvement and cognitive impairment. Therefore, sensitivity and specificity issues apply not only in distinguishing disease from health, but also in distinguishing impaired from unimpaired individuals within the MS group. A second potential difficulty in using screening instruments with MS is that when cognitive impairment does exist, it is apt to be relatively mild and may involve only one or a few discrete abilities that are inconsistent across affected individuals.

The MS patient group consisted of 40 subjects who had previously participated in the Heaton et al. (1985) study. All were outpatients who had clinically definite MS according to the diagnostic criteria proposed by Schumacher et al. (1965). Thirty-one (77.5%) were female, and at the time of their participation in the present study they had a mean age of 41.2 years (SD = 7.4) and a mean of 14.2 years (SD = 2.3) of education. Twenty had a relapsing-remitting disease course, and the other twenty had a chronic-progressive course. As in our previous study, the relapsing-remitting patients were tested during periods of remission.

The MS patients had been administered an expanded Halstead-Reitan Battery (HRB) approximately 12 months earlier as part of their participation in the previous study. The latter battery is quite comprehensive and has well-documented sensitivity to cerebral lesions involving various etiologies. Thus the patients' results on the previous testing were available as criterion measures of both general neuropsychological impairment and cognitive impairment. The group had a mean WAIS verbal IQ of 110.4 (SD = 9.0) and performance IQ of 103.1 (SD = 12.0). Their mean average impairment rating was 1.45 (SD = 0.68), which is considered impaired for a group with their demographic characteristics (Karzmark et al., 1984).

In the Heaton et al. (1985) study, blind clinical ratings were performed on the neuropsychological data of all 200 patients and controls. Separate ratings considered global neuropsychological functioning, cognitive functioning, sensory functioning, and motor functioning. These ratings used a nine-point scale, ranging from above average to severely impaired; a score of four marked the beginning of the impaired range and indicated very mild impairment. The clinical ratings in the previous study had classified 32 (80%) of our 40 patients as being neuropsychologically impaired and 22 (55%) as having cognitive impairment. Again based on clinical ratings of each subject's HRB data, this group's mean global neuropsychological impairment was in the mildly impaired range ($M$ = 4.8; SD = 1.3), whereas their mean cognitive impairment rating was in the very mildly impaired range ($M$ = 3.9; SD = 1.7).

The control group consisted of 90 subjects who had no history of neurologic illness, head trauma, or substance abuse. Fifty-six (62.2%) were female. This group had a mean age of 43.9 years (SD = 14.4) and a mean education of 14.3 years (SD = 2.8). There were no significant differences between the two groups with respect to sex distribution [$X^2$ (1) = 2.3], age [$t(128)$ = 1.1], or education [$t(128)$ = 0.3].

All screening tests were administered individually in a single session. The examiners were blind to the previously obtained HRB results of the MS patients.

The MMS is a very brief 30-point scale, based on 11 items that assess the following: Orientation to place and time, learning and delayed recall of three objects, attention and calculation, naming of two objects, repeating one statement, following a three-step command, reading one statement, writing one statement, and copying intersecting pentagons. The authors have suggested a cutoff score of less than 21 as indicating significant cognitive impairment (Folstein et al., 1975). The CCSE also uses a 30-point scale, with any score less than 20 being considered evidence of diminished cognitive capacity (Jacobs et al., 1977). This exam includes assessment of orientation to place and time, immediate memory for digits, short-term memory for digits after brief distraction, attention and calculation, delayed recall of four words, and simple verbal reasoning (similarities and opposites).

The published diagnostic cutoff scores for the MMS and CCSE were selected with the goal of establishing a false-positive rate of essentially zero; that is, in the initial studies of these instruments no normal subjects scored below the cutoffs. This is a more conservative procedure than is used with most neuropsychological tests, because ensuring a 100% specificity rate usually results in an unacceptably low sensitivity. More typically, a cutoff point of one or two standard deviations below the mean for normals is chosen, to make the scale more sensitive to pathology and in recognition of the commonly observed finding that a significant minority of subjects who have normal neuropsychiatric histories do show some neurocognitive impairment (Heaton et al., 1981). Thus for the NSB a cutoff of one standard deviation below the mean of the normative sample defines mildly impaired performance. In the present study it would not be appropriate to focus exclusively on much more conservative cutoffs for the MMS and CCSE than for the NSB. Therefore, in addition to using the standard cutoffs for the former two exams, we established alternative cutoffs in the same manner as we had for the NSB. This was possible because the normal standardization group for the NSB ($N$ = 130) also had been administered both the MMS and the CCSE. For the MMS, therefore, the NSB-comparable cutoffs for impairment were less than 29 for subjects below the age of 50 years, and less than 28 for subjects who are 50 and older. For the CCSE, these respective cutoffs are less than 27 and less than 25. With each test this resulted in a false-positive rate of about 15% in the NSB normative sample.

The NSB provides a relatively brief, standarized assessment of a variety of neuropsychological functions: psychomotor speed, sequencing efficiency, visual attention, verbal learning and delayed recall, nonverbal learning and delayed recall, visuoconstructional skills, expressive and receptive language abilities, and reading comprehension. The 18 subtests in the NSB were adapted directly or in abbreviated form from previously published sources. Included are two widely used neuropsychological screening tests that have previously demonstrated validity for detecting cerebral disorders: the Symbol Digit Modalities Test (Smith, 1973) and Parts A and B of the Trail Making Test (Armitage, 1946); as in the Heaton et al. (1985) study, a Trails B minus Trails A difference score was used to provide a more pure measure of cognitive efficiency which is not confounded by sensorimotor impairment. Our Numerical Attention Test is a one-page digit cancellation task (Lezak, 1976); this yields time and error scores reflecting adequacy of visual attention. Learning efficiency (up to three trials to reach criterion) and memory (percentage forgetting after a 20-minute delay) are assessed for verbal and nonverbal materials, respectively, using a story from the Wechsler Memory Scale (Wechsler, 1945) and part of the Rey-Osterrieth Complex Figure (Lezak, 1976). Visuoconstructional abilities are assessed by requiring the subject to copy the latter figure. A Speech Articulation rating was taken directly from the Multilingual Aphasia Examination (Benton and Hamsher, 1976), and other language assessments were abbreviated from that examination: Visual Naming, Aural Comprehension, and Reading Comprehension. Finally, the NSB also includes one-minute assessments of oral and written fluency, as well as an abbreviated version of the Commands with Auditory Sequencing subtest of the Western Aphasia Battery (Kertesz and Poole, 1974).

The NSB yields 18 subtest scores reflecting the adequacy of the foregoing skills. For each of these 18 subtest measures, cutoffs were developed for establishing two levels of impairment; called mildly impaired and very impaired, these respective cutoffs corresponded to the fifteenth and fifth percentiles of the normative sample. The cutoffs were based on the score distributions of 130 neurologically normal subjects who had a mean age of 52.5 years (SD = 17.9) and a mean education of 14.0 years (SD = 2.9). For subtest scores that showed significant age effects in the normative sample, separate cutoffs were developed for the younger (<50 years old; $n$ = 50) and older (≥50 years old; $n$ = 80) subjects. Further details regarding the NSB subtests and normative data are available from the senior author of this chapter.

Two NSB summary scores also have been developed: a total summary score (using all 18 subtest scores) and a more "pure" cognitive score which includes 11 NSB measures that do not involve motor efficiency with the upper extremities. (See Table 9–1 for the components of these two summary scores.) Each summary score is based on the number of its component measures that are classified as impaired, with one point given for a mildly impaired result (bottom fifteenth percentile) and two points given for a very impaired result (bottom fifth percentile for normals). Thus the NSB total summary score is based on 18 individual test measures and

**Table 9–1**  MS and Control Group Means (SDs) and Comparisons on Scores from NSB, MMS, and CCSE

|  | Control Group (n = 90) | MS Group (n = 40) | t | p |
|---|---|---|---|---|
| *MMS* | 29.2(1.1) | 29.0(1.4) | 1.3 | NS |
| *CCSE* | 28.1(2.0) | 27.1(2.8) | 2.3 | .02 |
| *NSB Summary Scores* |  |  |  |  |
| Total Summary Score | 2.3(2.7) | 8.9(6.5) | −8.1 | .0001 |
| Cognitive Summary Score | 1.5(1.8) | 3.2(3.3) | −3.7 | .0001 |
| *NSB Subtests* |  |  |  |  |
| Symbol Digit Modalities[a] | 55.7(10.1) | 41.0(12.5) | 7.1 | .0001 |
| Trails A[a] | 26.3(12.5) | 39.0(19.0) | −4.5 | .0001 |
| Trails B[a] | 58.3(26.5) | 82.8(62.0) | −3.2 | .002 |
| Trails B−A[b] | 31.9(22.9) | 43.8(46.8) | −1.9 | .05 |
| Numerical Attention (Time)[a] | 151.7(33.3) | 214.6(61.1) | −7.6 | .0001 |
| Numerical Attention (Errors)[a,b] | 4.6(5.1) | 5.0(6.1) | −0.4 | NS |
| Verbal Learning[a,b] | 7.5(3.2) | 6.1(3.5) | 2.2 | .03 |
| Verbal Memory[a,b] | 5.6(7.6) | 13.1(12.2) | −4.3 | .0001 |
| Figure Copying[a] | 16.7(2.2) | 15.8(2.8) | 1.9 | NS |
| Figure Learning[a] | 14.9(3.1) | 10.9(5.4) | 5.3 | .0001 |
| Figure Memory [a,b] | 5.9(8.5) | 6.8(7.8) | −0.6 | NS |
| Speech Articulation[a] | 8.0(0.0) | 7.6(0.8) | 4.8 | .0001 |
| Visual Naming[a,b] | 18.3(1.4) | 17.5(1.5) | 2.8 | .006 |
| Oral Fluency[a,b] | 12.2(3.7) | 11.9(4.2) | 0.5 | NS |
| Written Fluency[a] | 12.7(3.4) | 10.6(3.9) | 3.0 | .003 |
| Sentence Repetition[a,b] | 4.7(0.5) | 4.7(0.6) | 0.2 | NS |
| Aural Comprehension[a,b] | 11.8(0.5) | 11.9(0.3) | −1.3 | NS |
| Commands[a,b] | 22.4(1.3) | 21.4(2.1) | 3.6 | .0001 |
| Reading Comprehension[a,b] | 11.9(0.3) | 11.9(0.2) | −0.6 | NS |

[a]NSB subtests that contribute to total summary score.

[b]NSB measures that contribute to cognitive summary score.

has a possible range of 0–36. The cognitive summary score, based on 11 measures, has a possible range of 0–22. Again based on results of the normative sample, designated cutoffs define mildly impaired and very impaired summary scores.

Table 9–1 summarizes the results of the two subject groups on all the screening instruments. The MS group did not perform worse than the control group on the MMS. Most subjects in both groups obtained perfect scores on this test. Both groups also performed quite well on the CCSE, according to its published norms. The MS group mean was marginally worse than that of the controls on this ($p = .02$), however.

Highly significant group differences were obtained on the NSB total summary score and cognitive summary score ($p < .0001$), with the control group performing much better on both measures. The MS group mean on the total summary score is just within the very impaired range, which corresponds to the fifth percentile of the NSB normative sample. On the other hand, their mean on the cognitive summary score is at the juncture between the normal and mildly impaired ranges (about at the fifteenth percentile of the NSB normative sample). This suggests that much, but not all, of the MS group's neuropsychological impairment on the NSB occurred on subtests that have significant sensorimotor requirements. Inspection of the NSB subtest results in Table 9–1 provides further support for this conclusion. Large group differences were found on the Symbol Digit Modalities Test, the time component of the Numerical Attention Test, Parts A and B of the Trail Making Test, and Written Fluency; it is likely that the MS patients' sensorimotor deficits interfered on these. On the other hand, their poor nonverbal learning scores cannot be explained on this basis, because their normal Figure Copying involves the identical sensorimotor requirements. Similarly, some cognitive impairment was demonstrated on the Trail Making Test B minus A difference score. Also, the MS group's scores on Verbal Learning, Verbal Memory, Visual Naming, and Commands clearly reflect cognitive impairment. Finally, Table 9–1 shows that the MS group performed comparably to the controls on several components of the NSB: Oral Fluency, Sentence Repetition, Aural Comprehension, Reading Comprehension, Figure Copying, Figure Memory, and Numerical Attention errors.

Table 9–2 lists the percentages of subjects in the MS and control groups who were impaired according to the published norms for the MMS and CCSE and according to the norms on all three screening procedures that were based on the results of the NSB standardization sample. As in the initial studies with the MMS and CCSE, the published cutoff scores made no false-positive errors; that is, all subjects in our normal group were classified as normal. Unfortunately, however, all MS patients also were classified as normal by these cutoffs. Using the NSB-comparable cutoffs, the MMS still failed to show significantly more impairment in the MS group than in the controls, whereas significant group differences did emerge on the CCSE. A somewhat higher percentage of MS patients were impaired on the NSB cognitive summary score, and a majority were impaired on the NSB total summary score. In detecting neuropsychological impairment in the MS group, the Symbol Digit Modalities Test showed even greater sensitivity than the NSB total summary score; because of the substantial sensorimotor requirements of the former test, however, it is not possible to determine how much of the impairment shown by MS patients on this is due to cognitive deficits.

**Table 9-2** Percentages of Control and MS Subjects Classified as Impaired by the MMS, CCSE, and NSB Exams

| | Control Group ($n = 90$) | MS Group ($n = 40$) | $\chi^2$ | $p$ |
|---|---|---|---|---|
| *MMS* | | | | |
| NSB-comparable cutoff | 12.2 | 22.5 | 1.5 | NS |
| Published cutoff | 0.0 | 0.0 | 0.0 | NS |
| *Cognitive capacity* | | | | |
| NSB-comparable cutoff | 10.0 | 25.0 | 3.9 | .05 |
| Published cutoff | 0.0 | 0.0 | 0.0 | NS |
| *NSB summary scores* | | | | |
| Total | 12.2 | 62.5 | 32.5 | .0001 |
| Cognitive | 10.0 | 32.5 | 8.4 | .01 |
| *NSB subtests* | | | | |
| Symbol Digit Modalities | 8.9 | 80.0 | 62.4 | .0001 |
| Numerical Attention (Time) | 10.0 | 62.5 | 36.8 | .0001 |
| Trails A | 14.4 | 55.0 | 21.1 | .0001 |
| Trails B | 14.4 | 50.0 | 16.7 | .0001 |
| Verbal Memory | 11.1 | 45.0 | 16.9 | .0001 |
| Verbal Learning | 7.8 | 37.5 | 15.4 | .0001 |
| Figure Learning | 10.0 | 37.5 | 12.1 | .001 |
| Written Fluency | 12.2 | 35.0 | 7.8 | .01 |
| Commands | 10.0 | 30.0 | 6.8 | .01 |
| Speech Articulation | 11.1 | 25.0 | 3.1 | NS |
| Trails B − A | 15.6 | 22.5 | 0.5 | NS |
| Figure Copying | 16.7 | 22.5 | 0.3 | NS |
| Visual Naming | 10.0 | 20.0 | 1.6 | NS |
| Numerical Attention (Errors) | 16.7 | 20.0 | 0.0 | NS |
| Figure Memory | 11.1 | 17.5 | 0.5 | NS |
| Oral Fluency | 6.7 | 15.0 | 1.4 | NS |
| Aural Comprehension | 17.8 | 10.0 | 0.8 | NS |
| Sentence Repetition | 2.2 | 5.0 | 0.1 | NS |
| Reading Comprehension | 7.8 | 5.0 | 0.0 | NS |

With the MS patients it was possible to assess concurrent validity of the screening procedures, using the expanded HRB data as criterion measures. To begin this process, Table 9-3 shows the product-moment correlations between the screening exam scores and summary measures from the WAIS and HRB. On some of the measures high scores represent good performance, whereas on other measures a high score reflects greater impairment; nevertheless, all correlations in Table 9-3 are in the direction of positive association between degree of impairment on the different measures.

The MMS was modestly, but significantly, correlated with the Wechsler performance IQ, as well as with the HRB average impairment rating and clinician's cognitive rating; its correlations with verbal IQ and the clinicians' global impairment rating approached significance, whereas MMS scores were less associated with the motor and sensory ratings.

Compared with the MMS, the CCSE had substantially higher correlations with both IQ scores and with all HRB scores. A substantial advantage over the MMS also was apparent for both NSB summary scores. Of interest, however, is that the

**Table 9–3**   Correlations between Screening Exam Scores and Summary Scores on the WAIS and Halstead-Reitan Battery (HRB) for 40 MS Patients

| | WAIS Verbal IQ | WAIS Performance IQ | Average Impairment Rating | Clinician HRB Impairment Ratings | | | |
|---|---|---|---|---|---|---|---|
| | | | | Global | Cognitive | Motor | Sensory |
| MMS | .31 | .36[c] | −.33[c] | −.30 | −.47[b] | −.05 | −.20 |
| Cognitive capacity | .59[a] | .61[a] | −.70[a] | −.61[a] | −.65[a] | −.29 | −.47[b] |
| NSB total | −.61[a] | −.73[a] | .77[a] | .63[a] | .67[a] | .37[c] | .37[c] |
| NSB cognitive | −.58[a] | −.61[a] | .61[a] | .54[a] | .70[a] | .13 | .30 |

[a] $p < .001$.
[b] $p < .01$.
[c] $p < .05$.

NSB total summary score correlated significantly with all four clinician HRB impairment ratings, whereas the NSB cognitive summary score was significantly related only to the HRB cognitive and global ratings. This latter finding supports the separate use of the NSB cognitive score as being relatively independent of sensorimotor impairment in MS.

It should be recalled that, based on their previous performances on the expanded HRB, a clinician in the Heaton et al. (1985) study rated 80% of the present MS sample as having significant neuropsychological impairment of any type (sensorimotor and/or cognitive) and 55% as having significant cognitive impairment. Using these ratings as the "gold standard," sensitivity and specificity data were computed for all screening procedures. These data are presented in Table 9–4. All three *cognitive* screening measures show excellent specificity, but less than impressive sensitivity. The NSB cognitive summary score obtained somewhat

**Table 9–4**   Sensitivity and Specificity of Screening Exam Measures in Predicting Global Neuropsychological Impairment and Cognitive Impairment in 40 MS Patients

| | Any Neuropsychological Impairment | Cognitive Impairment |
|---|---|---|
| *MMS Exam* | | |
| Sensitivity | .28 | .36 |
| Specificity | 1.00 | .94 |
| *CCSE* | | |
| Sensitivity | .31 | .41 |
| Specificity | 1.00 | .94 |
| *NSB Total Summary Score* | | |
| Sensitivity | .72 | .77 |
| Specificity | .75 | .56 |
| *NSB Cognitive Summary Score* | | |
| Sensitivity | .41 | .55 |
| Specificity | 1.00 | .94 |

Note: Cutoffs for all screening exam measures are based on the results of the NSB standardization sample of 130 normals. Criterion classifications of global and cognitive impairment are based on blind clinical ratings of these subjects' scores on an expanded HRB.

higher sensitivity ratings than did the others in predicting both general neuropsychological impairment and cognitive impairment within this MS sample. Finally, while the NSB total summary score shows moderately good sensitivity and specificity in predicting global neuropsychological impairment, its specificity drops in predicting cognitive impairment.


## DISCUSSION AND CONCLUSIONS

Before considering the results of the screening exams in this study, we again emphasize the fact that MS is a particularly challenging disease for such procedures. Not all MS patients have cognitive deficits, and those who do vary widely with respect to the range of abilities that are affected (from one or two discrete deficits to fairly widespread neurocognitive impairment). The cognitive deficits also tend to be milder than those seen with other dementing illnesses. Finally, more severe sensorimotor deficits in MS complicate the interpretation of impairment on complex neuropsychological screening tests which have both cognitive and sensorimotor requirements. In view of these factors, screening tests that are relatively easy and cover a restricted range of abilities can be expected to perform less well with MS than with many other neurological diseases. Therefore, the results of comparisons among the three screening procedures in MS should not be generalized to conditions that typically have more severe and widespread effects on neurocognitive functioning.

Screening procedures cannot be expected to replace comprehensive neuropsychological test batteries. They cannot measure the range of abilities tapped by daylong examinations such as the expanded HRB, and in some situations a comprehensive assessment is needed. For example, in counseling patients about their everyday functioning it is desirable to have the fullest possible knowledge of their strengths and deficits. On the other hand, there are other situations in which it is unnecessary to obtain that much information or in which the use of a comprehensive battery would be too expensive or time consuming. In such situations the use of a briefer, yet valid assessment of neuropsychological functioning may be indicated.

The screening procedures used in this study showed many statistically significant differences between the MS and control groups. Also, the screening measures were moderately to highly correlated with the results of comprehensive neuropsychological testing in the MS group. However, the different screening procedures had varying outcomes in attempting to detect the cognitive and other neuropsychological deficits in the MS patients.

The MMS performed least well, overall. Although previous research has demonstrated its usefulness in detecting more severe, generalized cognitive deficits in other patient groups, this test appears to have inadequate sensitivity to the mild or discrete deficits that are caused by MS.

Although the CCSE has comparable brevity, it outperformed the MMS in this study. It was better at discriminating MS patients from normals, and it was more strongly correlated with results on the expanded HRB. Its sensitivity in predicting cognitive impairment in the MS patients was not impressive, but again it was better than that of the MMS.

Compared with the much briefer CCSE and MMS, the intermediate-length NSB provided more powerful discrimination between the MS and normal control groups. The NSB's correlations with the results of comprehensive neuropsychological testing also were the highest, yet were only marginally higher than those achieved by the CCSE. Compared with the CCSE, the NSB showed greater sensitivity in predicting cognitive impairment (.55 versus .41) and global neuropsychological impairment (.72 versus .31) in the MS patients. As with all the cognitive screening measures used in this study, the NSB cognitive summary score had almost perfect specificity (.94) in its predictions; that is, predictions of cognitive impairment by these measures virtually always were confirmed by the expanded HRB.

As was anticipated, the NSB total summary score was best at predicting general neuropsychological impairment, whereas the NSB cognitive summary score was the best predictor of cognitive impairment. We would argue that it is useful to have both capabilities in a neuropsychological screening battery. Again, however, it should be recognized that interpreting an MS patient's impairment on the NSB total summary score may not be straightforward; to a greater degree than with most neurologic conditions, an elevated NSB total summary score in an MS patient may reflect sensorimotor rather than cognitive impairment, and at least some of the former impairment may be due to central nervous system (CNS) involvement below the cerebral level. Nevertheless, in a previous study of 60 chronic-progressive MS patients, the NSB total and cognitive summary scores had virtually the same correlations with ratings of cerebral lesions demonstrated by magnetic resonance imaging (MRI) (Franklin et al., 1988).

The results in Table 9–4 with regard to the NSB cognitive summary score may underestimate the NSB's actual sensitivity to cognitive impairment in MS. This score is a sum of the impaired scores on 11 NSB measures that have minimal sensorimotor components. It is similar to the Halstead Impairment Index of the HRB, in that its sensitivity depends on a sufficient range of abilities being impaired. Such summary scores do not perform as well when patients have only one or a few discrete deficits, as is not uncommon with MS, even when these deficits are detected by the test battery. In this situation a clinician has a major advantage over summary scores because he or she can use multiple levels of inference in identifying and interpreting impairment (Heaton et al., 1981). In the present study the HRB criterion ratings of cognitive impairment were made using the clinical method, whereas the NSB predictions used the simpler and perhaps less sensitive sum of impaired test measures. Further research on the sensitivity of the NSB to cognitive impairment should employ clinical ratings of the NSB data and should investigate the reliability and validity of such ratings, as has been done with the HRB (Heaton et al., 1981; Grant et al., 1982).

Another factor that may limit the NSB's sensitivity to cognitive impairment is the absence of a subtest that measures conceptual or abstraction skills. We did explore this by extracting the results on the Wisconsin Card Sorting Test from the expanded HRB and including them in the NSB cognitive summary score. This did not result in an increased sensitivity estimate for the latter score.

An important advantage of the NSB over the other screening instruments used in this study is that it yields subtest scores reflecting adequacy of a variety of individual neuropsychological abilities (albeit a less extensive variety than is the case for comprehensive batteries). This permits the clinician to comment on a given patient's pattern of strengths and deficits and to consider that pattern in relation to questions regarding lesion location and implications for everyday functioning. Similarly, the researcher can use these data to elucidate patterns of strengths and deficits in various patient groups. In the current study, the MS patient group did relatively well on subtests that measure oral fluency, verbal repetition, auditory comprehension, reading comprehension, and visuoconstructional skills. As the only possible exception to the absence of dysphasia in this group, there was evidence of a subtle naming deficit. (Impairment of written fluency in this group almost certainly is due to motor deficits rather than language deficits; also, their articulation impairment is due to dysarthria in some patients, rather than to paraphasic errors.) The MS group showed definite impairment on subtests that measure psychomotor efficiency, new learning, delayed retention of recently learned information, and ability to follow complex sequential procedures. Finally, the data regarding concentration and attention must be considered inconclusive; that is, the MS patients tended to be quite slow on the Numerical Attention Test (possibly because of motor impairment), but they were not error-prone. In general, these results on the NSB are consistent with those found in other studies of MS using more comprehensive testing: There is a relative absence of cortical deficits such as aphasia and constructional apraxia, and the deficits they showed are similar to those seen in other neurologic conditions that primarily affect subcortical brain structures (Rao, 1986).

## ACKNOWLEDGMENT

The authors gratefully acknowledge the assistance of Nanci S. Avitable in analyzing the data in this study.

## REFERENCES

Armitage, S.G. (1946). An analysis of certain psychological tests used for the evaluation of brain injury. *Psychol. Mono.,* **60,** Whole No. 277.

Benton, A.L., and Hamsher, K.deS. (1976). *Multilingual Aphasia Examination.* Iowa City, Iowa: Department of Neurology, University Hospitals.

Folstein, M.F., Folstein, S.E., and McHugh, P.R. (1975). "Mini-Mental State": A practical method for grading the cognitive state of patients for the clinician. *J. Psychol. Res.,* **12,** 189–98.

Franklin, G.M., Heaton, R.K., Nelson, L.M., Filley, C.M., and Siebert, C. (1988). Correlation of neuropsychological and magnetic resonance imaging findings in chronic/progressive multiple sclerosis. *Neurology,* **38,** 1826–29.

Grant, I., Heaton, R.K., McSweeny, A.J., Adams, K.M., and Timms, R.M. (1982). Neuropsychological findings in hypoxemic chronic obstructive pulmonary disease. *Arch. Int. Med.,* **142,** 1470–76.

Heaton, R.K., Grant, I., Anthony, W.Z., and Lehman, R.A.W. (1981). A comparison of clinical and automated interpretation of the Halstead-Reitan Battery. *J. Clin. Neuropsychol.,* **3**, 121–41.

Heaton, R.K., Nelson, L.M., Thompson, D.S., Burks, J.S., and Franklin, G.M. (1985). Neuropsychological findings in relapsing-remitting and chronic-progressive multiple sclerosis. *J. Consult. Clin. Psychol.,* **53**, 103–10.

Heaton, R.K., and Pendleton, M.G. (1981). Use of neuropsychological tests to predict adult patients' everyday functioning. *J. Consult. Clin. Psychol.,* **49**, 807–21.

Jacobs, J.W., Bernhard, M.R., Delgado, A., and Strain, J.J. (1977). Screening for organic mental syndromes in the medically ill. *Ann. Int. Med.,* **86**,40–6.

Karzmark, P., Heaton, R.K., Grant, I., and Matthews, C.G. (1984). Use of demographic variables to predict overall level of performance on the Halstead-Reitan Battery. *J. Consult. Clin. Psychol.,* **4**, 663–65.

Kertesz, A., and Poole, A. (1974). The Aphasia Quotient: a taxonomic approach to the measurement of aphasic disability. *Can. J. Neurol. Sci.,* **1**, 7–16.

Lezak, M.D. (1976). *Neuropsychological Assessment,* 2nd ed. New York: Oxford University Press.

Nelson, A., Fogel, B.S., and Faust, D. (1986). Bedside cognitive screening instruments. *J. Nerv. Ment. Dis.,* **174**, 73–83.

Rao, S.M. (1986). Neuropsychology of multiple sclerosis: A critical review. *J. Clin. Exp. Neuropsychol.,* **8**, 503–42.

Schumacher, G.A., Beebe, G., Kibler, R.F., Kurland, L.T., Kurtzke, J.F., McDowell, F., Nagler, B., Sibley, W.A., Tourtellotte, W.W., & Wilman, T.L. (1965). Problems of experimental trials of therapy in multiple sclerosis: Report by the panel on the evaluation of experimental trials of therapy in multiple sclerosis. *Ann. N.Y. Acad. Sci.,* **122**, 552–68.

Smith, A. (1973). *Symbol Digit Modalities Test.* Los Angeles: Western Psychological Services.

Wechsler, D.A. (1945). A standardized memory scale for clinical use. *J. Psychol.,* **19**, 87–95.

# 10

# Clinical Perspectives in the Identification of Cognitive Impairment

GARY M. FRANKLIN, LORENE M. NELSON,
ROBERT K. HEATON, AND CHRISTOPHER M. FILLEY

Several factors may account for the persisting lack of awareness that functionally important cognitive disturbances can occur in multiple sclerosis (MS). First, the degree of cognitive impairment may not be related to the degree of neurologic (sensorimotor) disability (Heaton et al., 1985; Franklin et al., 1988). Second, patients with predominant periventricular demyelination, even with long-standing disease, may be considered mildly affected, or even "silent," with respect to neurobehavioral deficits (Gilbert and Sadler, 1983). Third, the bedside mental status examination (Peyser et al., 1980a; Heaton et al., 1985) and brief standardized mental status examinations, such as the Mini-Mental State (MMS) (Folstein, Folstein and McHugh, 1975), are insensitive to detecting mild to moderate neurocognitive impairment (Franklin et al., 1988; Nelson et al., 1986).

Other possible factors include: (1) a paucity of information on the true prevalence of cognitive impairment in MS, (2) difficulty experienced by clinical neurologists in interpreting the results of published neuropsychological studies which report testing methods largely unfamiliar to them, (3) a lack of procedures and guidelines for detecting or even predicting cognitive impairment in the office setting, and (4) a general sense among patients and clinicians that, if nothing can be done, the problem should not be addressed at all.

In this chapter we address these issues in the context of published studies and with the perspective of our clinical experience. The focus is on clinical relevance, and we present guidelines for the detection of cognitive impairment in the office, with an attempt to balance our views with the potential heuristic value and ethics of detecting such impairment.

## THE PREVALENCE OF COGNITIVE IMPAIRMENT IN MS

The true prevalence of cognitive impairment in MS is unknown, and estimates are critically dependent on the population studied and the method by which impairment is defined. Most population-based studies done to date have relied on relatively brief bedside mental status examinations. Kahana et al. (1971) reported that 2% of 295 MS patients identified in Israel had an organic mental syndrome at the onset of their illness. At a mean follow-up period of 17 years, 25% of these patients had some organic mental impairment. Kurtzke et al. (1972) reported that the prevalence of cognitive impairment was 2.9% among 527 men hospitalized for MS.

More recent applications of standardized neuropsychological test batteries have yielded higher prevalence rates in more selected referral center patient populations. In a consecutive series of 100 MS outpatients, Heaton et al. (1985) found cognitive deficits in 46% of relapsing-remitting and 72% of chronic-progressive MS patients. Rao et al. (1984) reported a 63% prevalence estimate in a sample of chronic-progressive patients. Both neuropsychological studies yielded higher estimates than studies using briefer bedside screening procedures, which suggests that the harder one looks, the more impairment one finds.

Brief mental status examinations generally classify as normal many patients who would test impaired on standard neuropsychological tests. Peyser et al. (1980b) found that the neurologic examiner misclassified 79% (22/28) of MS patients who were cognitively impaired on neuropsychological testing. Similarly, Heaton et al. (1985) found that the misclassification rate for the bedside mental status exam was 57%.

A similar misclassification problem is posed by the better standardized MMS (Folstein, et al., 1975). Using MMS cutoff scores standardized to a normal control group, Franklin et al. (1988) found that the MMS classified only 20% of patients with chronic-progressive MS as abnormal compared with a 45-minute neuropsychological screening battery (NSB, see Chapter 9), which classified 60% as abnormal. When previously published MMS cutoffs were used (DePaulo and Folstein, 1978), none of the MS patients were classified as impaired.

One might question the clinical relevance of cognitive deficits that can be detected only by lengthy neuropsychological test batteries. To address this issue, it is necessary to define the clinical questions that are being asked. Such questions can be classified broadly as relating to diagnostic and patient management and treatment issues. Diagnostic questions relate to the presence, extent, and progression of cerebral involvement. An extensive literature documents the diagnostic value of neuropsychological tests (e.g., Filskov and Boll, 1981), yet their role in diagnosing MS is ancillary in most cases. Most essential diagnostic questions regarding MS can be answered with a thorough history and neurologic examination, together with nonbehavioral laboratory tests such as magnetic resonance imaging (MRI), CSF analysis, and evoked potential studies. On the other hand, neuropsychological tests have a unique and indispensable role in answering questions about MS patients' capabilities and limitations in everyday functioning. Moreover, previous research has demonstrated that even relatively mild and subtle neuropsychological deficits can have an important impact on patients' daily living;

for example, the prospects for successful employment appear to be substantially reduced in patients who score in the mildly impaired range on the average impairment rating of the Halstead-Reitan Battery (HRB) (Heaton and Pendleton, 1981).

Even if the treating neurologist appreciates the goals and capabilities of neuropsychological testing in MS, questions remain about when to test and how much of such testing is indicated in individual cases. In the remainder of this chapter, we review some clinical associations and guidelines that may be useful in answering these questions.

## CLINICAL RELEVANCE OF COGNITIVE IMPAIRMENT IN MS

We have recently described 12 patients seen over a two years period whose cognitive function was significantly worse than any other MS-related neurologic disability (Franklin et al., 1989). Although the number of patients is limited, detailed study of their relatively isolated functional cognitive impairment enabled us to understand more clearly why cognitive impairment in MS is frequently overlooked by community neurologists and others caring for these patients. Moreover, their clinical characteristics allowed us to put the literature on the subject in a context that may be helpful for practitioners. Few of these patients presented with a chief complaint of difficulty with thinking. The principal problem in the two most cognitively impaired patients was gait apraxia. The following case history illustrates one of these patients who was followed in the community for "depression" over the preceding two-year period.

A 31-year-old woman entered our center with a four-year history of MS. Her primary complaints were of progressive gait difficulty and depression during the preceding two years. When asked, she acknowledged that she also had been experiencing difficulty with her memory. She had recently quit her job as an administrative assistant in a physician's office. The patient had been told that her mental problems were related to depression. Bedside mental status examination revealed poor concentration, abstraction, and calculations. The patient exhibited a severely apraxic gait with placing response. Other neurologic dysfunction was minimal. Her Kurtzke Expanded Disability Status Score (EDSS) was 3.5. A computerized tomographic (CT) scan revealed diffuse white matter attenuation and ventricular enlargement. The MRI scan showed confluent demyelination. An expanded HRB revealed severe impairment across a wide range of functions (especially recent memory) and, in this college graduate, a Wechsler full scale IQ (WAIS-R) of 82. She had been quite cooperative with the testing, and her pattern of neuropsychological results could not be explained on the basis of depression (Heaton and Crowley, 1981). The patient's cognitive abilities have continued to deteriorate over the ensuing 1.5 years. Her gait apraxia is now severe enough to require bilateral assistance. A recent isotope cisternogram revealed no evidence of spinal fluid flow disturbance.

The patient's gait became nearly crablike and was strikingly different from other MS patients' difficulties with gait secondary to pyramidal, cerebellar, or sensory deficits. In addition to this gait apraxia, she exhibited frontal lobe release signs primarily seen in the lower extremities. These included placing and grasping in the feet. The grasping response was strong enough to overcome the Babinski sign, present bilaterally, but only with lateral plantar stimulation.

Ten of the twelve patients exhibited frontal release signs predominant in the lower extremities. These signs are characterized by a gait that is typically wide-based, with the feet appearing to be "magnetized" to the ground. An associated finding is grasping of the foot when the plantar surface is stimulated. Such grasping is likely responsible for the "magnetic" appearance of the feet during gaiting. A similar pattern of gait apraxia and lower extremity frontal release has been described in normal pressure hydrocephalus (Messert and Baker, 1966), but only rarely in MS (McLardy and Sinclair, 1964). Frontal release signs would be difficult to observe in MS patients who have significant cerebellar ataxia or spasticity. The most reasonable explanation for these signs in MS is the predominant periventricular demyelination seen both pathologically (Brownell and Hughes, 1962) and by MRI (Young et al., 1981; Lukes et al., 1983). Significant involvement of the frontal lobes in MS was also recently suggested by Vowels and Gates (1984).

We do not know the true prevalence of frontal release signs in MS patients and whether these signs occur more frequently in cognitively impaired patients. Our clinical experience, however, has been that nearly every MS patient with an apraxic gait disorder has significant cognitive impairment. Those patients who have placing or grasping but without clear gait apraxia seem to have lesser degrees of cognitive impairment. We have developed a four-point scale (0–3) for functional cognitive disability (which considers neuropsychological test results in relation to everyday functioning; Table 10–1) as well as for frontal lobe release signs (Table 10–2). The degree of functional cognitive disability was highly correlated with the degree of frontal release in our patient group ($r = .90$, $p < .001$).

*It is important to note that cognitive impairment may be unrelated to neurologic disability status, disease course, or disease duration in individual patients.* Although clinical course (chronic-progressive disease) and longer disease duration were associated with the occurrence of cognitive dysfunction in a large consecutive sample of patients (Heaton et al., 1985), these clinical parameters are not useful as predictors of cognitive dysfunction in a given patient. The mean age of our patient group was 38.6 years, and the mean Kurtzke EDSS (Kurtzke, 1983) was only 3.2. The Kurtzke scale is heavily weighted for brain-stem, cerebellar, and spinal cord disability; it is, therefore, not surprising that the EDSS might be an unreliable predictor of disability if cognitive impairment were the predominant functional problem. Van den Burg et al. (1987) recently investigated 40 mildly disabled MS patients whose mean EDSS was 2.6. These patients scored significantly worse in tests of memory compared with normal controls, and 17.5% of these patients were judged to be cognitively impaired. Peyser et al. (1980a) analyzed a group of MS patients by cluster analysis and discovered that one subgroup was cognitively impaired but

**Table 10–1**   Cognitive Function Scale

---

Grade 0—Normal function

Grade 1—Mild alteration of living pattern due to neurocognitive deficit; continues to work or function independently

Grade 2—Moderate alteration of living pattern due to neurocognitive deficit; unable to work because of cognitive impairment

Grade 3—Severe alteration of living pattern due to neurocognitive deficit; unable to function independently

---

**Table 10-2**   Frontal Lobe Release Signs

Grade 0—No signs
Grade 1—Mild lower extremity placing without gait apraxia
Grade 2—Clear lower extremity placing with mild to moderate gait apraxia
Grade 3—Severe gait apraxia; may require aids

had little other neurologic disability (mean EDSS = 2.2). It cannot, therefore, be assumed that a patient with minimal sensory and motor impairment will not be at risk for cognitive impairment. Minimal neurologic disability can be accompanied by severe cognitive dysfunction.

The EDSS is still the "gold standard" for following the clinical course of patients in clinical trials and in large MS clinics. But it is not adequate for following the course of cognitive function, and frontal lobe release signs are currently not specifically addressed among the Kurtzke functional systems. We recommend either expansion of the scale to include these functions more adequately or adaptation of scales similar to those described in Tables 10-1 and 10-2, after more detailed reliability and validity testing in larger and more representative MS populations. Even these scales, however, would not be adequate for the longitudinal assessment of cognitive function in MS clinical trials. The addition of a standardized battery, such as the NSB (see Chapter 9), at baseline and yearly intervals, would greatly improve upon the current paucity of such testing in MS clinical trials.

Fifty percent of our highly selected patient group (6/12) presented with serious cognitive disturbance within five years of disease onset, including the two most globally impaired patients. Prior reports have documented that severe, early dementia (diagnosed clinically) could occur in MS (Bergin, 1957; Koenig, 1968; Young, et al., 1976). Cognitive impairment in MS identified by standardized neuropsychological tests has also been reported early in disease course (Peyser et al., 1980a; Grant et al., 1984; and Lyon-Caen et al, 1986) or in the presence of mild neurologic disability (Van den Burg et al, 1987).

Two-thirds of our selected group of 12 patients would have been considered to have a relapsing-remitting disease course and half of these had lengthy disease durations of 6–20 years. This raises the issue of whether some patients who otherwise appear benignly affected by MS and whose lesions may have been considered clinically silent in the past (Gilbert and Sadler, 1983) might have significant cognitive impairment. On the other hand, it is also clear that MS patients with chronic-progressive disease tend to have more severe impairment on neuropsychological testing than those with relapsing-remitting disease (Heaton et al., 1985). One must keep in mind, however, that even patients with the chronic-progressive disease course may be spared from cognitive dysfunction. In fact, Heaton et al. (1985) found that 28% of those with a chronic-progressive disease course tested normally on the cognitive components of the expanded HRB.

We found no correlation between degree of functional cognitive impairment (Table 10–1) and disease duration in our selected case series. Heaton et al. (1985), however, found a significant but low correlation between cognitive impairment and disease duration ($r = 0.22$, p $< .05$) in 100 unselected MS outpatients. A similarly low correlation ($r = .25$, $p < .04$) between extent of involvement shown by MRI and disease duration was recently described by Stevens et al. (1986). These weak, albeit statistically significant, correlations again suggest that disease duration is not an accurate predictor of the degree of cognitive dysfunction or cerebral MRI lesion burden in an individual patient.

*Cognitive symptoms, like other neurologic symptoms seen in MS, can present with relapse and remission, relapse and progression or chronic progression.* One of our patients presented with a six-week history of severe disorganization of thinking. An expanded HRB documented an isolated deficit in nonverbal memory. Her neurological examination was otherwise normal, save for minor sensory deficits. Three months after presentation, and without treatment intervention, the patient's cognitive symptoms had cleared completely and a repeat HRB was entirely normal. A second patient with relapsing-progressive cognitive symptoms responded to cyclophosphamide treatment, stabilizing and remaining at work over a two-year period of treatment. Although treatment with immunosuppressive agents is still largely experimental and confined to chronic-progressive disease, it is clear that such intensive treatment approaches should be just as rigorously applied to progression in the cognitive sphere as it has been to progression of sensorimotor deficits.

*The routine bedside mental status examination is not predictive of cognitive impairment in MS.* As mentioned earlier, both Peyser et al. (1980b) and Heaton et al. (1985) have reported insensitivity of the bedside mental status examination as compared to standardized neuropsychological tests. This insensitivity of brief screening procedures may at least partly be explained on the basis of MS being a disease of the subcortical white matter which does not primarily involve the cerebral cortex (Filley et al., 1989; see Chapter 9). On the other hand, the bedside mental status examination is also insensitive to mild cortical involvement because of the inclusion of easy test items which sample a very narrow range of cognitive abilities. Whereas the bedside mental status examination focuses on memory and language skills, MS dementia may be dominated by difficulty with concept formation, complex problem solving, new learning, psychomotor efficiency, and attention and concentration (Peyser et al., 1980b; Rao, 1986; Filley et al., 1989). These latter skills are not adequately tested in the routine bedside mental status examination portion of the neurologic examination. The addition of a formal neuropsychological screening battery (see Chapter 9), possibly with the addition of a test of concept formation such as the Wisconsin Card Sorting Test (Rao et al., 1987), should be a useful supplement to the standard bedside MSE testing procedure.

*Ventricular enlargement, corpus callosum atrophy or moderate to severe periventricular demyelination may predict cognitive impairment in MS.* Specific findings on a cranial MRI scan may be a clue to the presence of significant, albeit clinically inapparent, cognitive dysfunction in MS. Previous investigations have found correlations with both enlarged ventricular size (Rao et al., 1985; Rabins et al., 1986) and atrophy of the corpus callosum (Huber et al., 1987). We have recently found a significant correlation ($r = 0.35$, $p < .01$) between cerebral lesion burden on an MRI and a cognitive summary score on the NSB in 60 patients with chronic-progressive MS (Franklin et al., 1988). Higher degrees of correlation will probably be attained with improved quantification of lesion burden (see Chapter 7) and with more comprehensive testing for detection of subcortical dementia in MS.

*Major depressive disorder refractory to therapy or bipolar disorder may herald cognitive impairment in MS.* Recent evidence suggests that affective disorder may be an organic concomitant of MS, possibly related to a substrate of cognitive dysfunction and specific patterns of subcortical demyelination (Grant, 1986; Rabins et al., 1986). One of our patients was brought to our attention because of subacute symptoms of depression that had been refractory to counseling and antidepressant medication. A second patient was diagnosed as having a manic-depressive psychosis during a period of acute MS relapse involving cognitive dysfunction. Schiffer et al. (1983) reported more depressive episodes in MS patients with cerebral involvement than in those without such involvement. Depression may also precede the diagnosis of MS itself (Whitlock and Siskind, 1980). A rapidly cycling bipolar illness in association with MS has been previously reported (Kellner et al., 1984). Other acute psychotic episodes (schizophrenic reactions) have also rarely been described in association with MS (Grant, 1986). There is, as yet, no clear association between localization of cerebral lesions and either depression or psychosis in MS.

In summary, the natural history of cognitive dysfunction is as varied as the occurrence of sensorimotor deficits in MS. The clinical findings that may best predict cognitive impairment in MS are (1) gait apraxia and/or frontal release signs predominant in the lower extremities, (2) a chronic-progressive disease course, (3) moderate to severe periventricular demyelination, ventricular enlargement, or corpus callosum atrophy on MRI scan, and (4) depression that appears refractory to treatment, or bipolar illness. Age, disease duration, and neurologic disability status are poor predictors of cognitive impairment in individual patients with MS. Although, in our experience, patients often do not complain de novo of difficulty thinking, when asked in some detail, some will complain of trouble thinking, particularly in relation to memory, complex problem-solving skills, or attention and concentration. The majority, however, are not specific and simply complain of fogginess, disorientation, or a sense of being confused, especially during periods of fatigue. Many have had cognitive difficulties for months or years without such dysfunction being discovered. If the clinician, however, suspects underlying cognitive dysfunction, an approach to the problem might be difficult given that (1) the patient or his or her family may not realize that a problem exists, (2) there is currently no cure for MS, and (3) the practical outcome of discovering cognitive dysfunction is unclear. The following section focuses on the issue of the usefulness of detecting cognitive impairment in MS and outlines specific clinical, rehabilitation, and social indications for neuropsychological testing.

## GUIDELINES FOR NEUROPSYCHOLOGICAL ASSESSMENT OF THE MS PATIENT

The issue of neuropsychological assessment in MS is difficult, given that most patients (and even some clinicians) believe that mentation is spared in MS. To some patients, the knowledge that they are at risk for cognitive impairment is very threatening; other patients are actually relieved to know that there is a physical cause for the changes in cognition they have experienced.

There are several reasons why clinicians should consider neuropsychological

**Table 10–3**   Indications for Neuropsychological Assessment

| | Tests Indicated | Counsel Then Decide | Tests Not Indicated |
|---|:---:|:---:|:---:|
| *Patient, family, or employer observes cognitive dysfunction* | | | |
| Patient complains that cognitive dysfunction affects function at work or home. | X | | |
| Patient denies concern about cognitive difficulties, and there is no clinical evidence of such difficulty. | | | X |
| Patient's employer reports reduced work capacity. | X | | |
| Patient is concerned about his or her potential for cognitive dysfunction, but as yet has not experienced difficulties. | | X | |
| Patient is seeking vocational counseling to obtain employment suitable to his or her ability level. | X | | |
| Patient is seeking disability benefits. | | X | |
| Patient is a rehabilitation candidate, but complains of cognitive difficulties that are likely to affect his or her ability to carry out requisite components of rehabilitation program. | X | | |
| Patient is a candidate for immunosuppressive therapy, may or may not complain of cognitive difficulties, and clinician desires baseline cognitive test battery for later comparison. | X | | |
| Patient is thought by others (family, employer) to have some cognitive impairment, but patient denies that he or she has any difficulties in this area. | | X | |
| Patient has relapsing-remitting disease with very little objective neurologic deficit, but reports some difficulty with cognitive tasks. | X | | |
| Patient has noted cognitive impairment, but deficits are not likely to be functionally significant because patient functions in a low-demand environment. | | X | |
| Patient has MS of long duration and is severely physically disabled (custodial); other deficits have more functional impact than impaired cognition. | | | X |
| Patient reports cognitive deficits that are subtle or fluctuating and may have functional consequences. | X | | |
| *Neuro exam and/or imaging procedure suggest cognitive impairment* | | | |
| Neurology exam (e.g., frontal release signs, mental status exam impaired) and/or imaging procedure (MRI, CT) suggest the possibility of cognitive involvement, but there is no other evidence of functionally significant cognitive changes, family difficulties, or work disruption. | | X | |
| Neurology exam and/or imaging procedure suggest cognitive impairment, patient is a candidate for | X | | |

**Table 10-3**    Indications for Neuropsychological Assessment

| | Tests Indicated | Counsel Then Decide | Tests Not Indicated |
|---|---|---|---|
| immunosuppressive therapy, and clinician desires baseline cognitive battery for later comparison. | | | |
| Neurology exam and/or imaging procedure suggest the possibility of cognitive impairment in a patient with relapsing-remitting disease who has little other evidence of objective neurologic deficits. | | X | |
| Neurology exam and/or imaging procedure suggest the possibility of cognitive impairment in a patient who exists in a low-demand environment; neither the patient nor his or her family report cognitive impairment of a functionally significant nature. | | | X |
| Neurology exam and/or imaging procedure suggest the possibility of cognitive impairment in a patient who is severely disabled (possibly custodial), in whom other neurologic deficits have as much functional significance as cognitive impairment. | | | X |
| Patient has a history of unexplained or treatment-resistant bipolar or other affective disorder which may have resulted from MS lesions. | X | | |

assessment of the MS patient. In the case of a particular patient, knowing his or her cognitive strengths and weaknesses may provide the opportunity to: (1) improve accuracy in reporting the contribution of cognitive abilities to vocational and disability determination agencies, (2) provide more appropriate rehabilitation that targets neurocognitive deficits and compensation strategies in addition to physical disabilities, (3) improve understanding on the part of the family and employer, (4) consider the patient for immunosuppressive treatment, and (5) relieve the patient's anxiety about ill-defined cognitive difficulties. In deciding whether and when to test, however, and especially in communicating the results, particular care should be taken with individuals who are newly diagnosed, who have poor coping skills, who deny the presence of cognitive deficits, and those in whom recovery from cognitive deficits is unlikely. The following indications for neuropsychological assessment are intended only as a point of departure for clinicians; in any given case the approach should be modified to fit the patient's circumstances.

Table 10–3 suggests some guidelines for deciding whether to obtain neuropsychologic assessment. The first part of Table 10–3 focuses on situations that would be apparent to the observant family, employer, or patient and the second part focuses on situations that would primarily be noted by the attending physician. Table 10–4 recommends instances in which a comprehensive neuropsychological screening battery might be more appropriate than a screening battery. Test batteries

**Table 10-4** Specific Indications for the Screening Battery and the Comprehensive Battery

| | Screening Battery[a] | Screening Battery +[b] | Comprehensive Battery[c] |
|---|:---:|:---:|:---:|
| *Disability determinations* | | | |
| Cognitive impairment is suspected on the basis of patient report, employer or family complaint, neuro exam, and/or imaging procedures. | | X | |
| Cognitive impairment is not documented; patient does not report cognitive difficulties. | X | | |
| *Patient is a candidate for immunosuppressive therapy* | | | |
| Cognitive impairment is suspected on the basis of patient report, employer or family complaint, neuro exam, and/or imaging procedures; cognition is the primary target of therapy. | | | X |
| Cognitive impairment is suspected on the basis of patient report, employer or family complaint, neuro exam, and/or imaging procedures; cognition is not the primary target of therapy. | X | | |
| Cognitive impairment is not strongly suspected and patient does not report cognitive difficulties, but patient has chronic-progressive MS. | X | | |
| *Patient is a candidate for rehabilitation program* | | | |
| Cognitive impairment is suspected on the basis of patient report, employer or family complaint, neuro exam, and/or imaging procedures. | | | X |
| Cognitive impairment is not documented; patient does not report cognitive difficulties. | | X | |
| *Patient is seeking vocational counseling* | | | |
| Cognitive impairment is suspected on the basis of patient report, employer or family complaint, neuro exam, and/or imaging procedures. | | | X |
| Cognitive impairment is not documented; patient does not report cognitive difficulties. | | X | |
| To confirm presence/absence of cognitive deficits in patients with little or no functional impact | X | | |
| To counsel patients and/or family members when functional impact of cognitive deficits may be significant | | X | |
| *Patient is seeking or obtaining psychiatric treatment* | | | |
| Presenting psychiatric complaints are apparently unrelated to MS, and there is no clinical evidence or suspicion of cognitive impairment. | X | | |
| Patient's psychosocial difficulties are not clearly attributable to situational factors or long-standing personality characteristics. | | X | |
| Patient is not making expected progress in psychotherapy, seems to be somewhat forgetful, inattentive, or conceptually unfocused/dull. | | | X |
| Patient has an affective disorder with poor response to pharmacotherapy. | | X | |

[a]"Screening Battery" is NSB.

[b]"Screening Battery +" is NSB, with a consideration to order the comprehensive battery if the screening battery indicates cognitive impairment.

[c]"Comprehensive Battery" is the expanded HRB.

utilized for MS should assess relative strengths as well as deficits. Patients will often have isolated or spotty deficits in the context of generally good cognitive functioning. A balanced interpretation of strengths and deficits is critical to patient advocacy and treatment in the following situations:

1. *Vocational counseling.* Adjustment of employers' expectations regarding performance and specific adaptations to minimize the impact of cognitive deficits at work can be crucial for maintaining employment. Supervisors are often relieved to know that they can help a valued employee maintain productivity.

2. *Individual and family counseling.* Patients and families are often relieved to discover that cognitive and behavioral problems may be related to the organic disease process, and that they involve a relatively restricted range of cognitive functions. Family members, especially spouses, children, and parents, will be less likely to inappropriately ascribe altered personality patterns solely to interpersonal conflict.

3. *Rehabilitation.* Therapists can be advised of the nature of cognitive deficits, and their treatment approach can be altered to maximize success (e.g., providing more redundancy and encouraging tape recording and/or note taking in the case of a memory deficit). Conversely, expectations for improvement of physical functioning may have to be lowered in the face of moderate to severe cognitive impairment. Of special interest is the relatively new field of cognitive retraining (Ben-Yishay and Diller, 1983). Applying these techniques in a fluctuating and sometimes progressive disease like MS may tax the limits of this treatment modality. Application to patients who are either relatively stable over time or who have good overall cognitive function in conjunction with spotty deficits may prove rewarding.

4. *Disability determination.* The Social Security Administration currently recognizes an assignment of disability specifically related to motor, sensory, fatigue, or cognitive impairments in MS. Criteria for impairment would be applicable to private disability coverage as well. Aggressive early advocacy on the part of attending physician or psychologist can avoid months or years of income loss, particularly in socially isolated patients who do not have the cognitive wherewithal to recover their just entitlement.

5. *Clinical trials.* Cognitive deficits comprise a major sphere of functional disability in MS; therefore, outcome measures in clinical trials should incorporate sensitive tests of cognitive function. A neuropsychological screening battery (see Chapter 9), rather than a comprehensive battery, may be adequate to this task and more reasonable in the face of a plethora of other neurologic outcome measures used in MS clinical trials.

In summary, the discovery of cognitive deficits could pose a threat to the well-being of the MS patient. It is important to approach neuropsychological assessment in a manner that recognizes the psychosocial and therapeutic impact of such an assessment in each individual. Neuropsychological deficits observed in a standardized test setting should be neither downplayed or exaggerated, recognizing that the functional impact of the cognitive deficits may vary, depending on the patient's premorbid level of functioning, coping abilities, employment setting, and social support network. Patients who are newly diagnosed often will find the prospect of cognitive deficits potentially devastating, while patients with longer disease duration who have observed fleeting or mild deficits may actually be relieved to ascribe these problems to MS. An advocacy plan and awareness of possible treatment implications should be foremost in the clinician's mind even before testing is undertaken. Counseling should precede testing, especially in newly diagnosed patients or in those patients in whom the reason for testing is unclear. Posttesting counseling also is frequently important, particularly to focus on cognitive strengths and the interpretation of results best suited to the needs of the individual patient.

## REFERENCES

Ben-Yishay Y., and Diller, L. (1983). Cognitive rehabilitation. In: M. Rosenthal, E.R. Griffith, M.R. Bond, and J.D. Miller, eds., *Rehabilitation of the Head Injured Adult*, pp. 367–80. Philadelphia: F.A. Davis.

Bergin, J.D. (1957). Rapidly progressing dementia in disseminated sclerosis. *J. Neurol. Neurosurg. Psychiat.*, **20**, 285–92.

Brownell, B., and Hughes, J.F. (1962). The distribution of plaques in the cerebrum in multiple sclerosis. *J. Neurol. Neurosurg. Psychiat.*, **25**, 315–20.

DePaulo, J.R., and Folstein, M.F. (1978). Psychiatric disturbance in neurological patients: Detection, recognition and hospital course. *Ann. Neurol.*, **4**, 225–28.

Filley, C.M., Heaton, R.K., Nelson, L.M., Burks, J.S., and Franklin, G.M. (1989). A comparison of dementia in Alzheimer's disease and multiple sclerosis. *Arch. Neurol.*, **46**, 157–61.

Filskov, S.B., and Boll, T.J. (1981). *Handbook of Clinical Neuropsychology*. New York: Wiley.

Folstein, M.F., Folstein, S.E., and McHugh, P.R. (1975). Mini-Mental State: A practical method for grading the cognitive state of patients for the clinician. *J. Psychiat. Res.*, **12**, 189–98.

Franklin, G.M., Heaton, R.K., Nelson, L.M., Filley, C.M., and Seibert, C. (1988). Correlation of neuropsychological and MRI findings in chronic/progressive multiple sclerosis. *Neurology*, **38**, 1826–29.

Franklin, G.M., Nelson, L.M., Filley, C.M., and Heaton, R.K. (1989). Cognitive loss in multiple sclerosis: Case reports and review of the literature. *Arch. Neurol.*, **46**, 162–67.

Gilbert, J.J., and Sadler, M. (1983). Unsuspected multiple sclerosis. *Arch. Neurol.*, **40**, 533–36.

Grant, I. (1986). Neuropsychological and psychiatric disturbances in multiple sclerosis. In W.I. McDonald and D.H. Silberberg, eds., *Multiple Sclerosis*, pp. 134–52. London: Butterworths.

Grant, I., McDonald, W.I., Trimble, M.R., Smith, E., and Reed, R. (1984). Deficient learning and memory in early and middle phases of multiple sclerosis. *J. Neurol. Neurosurg. Psychiat.*, **47**, 250–55.

Heaton, R.K., and Crowly, T.J. (1981). Effects of psychiatric disorders and their somatic treatments on neuropsychological test results. In S.B. Filskov, and T.J. Boll, eds., *Handbook of Clinical Neuropsychology*, pp. 481–525. New York: Wiley.

Heaton, R.K., Nelson, L.M., Thompson, D.S., Burks, J.S., and Franklin, G.M. (1985). Neuropsychological findings in relapsing-remitting and chronic-progressive multiple sclerosis. *J. Consult. Clin. Psychol.*, **53**, 103–10.

Heaton, R.K., and Pendleton, M.G. (1981). Use of neuropsychological tests to predict adult patients' everyday functioning. *J. Consult. Clin. Psychol.,* **49**, 807–21.

Huber, S.J., Paulson, G.W., Shuttleworth, E.C., Chakeres, D., Clapp, L.E., Pakalnis, A., Weiss, K., and Rammohan, K. (1987). Magnetic resonance imaging correlates of dementia in multiple sclerosis. *Arch. Neurol.,* **44**, 732–36.

Kahana, E., Leibowitz, U., and Alter, M. (1971). Cerebral multiple sclerosis. *Neurology,* **21**, 1179–85.

Kellner, C.H., Davenport, Y., Post, R.M., and Ross, R.J. (1984). Rapidly cycling bipolar disorder and multiple sclerosis. *Am. J. Psychiat.,* **141**, 112–13.

Koenig, H. (1968). Dementia associated with the benign form of multiple sclerosis. *Trans. Am. Neurol. Assoc.,* **93**, 227–28.

Kurtzke, J.F. (1983). Rating neurologic impairment in multiple sclerosis: An expanded disability status scale (EDSS). *Neurology,* **33**, 1444–52.

Kurtzke, J.F., Beebe, G.W., Nagler, B., Auth, T.L., Kurland, L.T., and Nefzger, M.D. (1972). Studies on the natural history of multiple sclerosis: Clinical and laboratory findings at first diagnosis. *Acta Neurol. Scand.,* **48**, 19–46.

Lukes, S.A., Crooks, L.E., Aminoff, M.J., Kaufman, L., Panitch, H.S., Mills, C., and Norman, D. (1983). Nuclear magnetic resonance imaging in multiple sclerosis. *Ann. Neurol.,* **13**, 592–601.

Lyon-Caen, O., Jouvent, R., Hauser, S., Chaunu, M.-P., Benoit, N., Widlocher, D., and Lhermitte, F. (1986). Cognitive function in recent-onset demyelinating diseases. *Arch. Neurol.,* **43**, 1138–41.

McLardy, T., and Sinclair, A. (1964). A case of presenile fulminating multiple sclerosis (with pathogenic considerations). *Confin. Neurol.,* **24**, 417–24.

Messert, B., and Baker, N.H. (1966). Syndrome of progressive spastic ataxia and apraxia associated with occult hydrocephalus. *Neurology,* **16**, 440–52.

Nelson, A., Folgel, B.S., and Faust, D. (1986). Bedside cognitive screening instruments. *J. Nerv. Ment. Dis.,* **174**, 73–83.

Peyser, J.M., Edwards, K.R., and Poser, C.M. (1980a). Psychological profiles in patients with multiple sclerosis: A preliminary investigation. *Arch. Neurol.,* **37**, 437–40.

Peyser, J.M., Edwards, K.R., Poser, C.M., and Filskov, S.B. (1980b). Cognitive function in patients with multiple sclerosis. *Arch. Neurol.,* **37**, 577–79.

Rabins, P.V., Brooks, B.R., O'Donnell, P., Pearlson, G.D., Moberg, P., Jubelt, B. Coyle, P., Dalos, N., and Folstein, M.F. (1986). Structural brain correlates of emotional disorder in multiple sclerosis. *Brain,* **109**, 585–97.

Rao, S.M. (1986). Neuropsychology of multiple sclerosis: A critical review. *J. Clin. Exp. Neuropsychol.,* **8**, 503–42.

Rao, S.M., Glatt, S., Hammeke, T.A., McQuillen, M.P., Khatrri, B.O., Rhodes, A.M., and Pollard, S. (1985). Chronic progressive multiple sclerosis: Relationship between cerebral ventricular size and neuropsychological impairment. *Arch. Neurol.,* **42**, 678–82.

Rao, S.M., Hammeke, T.A., McQuillen, M.P., Khatri, B.O., Lloyd, D. (1984). Memory disturbance in chronic progressive multiple sclerosis. *Arch. Neurol.,* **41**, 625–31.

Rao, S.M., Hammeke, T.A., and Speech, T.J. (1987). Wisconsin Card Sorting Test performance in relapsing-remitting and chronic-progressive multiple sclerosis. *J. Consult. Clin. Psychol.,* **55**, 263–65.

Schiffer, R.B., Caine, E.D., Bamford, K.A., and Levy, S. (1983). Depressive episodes in patients with multiple sclerosis. *Am. J. Psychiat.,* **140**, 1498–1500.

Stevens, J.C., Farlow, M.R., Edwards, M.K., and Yu, P. (1986). Magnetic resonance imaging: Clinical correlation in 64 patients with multiple sclerosis. *Arch. Neurol.,* **43**, 1145–48.

van den Burg, W., van Zomeren, A. H., Minderhoud, J.M., Prange, A.J.A., and Meijer,

N.S.A. (1987). Cognitive impairment in patients with multiple sclerosis and mild physical disability. *Arch. Neurol.,* **44,** 494–501.

Vowels, L.M., and Gates, G.R. (1984). Neuropsychological findings. In A.F. Simons, ed., *Multiple Sclerosis: Psychological and Social Aspects,* pp. 82–90. London: Heinemann.

Whitlock, F.A., and Siskind, M.M. (1980). Depression as a major symptom of multiple sclerosis. *J. Neurol. Neurosurg. Psychiat.,* **43,** 861–65.

Young, A. C., Saunders, J., and Ponsford, J.R. (1976). Mental changes as an early feature of multiple sclerosis. *J. Neurol. Neurosurg. Psychiat.,* **39,** 1008–13.

Young, I.R., Hall, A.S., Pallis, C.A., Legg, N.J., Bydder, G.M., and Steiner, R.E. (1981). Nuclear magnetic resonance imaging of the brain in multiple sclerosis. *Lancet,* **2,** 1063–66.

# III
# Affective Disturbance in Multiple Sclerosis

# Introduction

MOLLY HARROWER

My initial reaction to the chapters that comprise this section was an inevitable comparison between the current state of the art and that prevailing in the 1950s and 1960s. During this early period, I conducted various psychological projects relating to multiple sclerosis (MS) patients in response to an invitation by Sylvia Lawry, the founder of the National Multiple Sclerosis Society. My early opportunities to work with MS patients serve as a backdrop against which the work epitomized in the following chapters may be seen.

In 1949 I was asked to conduct psychologically oriented interviews of a number of MS patients in south Florida. With no special format in mind, I followed the lead of each patient as they described how their lives had been affected by their illness. The results of these interviews found expression in an article (Harrower and Kraus, 1951) and two manuals: one directed to MS patients themselves (Harrower, 1953) and the other to physicians and caregivers (Harrower and Herrmann, 1953). In the latter, three difficulties in adjustment were identified that seemed to relate specifically to the experienced world of the MS patient as distinct from the handicapped in general.

The first was called the concept of *marginality,* which epitomizes the period at the beginning of the MS illness when the patient can neither live within the world of the healthy individual nor find his or her place as an accepted and recognized invalid. Shall he continue to play a role as a normal citizen? Shall she struggle to outwit minor symptoms without expectation of special consideration? Or shall he accept his handicap and move consciously into the framework of the invalid?

A second difficulty experienced by MS patients can be described as feelings of *uncertainty* which accompany a delayed, tentative, or questionable diagnosis. Recent comments from patients are as vivid as those in my earlier studies. One patient indicated that "waiting for a test result goes beyond the pale, white-faced, clammy torture." Another comments, "The patient may ache as much in his mind as he does in his body for fear that others will suppose him a fraud when in fact he is seriously ill" (Hackney, 1988a,b).

The third characteristic problem relates to *loss of control*, be it from bladder incontinence or from inappropriate laughing and crying. These loomed large as experienced difficulties. Not only was the awareness of loss of control a distressing psychological experience in itself, but so, too, was the concern that the patient may be reflecting through behavior an inappropriate or diametrically opposite impression from that which he would wish to give.

This incongruity between the MS patients' actual feeling state and the unwanted, uncontrolled emotional display is addressed by Rabins in Chapter 11. He has disentangled for the reader the various clinical pictures that have appeared under the heading of euphoria. He has also clearly demonstrated that euphoria is, in all probability, closely linked to the presence of brain involvement. Rabins recognizes the difficulties this symptom complex may evoke in the families of MS sufferers. Noting that the emotional symptoms of MS are sometimes among the most disabling aspects of the disease, Rabins challenges clinicians to develop effective treatments for euphoria.

In Chapter 12, Schiffer presents a lucid discussion of the range of affective changes in MS, along with an analysis of the biologic factors that may contribute to their etiology. His chapter has a particularly useful section that provides suggestions concerning appropriate psychological treatment for MS patients who have varying degrees of psychological insight. He describes three levels of psychological awareness: (1) patients who are unable to confront any psychological issue concerning their feelings, (2) patients who tend to focus their attention on events and people in the environment, such as job or family structures, and (3) patients who are able to "examine their feelings and their life histories and to consider the meaning of these events." Such people are in a minority, but they are amenable to an insight-oriented treatment approach.

Warren's review (Chapter 13) of the role of stress in MS systematically covers the extant literature in this controversial area and presents new findings from her own group at the University of Alberta. Her discussion of methodological issues and directions for future research is invaluable. Our early study of residual stress following combat fatigue in World War II pilots (Harrower and Grinker, 1946) may have implications for treating stress in MS patients. We showed that experimental stress, that is, slides of combat scenes, produced emotional disturbance far beyond what could have been anticipated, requiring alterations of the experimental material and experimental procedure. But even more interesting, these pilots requested permission to attend subsequent showings, finding that these later exposures had a therapeutic effect.

From this discussion it is obvious that my primary interest in these chapters is concerned with the role of psychotherapy in the treatment of the MS patient. In 1954, I wrote: "Those of us who have worked actively in a counseling or therapeutic capacity with patients suffering from multiple sclerosis have seen the extent to which the adjustment of acute personal problems may contribute not so much to the disease per se, but to the functioning of that individual in a less self-destructive and more creative manner. If research funds were available, an important piece of quantitative work to be done would be the systematic and careful contrasting of a group of patients exposed to psychotherapy as opposed to a matched group who had received no such help."

One of my major problems in the 1950s and 1960s was to convince the "establishment" of the usefulness of various kinds of psychotherapeutic endeavor. The latest information from the National Multiple Sclerosis Society indicates that there are 425 counseling groups led by professionals, and approximately 1000 self-help groups in existence (Nielsen, 1988, personal communication). Time marches on.

## REFERENCES

Hackney, A. (1988a). Book review of *Pursuit of Hope* by Miriam Ottenburg in *Outlook*. New York: National Multiple Sclerosis Society.

Hackney, A. (1988b). Book review of *You Can Make It Back: Coping With Serious Illness* by Paul Levitt and Elissa Guralnick in *Outlook*. New York: National Multiple Sclerosis Society.

Harrower, M. (1953). *Mental Health and MS*. New York: National Multiple Sclerosis Society.

Harrower, M. (1954). Psychological factors in multiple sclerosis. *Ann. N.Y. Acad. Sci.,* **58,** 715–19.

Harrower, M., and Grinker, R. R. (1946). The stress tolerance test. *Psychosom. Med.,* **8,** 3–15.

Harrower, M., and Herrmann, R. (1953). *Psychological Factors in the Care of Patients with Multiple Sclerosis*. New York: National Multiple Sclerosis Society.

Harrower, M., and Kraus, J. (1951). Psychological studies on patients with multiple sclerosis. *Arch. Neurol. Psychiat.,* 66, 44–57.

# 11

# Euphoria in Multiple Sclerosis

PETER V. RABINS

Charcot (1873) included "foolish laughter without cause" among the emotional changes seen in multiple sclerosis (MS) patients. Since this first clinical description of euphoria in MS over 100 years ago, elevated mood has been one of the most controversial psychological aspects of MS. It has been reported to be both rare and common, both a psychogenic reaction to the illness and a result of direct brain damage. This chapter reviews the published literature on euphoria in MS and presents data from a longitudinal study conducted at our institution. It does not address, except in passing, sustained euphoria as a manifestation of mania or as a side effect of steroid usage.

Two studies published in the 1920s formulated many of the themes related to euphoria and developed hypotheses that are still being studied. Brown and Davis (1922) described euphoria as common, finding it in 10 of 14 (71%) patients with "mental symptoms." By their description, many of these individuals had a "slight elevation of mood." They contrasted this with the delusions of grandeur seen in "the terminal stage [of MS] associated with considerable dementia." They noted that "even in [depressed] cases, euphoria tends to develop as the disease progresses." While unsure of the cause of the euphoria, they placed it among the symptoms attributed to organic lesions.

Soon thereafter, Cottrell and Wilson, in an influential paper published in 1926, reported on 100 patients whom they had systematically examined. They identified four feeling states of well-being. In *euphoria sclerotica* the patient's mood is persistently cheerful. They characterized this as a state of "mental well-being." In *eutonia sclerotica* the patient is unaware or unconcerned about his physical disability. Cottrell and Wilson considered this a state of "physical well-being" and considered eutonia a "fundamental," that is, unique, symptom of MS. They distinguished eutonia from *spes sclerotica,* an "optimism as to the future and the prospects of ultimate recovery which is out of place and incongruous." Finally, they noted that some individuals are *emotionally labile.*

Of Cottrell and Wilson's subjects, 63% were euphoric and 10% depressed. Overall, 84% of their cases had a shift in outlook toward increased optimism and 25% had experienced increased variability of mood since the onset of their illness; 84% of their subjects had eutonia and another 4% had mixed feelings of well-being and "ill-being." In sum, 96% of their subjects had symptoms of "emotional overreaction."

These high prevalence rates contrasted with a 17% rate of explosive laughter and emotional instability reported by Sachs and Friedman (1922), a 24% rate reported by Poser (1978), and a 25.9% rate reported by Surridge (1969). Nonetheless, the high rates of euphoria found by Brown and Davis (1922) and Cottrell and Wilson (1926) found their way into the mythology of MS and are still well known in spite of the rarity of studies that have found rates as high as theirs. While an occasional study can be cited that finds high rates of euphoria [e.g., Thygesen (1953) reported that 77% of 60 patients experienced euphoria when followed for an 18-month period], others can be found in which euphoria is rare (Braceland and Griffin, 1950). The study of Braceland and Griffin is of note, as they found that only a small percentage of MS patients were euphoric but that those who were had widespread brain involvement. Nonetheless, they suggested that euphoria was a defense mechanism that provided psychological stability.

A particularly well-designed study of emotional disorder in MS patients was reported 20 years ago by Surridge (1969). Among the methodological strengths of his study were the inclusion of all patients in an MS case register rather than examination of patients coming into a clinic for treatment, the use of another informant, and the comparison to a control group of neurologically ill individuals with muscular dystrophy (MD). Surridge found similar rates of depression in the MS and MD groups (27% vs. 13%, respectively, which was not significantly different statistically). In contrast, he found that 26% of the MS patients were euphoric, while none of the MD patients were. This was a statistically significant difference. Importantly, Surridge noted that many of the subjects who initially appeared euphoric often appeared less so as the interview proceeded. He concluded that "instability of the outward appearance of mood" rather than lability per se was common. Surridge demonstrated that 26 of the 28 euphoric patients had evidence of cognitive disorder and that the euphoric patients had more extensive neurologic disability. He concluded that it is the extent of brain involvement that determines euphoria in MS and, by implication, that structrual brain involvement is the cause of the euphoria.

Several methodological issues have plagued studies of euphoria in MS and are yet to be fully resolved. The first problem is the definition of euphoria. Many authors have not described what they mean by euphoria or operationalized its definition. Few, for example, have followed the example of Cottrell and Wilson (1926) in distinguishing between a sustained cheerful mood and the unconcern and unawareness they called eutonia.

Another issue complicating the study of euphoria is the frequency of emotional lability and emotional incontinence. In the latter, patients suffer sudden outbursts of crying or laughter. They generally report that their emotional state is not consonant with their emotional expression, even if the episode is precipitated by an upsetting or happy event. This condition is associated with lesions, usually bilateral, of corticobulbar fibers. Emotional lability, on the other hand, is characterized by wide swings of mood which are experienced by patients as feelings of happiness and sadness. Its frequency as a symptom of MS was noted by Charcot (1873). As noted, Surridge (1969) emphasized that many of the patients he called euphoric reported low or depressed mood when specifically asked; he suggested that outward expression of emotional state in MS patients and their inner experience of mood often differ.

In summary, reported prevalence rates of euphoria in MS range from 0 to 90%. A median figure of 25% can be cited, but it is likely that many of these patients are eutonic rather than euphoric and that many others have the outward appearance of euphoria but the internal experience of a normal or sad mood.

In a previously published study (Rabins et al., 1986), we examined mood, degree of physical handicap, and functional disability in a group of 87 MS patients who filled out questionnaires measuring these variables once per month for 12 months. The patients included in this study were a consecutive series of clinic attenders. Patients were excluded if they were so severely cognitively impaired that they were unable to understand the purpose of the study (and thus were unable to give informed consent) or were unable to fill out the questionnaires on a monthly basis. CT head scans were performed on 38 of the 82 individuals in the study. There was no difference in age, sex distribution, length of illness, or severity between those who did and did not undergo CT scanning.

To measure euphoria we asked the treating neurologist to identify patients whom they considered clinically euphoric. We instructed them to use the definitions of Cottrell and Wilson (1926), designating as euphoric those individuals who fulfilled the definitions of either euphoria sclerotica or eutonia sclerotica.

Using these criteria the neurologist identified 48% of the patients as euphoric, a prevalence rate between those of Cottrell and Wilson (1926) and Surridge (1969).

To examine the hypothesis that euphoria is related to the degree of brain involvement, we examined correlations between euphoria and several measures of brain disease. Euphoric patients were more likely to be designated as having evidence of brain involvement in contrast to spinal cord involvement only ($p = .006$). [The study was done before the availability of magnetic resonance imaging (MRI) scanning, a clear limit to this designation.] The euphoric patients were also more likely to have relapsing-progressive or progressive MS as opposed to the relapsing-remitting form ($p < .0001$), to have enlarged ventricles on CT head scan ($p = .04$), to be more physically disabled ($p = .05$), to be more functionally disabled ($p = .01$), and to have lower scores on the Mini-Mental State (MMS) test, a measure of cognition ($p = .04$).

These results are summarized in Table 11-1 and show that euphoria is seen predominantly in patients with extensive brain involvement. Overall, euphoric patients scored similarly to noneuphoric subjects on the General Health Questionnaire (GHQ), the measure of emotional distress used in this study. This supports

**Table 11-1**  Correlates of Euphoria in MS Patients

MS patients with "euphoria" are more likely than noneuphoric patients to have:
  Brain involvement
  Relapsing-progressive or progressive MS
  Enlarged ventricles

As a group they have:
  Poorer scores on cognitive testing
  More neurological abormalities
  More functional and social disability

Surridge's statement that many patients who appear euphoric are actually experiencing depressive and euthymic mood symptoms; this suggests that the "euphoria" described in MS patients is not a sustained mood state such as that experienced in the manic phase of bipolar affective disorder. These results support the hypothesis proposed by Brown and Davis (1922), Surridge (1969), Ombredane (1929), and others that euphoria results directly from the extent of brain involvement and is not a defense against accepting the severity of the illness. We hypothesize that this syndrome is one aspect of the so-called frontal lobe disconnection syndrome which results from periventricular involvement of pathways coursing toward and coming from the frontal lobes.

We also examined the relationship between euphoria and emotional lability. Emotional lability scores were calculated by taking the mean of the squares of the successive difference of each mood measurement. We found no relationship between mood lability and euphoria, suggesting that they are distinct phenomena. We did not specifically examine patients for the presence of emotional incontinence and so cannot examine any relationship between it and euphoria. No patients in the study had been diagnosed as having bipolar disorder, and none was considered by either the treating neurologist or the principal author to be suffering from a sustained mood state that would be called manic. Subjects on steroids were no more likely to be identified as euphoric than those not on steroids.

This review of the literature and the results of our study suggest several conclusions:

1. Euphoria has multiple meanings. Future studies of euphoria in MS must develop careful descriptions along with reliable and valid measures of the various euphoric mood states. Cottrell and Wilson's (1926) distinction between eutonia and euphoria is of both clinical and theoretical relevance, and the two states should be studied separately.
2. When a distinction is made between true euphoria, that is, a sustained mood state in which the individual experiences a persistent elevation of mood, and eutonia, a state in which patients seem to lack cognizance of the severity of their physical condition, the prevalence of euphoria is low. Fewer than 10% of MS patients experience a persistent elevation of mood.
3. Euphoric mood in MS patients, as defined in its broader sense, correlates with the extent of brain involvement, particularly of periventricular structures. Furthermore, the presence of euphoria correlates with the presence of

dementia. This suggests that euphoria reflects a neurologically based inability to appreciate the severity of deficit rather than a psychogenic denial stage.


## CLINICAL IMPLICATIONS

The recognition that some patients have a lack of concern about their state has relevance both to the treatment of MS patients and to their families. Eutonia or euphoria might lead some patients to be less motivated to change and participate fully in a program designed to readapt them to new functional levels. We suggest that patients who are not fully or actively participating in rehabilitation be examined for the prevalence of eutonic or euphoric states. We do not suggest that patients with these symptoms cannot be rehabilitation candidates, but rather, that the treatment plan must take this into consideration.

The symptom complex of euphoria and eutonia can also be a source of demoralization for the families of patients. The lack of concern characteristic of these states can frustrate family members who are themselves struggling against the symptoms of the illness. By recognizing that the combination of eutonia and euphoria is present, the clinician can directly discuss the issue with the patient and family and try to help the patient deal more effectively with his or her disability. It is imperative that the patient not be blamed for lack of initiative or lack of appreciation, but rather that it be seen as another manifestation of the disease that requires its own treatment.

There is no literature on the effective treatment of euphoria in MS. Its recognition should lead clinicians to try a variety of treatment strategies. It is possible that patients can be taught to appreciate the extent of their defects; the preservation of many intellectual skills in MS patients could then be used to overcome this disability.

Finally, the measurement of eutonia and euphoria and of the associated dementia should be included in MS treatment studies, as should the prevention of their development. This is important because the emotional symptoms of MS are sometimes among the most disabling aspects of the disease. Because there can be dissociations among the motor, cognitive, and emotional symptoms of MS, specific treatments might improve or prevent disorder in one of these realms more than another.


## REFERENCES

Braceland, F.J., and Griffin, M.E. (1950). The mental changes associated with multiple sclerosis (an interim report). *Res. Publ. Assoc. Res. Nerv. Ment. Dis.,* **28,** 450–55.

Brown, S., and Davis, T.K. (1922). The mental symptoms of multiple sclerosis. *Arch. Neurol. Psychiat.,* **7,** 629–34.

Charcot, J.M. (1873). *Lectures on the diseases of the nervous system.* London: New Sydenham Society.

Cottrell, S.S., and Wilson, S.A.K. (1926). The affective symptomatology of disseminated sclerosis. *J. Neurol. Psychopathol.,* **7,** 1–30.

Ombredane, A. (1929). Sur les Troubles Mentaux de la Sclerose en Plaques. These de Paris, cited in Surridge (1969).

Poser, C.M. (1980). Exacerbations, activity, and progression in multiple sclerosis. *Arch. Neurol.,* **37,** 471–74.

Rabins, P.V., Brooks, B.R., O'Donnell, P., Pearlson, G.D., Moberg, P., Jubelt, B., Boyle, P., Dalos, N., and Folstein, M.F. (1986). Structural brain correlates of emotional disorder in multiple sclerosis. *Brain,* **109,** 585–97.

Sachs, B., and Friedman, E.D. (1922). General symptomatologic and differential diagnosis of disseminated sclerosis. *Arch. Neurol. Psychiat.,* **7,** 551–60.

Surridge, D. (1969). An investigation into some psychiatric aspects of multiple sclerosis. *Br. J. Psychiat.,* **115,** 749–64.

Thygesen, P. (1953). *The Course of Disseminated Sclerosis: A Close-up of 105 Attacks.* Copenhagen: Rosenkilde and Bagger.

# 12
## Disturbances of Affect

RANDOLPH B. SCHIFFER

### HISTORICAL NOTES

The clinical association between multiple sclerosis (MS) and a variety of affective disturbances has been known since the time of Charcot (1881). In this sense, it may well represent the first observation of a neurologic disease that affects the neural substrate of the emotions. The *significance* of this association, however, has continued to be elusive for both investigators and clinicians.

Charcot himself appears to have been quite descriptive in his approach to the affective symptomatology observed among patients suffering from MS. He described these syndromes (apathy, pathological weeping and laughter, depression, mania) alongside vertigo and paresis of the extremities, implying that he considered them all signs of nervous system involvement by the disease. His perspective seems quite modern.

This "Charcot position" concerning affective symptomatology is reminiscent of a position taken by some more resent psychiatric observers that MS may *present* initially as an affective disorder (Goodstein and Ferrell, 1977). If the demyelination of MS causes mood disturbances, there should be nothing surprising in such observations. It would be misleading, however, to suggest that this represents a common diagnostic error. Patients with early MS *are* often referred to psychiatrists, but usually with the diagnosis of conversion disorder. In addition, I suspect that the patients described in reports such as Goodstein and Ferrell's actually had other neurologic manifestations of the disease at the time they presented with affective symptoms, which would have been evident on more careful neurologic evaluation.

The extreme development of this "Charcot position" appeared in Cottrell and Wilson's 1926 paper, which has been described in detail by Rabins in the preceding chapter. Briefly, these authors concluded that 100% of their MS patients had experienced affective alteration as a direct sign or symptom of the disease. They concluded that alteration in experienced mood or expressed affect was a "basal" sign of the disease, more reliable in diagnosis than more traditional neurologic findings such as spasticity or weakness.

During the middle years of this century, a different view of the possible link between affective disturbance and MS came from psychoanalytic psychiatry. Instead of viewing emotional disturbances as the product of central nervous system (CNS) pathology, several American authors suggested that emotional stress might have caused the neurologic disease (Langworthy, 1948; Philippopoulos et al., 1958; Mei-Tal et al., 1970; Warren et al., 1982; Grant, 1987). Some of these reports were anecdotal and speculative. Still, when community or mixed neurologic control groups are used in such research, the finding seems to persist that MS patients report a higher degree of emotional distress, or at least distressing life events, before the onset of symptomatic disease. Structural design difficulties inherent in the performance of retrospective studies of this sort probably make firm conclusions impossible. For example, determining the date of MS onset by using the first recalled symptom is questionable. In addition, an anamnestic effect by which patients' recollections are galvanized to life events preceding disease symptoms may also be at work. Observer bias may also be a factor in those studies that have involved interviewer assessments.

A second possible association between affect and MS, that stressful life experiences or emotions might precipitate an MS exacerbation in someone who already has the disease, is reviewed in Chapter 13 and is not discussed here.

A third possibility is that affective disturbance, particularly depression, occurs as a psychological reaction to a very upsetting disease. Historically, this position has been the most recent to receive attention in the literature. As noted in Chapter 11, Surridge (1969) found that 26% of his MS patients demonstrated some degree of depression, compared with 12.9% of his muscular dystrophy controls. The difference was not statistically significant, but Surridge's assertion that the quality of the MS depressions was primarily "reactive" was significant. In favor of such a contention has been evidence that depressive episodes coincide with clinical neurologic exacerbations in many cases (Dalos et al., 1983). Potentially adverse evidence for this point of view is the emerging consensus that frequency or severity of depressive episodes among MS patients are quite independent of disease severity as measured by Kurtzke scores (Rabins et al., 1986; Joffe et al., 1987). It might be that "reactive" psychological explanations for the affective disorders in MS will be difficult or impossible to prove and that they will be indicated only by the absence of the demonstration of convincing biologic mechanisms.

## EPIDEMIOLOGIC STUDIES—DEPRESSION

An important research approach to the connection between affective disorders and neurologic diseases in recent times has been the controlled epidemiologic study.

The reasoning implicit in such studies of MS has been that if there is a greater prevalence or incidence of a specific affective disorder among MS patients, there must be an underlying neurobiological disturbance that accounts for both sets of symptoms.

For depressive spectrum disorders, the first such controlled study was conducted by Baldwin (1952). She administered the Minnesota Multiphasic Personality Inventory (MMPI) to 34 women with MS and 34 normal controls. The MS patients demonstrated not only significantly higher scores on the Depression Scale of the MMPI, but also on seven other scales. The MMPI is a poor instrument for assessing prevalence of depressive disorders among medical patients, but this was the first controlled study to provide evidence of a relationship between MS and depression.

At about the same time as Baldwin's investigation, Pratt (1951) reported the results of his controlled interview study. Pratt interviewed 100 randomly selected MS patients using the same questionnaire used by Cottrell and Wilson 30 years before. One hundred control patients with mixed neurologic diseases affecting the CNS served as controls. He did not find more frequent reports of depressive feelings among the MS patients, although significantly more reports of euphoria and pathological laughing and weeping were found in this group.

Whitlock and Siskind (1980) extended the methodology used in these earlier reports to include an anamnestic assessment of previous depressive episodes in an MS cohort. These authors interviewed 30 MS patients and 30 mixed neurologic controls and found that not only were the MS patients more depressed at time of interview compared with controls, but that eight of the MS patients had histories of depressive episodes prior to clinical onset of their MS. None of the controls had such a history. The authors were unsure as to what to make of this finding and speculated that some of the earlier depressive episodes may have been initial MS symptoms.

The relevance of neurologic exacerbations to mood disturbance was considered in a controlled, prospective study undertaken by Dalos and colleagues (1983). These investigators followed 64 MS patients for one year using the self-report General Health Questionnaire (GHQ). The patients were simultaneously followed neurologically. Twenty-three spinal-cord-injured patients served as controls. Twelve of the MS patients experienced neurologic exacerbations during the study, and during these exacerbations, prominent elevations of scores were seen on all four subscales of the GHQ, including depression, social, anxiety, and somatic. Baseline scores on these scales were also elevated for the MS patients, but the authors drew attention to the importance of disease activity for at least some of the emotional distress experienced by the subjects.

A major design flaw in all of these studies has been the unblinded condition of the interviewers or investigators. That is, those clinicians who dealt with the research patients were also the investigators who, presumably, brought certain biases to the study. One epidemiologic study that has circumvented this problem was conducted by our group at the University of Rochester (Schiffer and Babigian, 1984). In this study, we used a computerized psychiatric register to ascertain types of diagnoses among 368 patients with MS, 402 with temporal lobe epilepsy, and

124 with amyotrophic lateral sclerosis. During a 13-year period, 62% of the MS patients had received a depressive spectrum diagnosis from psychiatric clinicians who were not part of an investigation and who presumably would have been blind to our hypotheses.

Another important conceptual problem for such epidemiologic studies has been the comparison group. It is not surprising that individuals with a chronic and threatening neurologic disease might demonstrate more depressive episodes than matched normal controls. But what is the appropriate comparison group? In an effort to address this problem, Minden and her colleagues (1987) compared scores on the Beck Depression Inventory for 50 randomly selected MS patients with published scores on this inventory among various general medical populations. The MS cohort still demonstrated higher scores on this inventory than most of the medical comparison groups.

To summarize the epidemiologic research concerning depressive disorders and MS, most of the controlled studies have indicated greater incidence and prevalence of depressive features among MS patients when compared with other neurologic controls. All studies are flawed by one or more design problems having to do with selection, observer bias, psychiatric diagnostic criteria, or comparability of control groups. It seems likely that a definitive study in this area will be difficult or impossible to perform and that the question of a specific connection between MS and depressive disorders will await the elucidation of a plausible neurobiologic mechanism (see the following).

## EPIDEMIOLOGIC STUDIES—BIPOLAR DISORDER

All affective syndromes defined clinically are probably heterogeneous with regard to underlying neurobiologic mechanisms, but there is some reason to believe that bipolar disorder may be a more homogeneous syndrome than unipolar disorder. For example, data from restriction fragment length polymorphism studies of genomes from various families implicate vulnerability genes from chromosome X and chromosome 11 in some bipolar pedigrees (Baron et al., 1987; Egeland et al., 1987). It is interesting, therefore, to note that there are a number of anecdotal reports concerning the coexistence of mania and MS within individual patients (Kellner et al., 1984; Peselow et al., 1981; Mapelli and Ramelli, 1981; Solomon, 1978; Kemp et al., 1977). Our group has reported a lifetime risk for bipolar disorder among MS patients in Monroe County, New York, which is at least twice that seen among comparable populations free of neurologic disease (Schiffer et al., 1986). Joffe and colleagues (1987) in Toronto have provided some confirmation of this report. In a standardized psychiatric assessment of 100 consecutive MS patients, using Research Diagnostic Criteria, these authors reported that 13% had past psychiatric histories that met criteria for bipolar disorder. These studies are smaller and fewer than the studies implicating an association between MS and unipolar disorder, but bipolar disorder is less common than unipolar depression. In addition, the clinical signs and symptoms of mania are less likely to be mistaken for such symptoms of the neurologic disease as fatigue, energy, and weakness. Taken together, it is reasonable to say that there is suggestive evidence for an association on clinical grounds between bipolar disorder and MS.

## EPIDEMIOLOGIC STUDIES—NEUROLOGICALLY BASED AFFECTIVE DISORDERS

Included under this rubric are those abnormalities of emotion that have been characterized variously by the terms lability, pathologic emotionality, euphoria, eutonia, *spes sclerotica,* and similar appellations. A more detailed discussion of these syndromes is found in Chapter 11. They differ from unipolar and bipolar affective disorders in certain respects. First, these syndromes appear to be directly attributable to structural brain disease, while this remains a moot point with regard to unipolar and bipolar disorders. Second, these disorders are not quite like the emotional disorders seen in psychiatric patients. Emotional lability, for example, is probably a misnomer for the abnormality of emotional regulation experienced by some MS patients. A true emotional lability, in which rapid oscillations of feeling state occur, may be seen in certain psychiatric patients with such syndromes as borderline personality disorder. In the emotional dysregulation syndrome experienced by MS patients, however, the experienced or subjective emotional state may not be so much affected as the *displayed* emotional state. It is as if a *disconnection* had arisen between neuronal centers involved in perceived emotion and those involved in displayed emotion, and no doubt this is what happens. Patients may weep or laugh with slight provocation, and without regard for their underlying mood state. We prefer the term *pathologic laughing and weeping* for this syndrome, to distinguish it from the true emotional lability seen among some psychiatric patients. There has been little epidemiologic research involving these disturbances of emotional regulation.

## MECHANISMS OF THE RELATIONSHIP BETWEEN AFFECTIVE DISORDERS AND MS

We are probably close to the limits of scientific benefit that can accrue from intergroup comparisons of patients with MS and affective disorders. The specification of the neurologic or psychologic link will more likely depend on future intragroup research. What is different about MS patients who develop affective disorders compared with those who do not? Is there some neurobiologic feature of the neurologic disease that could plausibly explain the associated mood disturbances?

With reference to unipolar disorders, there is some evidence that the neuroanatomic locus of disease activity is relevant as a risk factor for the development of a depressive illness. In a study at Rochester, we found that MS patients who seemed to have cerebral disease involvement on clinical grounds were more likely to have a history of depressive episodes than were patients with primarily spinal involvement (Schiffer et al., 1983). Rabins and his colleagues (1986) found similarly by CT scan that MS patients with cerebral involvement were more likely to score highly on the depression subscale of the GHQ than were patients with primarily spinal-cord involvement. These studies are limited by the fact that both clinical examination and CT scan are relatively crude techniques by which to judge cerebral MS activity.

In the first study to use magnetic resonance imaging (MRI) to address this problem, Honer and colleagues (1987) at the University of British Columbia scanned eight MS patients with psychiatric disorders and eight matched controls without such disorders. Six of the eight psychiatric patients had bipolar or unipolar disorder. They found that although the two groups did not differ with regard to total MS plaque volume, the psychiatric group had a greater proportion of plaques within temporal lobe structures. This result could be very interesting if replicated with larger numbers of patients and more homogeneous psychiatric diagnoses.

The possibility of a cognitive mediation in the depressive episodes of MS patients is suggested by evidence from Rao and his colleagues (1984). Results of their study suggested that MS patients with mild to moderate cognitive impairments on neuropsychological testing are more likely to report depression than patients without cognitive deficits or patients with severe cognitive impairment. In view of certain cognitive theories concerning the etiology of depression, it is conceivable that mildly impaired cognition might somehow predispose an individual to affective disturbance. Such an idea remains quite speculative now but deserves further investigation. An alternative explanation for this finding is that advancing structural brain damage from MS produces both the cognitive impairments and the mood disorder, but by separate mechanisms.

It is not clear whether bipolar disorder differs from unipolar disorder in terms of pathophysiology when these syndromes occur among MS patients. We have presented some preliminary evidence, however, to suggest a shared genetic vulnerability to the co-occurrence of MS and bipolar disorder within individuals (Schiffer et al., 1988). In a family history and genetic marker study of MS/bipolar, MS/unipolar, and MS/no affective disorder patients, we found a more prominent family history both for bipolar disorder and for MS within the MS/bipolar cohort. In addition, the bipolar patients seemed to demonstrate an increased frequency of the HLA (human leukocyte antigen) allele, DR2, and decreased frequencies of DR1 and DR4 compared with the unipolar and no affective disorder groups. These studies, too, are preliminary and will require confirmation in other MS populations. Still, one fact about the affective disorders seen in MS that might be well explained by a genetic model is the substantial number of affective episodes that seem to occur *prior to* the first MS symptom. These prior affective events pose somewhat of a problem for the neuroanatomic theories concerning an MS/affective connection.

What I have called the neurologically based affective disturbances of MS present less of a problem with regard to putative neurobiologic mechanisms. Similar forms of pathological laughing and weeping are seen in stroke, amyotrophic lateral sclerosis, and other diseases that damage subcortical forebrain structures. It is generally accepted that this produces a "disconnectionlike" loss of cortical modulation over brain-stem bulbar nuclei that produce affective display. What is *not* settled are the relevant tracts that are involved. One retrospective study implicated damage to the right hemisphere in right-handed persons as more likely to produce pathological emotionality (Sackheim et al., 1982), but other authors believe that bilateral damage is needed. Some very recent clinical research on stroke patients suggests that pontine brain-stem lesions, or lesions connecting the mid-right cerebral hemisphere with the pons, may be implicated in this syndrome (Tatemichi et al., 1987; Yarnell, 1987).

## TREATMENT OF AFFECTIVE DISORDERS

There are several reasons to consider that usual psychotherapeutic and psychopharmacological treatments might be less effective among MS patients than among general psychiatric patients, or that they might at least require modification. For psychopharmacological treatments, absorption and distribution kinetics might be quite different among MS patients. GI motility is altered among such patients, for example, and alterations of the blood-brain barrier function may also occur. Second, the side-effect spectrum of psychotropic drugs could reasonably be expected to be altered among MS patients, especially with regard to their ability to tolerate autonomic side effects. And lastly, it could well be the case that in MS, neurobiologic effector mechanisms for psychotropics could be altered if specific neuropathological processes are generating the affective disturbances. In psychotherapeutic terms, even greater departures from techniques that have been successful in psychiatric populations might be expected. The psychotherapeutic field in this disease is characterized by the complexity of the individual life history and conflicts for each patient, plus the additional problems of here-and-now alterations of bodily integrity over which the patient has only fantasied control.

Unhappily, relatively little clinical research has been done in the broad area of therapy for MS/affective disorders.

For unipolar depressive disorders, no properly controlled trials of antidepressants have appeared yet, although we have recently completed such a trial, and another is in progress in Canada. In our study, 28 MS patients who met Research Diagnostic Criteria for major depressive episode were randomized either to a desipramine plus psychotherapy treatment or to psychotherapy plus placebo. Fourteen patients were randomized to the placebo arm and fourteen to the desipramine arm of the study. Details of the study are in press, but we found a significantly greater rate of improvement in depression in the desipramine group compared with the placebo group. Our conclusion is that most MS patients can tolerate a therapeutic dosage of desipramine and that this drug is approximately as effective for depression associated with MS as for depression in general psychiatric populations.

It has been our clinical experience that the bipolar disorders among MS patients respond as well to lithium therapy as do bipolar disorders among general psychiatric patients. Controlled studies of this matter are not available, but uncontrolled observations such as those cited by Kellner et al. (1984) and by Kemp et al. (1977) would seem to corroborate this opinion.

With regard to the neurologically based affective disorders, the euphoria, eutonia, and related syndromes do not usually occasion therapeutic interventions, since both patient and family often find them pleasant. The pathological laughing and weeping, on the other hand, is often distressing and sometimes disabling. Our group (Schiffer et al., 1985) reported a double-blind, crossover study of low-dose amitriptyline that produced dramatic improvement when the syndrome was especially severe or when the syndrome included pathological laughing. These patients were not particularly depressed despite the paroxysmal weeping many of them experienced, and scaled measures of depression did not change during the study. No patient received more than 75 mg per day of amitriptyline. In cases of pathological laughing and weeping that do not improve with amitriptyline, we have found it useful first to consider whether an underlying major depressive syndrome may be present. When this is the case, longer therapeutic trials and higher doses of antidepressants are required. Rarely, a case of true pathological laughing and weeping is present but does not respond to amitriptyline. In these instances we have treated patients with levodopa. There are two uncontrolled reports of the successful use of levodopa in pathological emotionality (Wolf et al., 1979; Udaka et al., 1984), and it has been our experience that it does help.

We do not know the most helpful forms of psychotherapy for MS/affective patients. Again, our group has described three general psychotherapeutic positions which we have intended for use by the treating neurologist (Schiffer, 1987). We have suggested that neurologists should take their cues from the patients' levels of psychological mindedness. Some patients with neurologic disease and major depression are unable to confront any psychological issues concerning their feelings. For these, we have suggested a traditional "medical" stance on the part of the treating physician, labeling the mood disorder much like any other medical sign or symptom and prescribing antidepressants. We have labeled such an approach the "William Osler" therapy. Other patients have more insight into psychosocial conflicts relevant to their feelings but still fall short of the psychological mindedness which is prerequisite for true psychotherapy. These patients tend to focus their attention on events and people in the environment, such as job structure or family structures, and often real benefits can be reaped from working with such environmental factors. Since these interventions are more interpersonal and social by nature, we have labeled this approach the "Thorstein Veblen" posture. Lastly, there are patients with MS/depression who are able to examine their feelings and their neurologic disease in the global context of their life histories and to consider the meaning of these events. Such people are in a minority but are amenable to an insight-utilizing approach, which involves a reexamination of the current situation in the light of past conflict. It is our belief that patients who are able to do this are better off in the long run, without any necessary implication that psychotherapy affects the neurologic disease. We have labeled this approach, fittingly, the "Sigmund Freud" posture.

To summarize, the various affective disturbances associated with MS should prove to be both scientifically interesting and clinically relevant as we come to learn more about them. They may have much to teach us concerning the neurobiology of at least some affective disorders, and they are potentially treatable sources of dysfunction and disability for the patients who have them. Hopefully, future clinical and basic research will reveal the presence or absence of specific neurobiological connections between MS and affective disturbance, and we will become more effective in our treatments of these syndromes.

## ACKNOWLEDGMENT

Clinical research efforts related to this chapter were supported by NIH Grant RR000444 and New Investigator Research Award 1 R23NS20838-01 from NINDS.

## REFERENCES

Baldwin, M.V. (1952). A clinico-experimental investigation into the psychologic aspects of multiple sclerosis. *J. Nerv. Ment. Dis.,* **115**, 299–342.

Baron, M., Risch, N., Hamburger, R., Mandel, B., Kushaer, S., Newman, M., Drumer, D., and Belmaker, R.H. (1987). Genetic linkage between X-chromosome markers and bipolar affective illness. *Nature,* **326**, 289–92.

Charcot, S.M. (1881). *Lectures on the Diseases of the Nervous System Delivered at La Salpetrier.* London: New Sydenham Society 2.

Cottrell, S.S., and Wilson, S.A.K. (1926). The affective symptomatology of disseminated sclerosis: A study of 100 cases. *J. Neurol. Psychopathol.,* **7**, 1–30.

Dalos, N.P., Rabins, P.V., Brooks, B.R., and O'Donnell, P. (1983). Disease activity and emotional state in multiple sclerosis. *Ann. Neurol.,* **13**, 573–77.

Egeland, J.A., Gerhard, D.S., Pauls, D.L., Sussex, J.N., Kidd, K.K., Allen, C.R., Hostetter, A.M., and Housman, D.C. (1987). Bipolar affective disorders linked to DNA markers on chromosome 11. *Nature,* **325**, 783–87.

Goodstein, R.K., and Ferrell, R.B. (1977). Multiple sclerosis—presenting as depressive illness. *Dis. Nerv. Syst.,* **38**, 117–27.

Grant, I. (November 1987). Life events and onset and exacerbation of symptoms of multiple sclerosis. Presented at the Symposium on Mental Disorders, Cognitive Deficits, and Their Treatment in Multiple Sclerosis, Odense, Denmark.

Honer, W.G., Hurwitz, T., Li, D.K.B., Palmer, M., and Paty, D.W. (1987). Temporal lobe involvement in multiple sclerosis patients with psychiatric disorders. *Arch. Neurol.,* **44**, 187–90.

Joffe, R.T., Lippert, G.P., Gray, T.A., Sawa, G., and Horvath, Z. (1987). Mood disorder and multiple sclerosis. *Arch. Neurol.,* **44**, 376–78.

Kellner, C.H., Davenport, Y., Post, R.M., and Ross R.J. (1984). Rapidly cycling bipolar disorder and multiple sclerosis. *Am. J. Psychiat.,* **141**, 112–13.

Kemp, K., Lion, J.R., and Magram, G. (1977). Lithium in the treatment of a manic patient with multiple sclerosis: A case report. *Dis. Nerv. Syst.,* **38**, 210–11.

Langworthy, O.R. (1948). Relation of personality problems to onset and progress of multiple sclerosis. *Arch. Neurol. Psychiat.,* **59**, 13–28.

Mapelli, G., and Ramelli, E. (1981). Manic syndrome associated with multiple sclerosis: Secondary mania? *Acta Psychiatr. Belg.,* **81**, 337–49.

Mei-Tal, V., Meyerowitz, S., and Engel, G.L. (1970). The role of psychological process in a somatic disorder: Multiple sclerosis. *Psychosom. Med.,* **32**, 67–86.

Minden, S.L., Orav, J., and Reich, P. (1987). Depression in multiple sclerosis. *Gen. Hosp. Psychiat.,* **9**, 426–34.

Peselow, E.D., Deutsch, S.I., Fieve, R.R., and Kaufman, M. (1981). Coexistent manic symptoms and multiple sclerosis. *Psychosomatics,* **22**, 824–25.

Phillippopoulos, G.S., Wittkower, E.D., and Cousineau, A. (1958). The etiologic significance of emotional factors in onset and exacerbations of multiple sclerosis. *Psychosom. Med.,* **20**, 458–74.

Pratt, R.T.C. (1951). An investigation of the psychiatric aspects of disseminated sclerosis. *J. Neurol. Neurosurg. Psychiat.,* **14,** 326–35.

Rabins, P.V. Brooks, B.R., O'Donnell, P., Pearlson, G.D., Moberg, P., Jubelt, B., Boyle, P., Dalos, N., and Folstein, M.F. (1986). Structural brain correlates of emotional disorder in multiple sclerosis. *Brain,* **109,** 585–97.

Rao, S.M., Hammeke, T.A., McQuillen, M.P., Khatri, B.O., and Lloyd, D. (1984). Memory disturbance in chronic progressive multiple sclerosis. *Arch. Neurol.,* **41,** 625–31.

Sackheim, H.A., Greenberg, M.S., Weiman, A.L., Gur, R.D., Hungerbuhler, J.P., and Geschwind, N. (1982). Hemispheric asymmetry in the expression of positive and negative emotions. *Arch. Neurol.,* **39,** 210–18.

Schiffer, R.B. (1987). The spectrum of depression in multiple sclerosis: An approach for clinical management. *Arch. Neurol.,* **44,** 596–99.

Schiffer, R.B. Weitkamp, L.R., Wineman, N.M., and Guttormsen, S. (1988). Multiple sclerosis and affective disorder: Family history, sex, and HLA-DR antigens. *Arch. Neurol.,* **45,** 1345–48.

Schiffer, R.B., and Babigian, H.M. (1984). Behavioral disorders in multiple sclerosis, temporal lobe epilepsy, and amyotrophic lateral sclerosis: An epidemiologic study. *Arch. Neurol.,* **41,** 1067–69.

Schiffer, R.B., Caine, E.D., Bamford, K.A., and Levy, S. (1983) Depressive episodes in patients with multiple sclerosis. *Am. J. Psychiat.,* **140,** 1498–1500.

Schiffer, R.B., Herndon, R.M., and Rudick, R.A. (1985). Treatment of pathologic laughing and weeping with amitriptyline. *N. Engl. J. Med.,* **312,** 1480–82.

Schiffer, R.B., Winemen, N.M., and Weitkamp, L.R. (1986). Association between bipolar affective disorder and multiple sclerosis. *Am. J. Psychiat.,* **143,** 94–5.

Solomon, J.G. (1978). Multiple sclerosis masquerading as lithium toxicity. *J. Nerv. Ment. Dis.,* **166,** 663–65.

Surridge, D. (1969). An investigation into some psychiatric aspects of multiple sclerosis. *Br. J. Psychiat.,* **115,** 749–64.

Tatemichi, T.K., Nichols, F.T., and Mohr, J.P. (1987). Pathological crying: A pontine pseudobulbar syndrome. *Ann. Neurol.,* **22 (Suppl. 1),** 133.

Udaka, F., Yamao, S., Nagata, H., Nakamura, S., and Kumeyama, M. (1984). Pathological laughing and crying treated with levodopa. *Arch. Neurol.,* **41,** 1095–196.

Warren, S., Greenhill, S., and Warren, K.G. (1982). Emotional stress and the development of multiple sclerosis: Case-control evidence of a relationship. *J. Chron. Dis.,* **35,** 821–31.

Whitlock, F.A., and Siskind, M.M. (1980). Depression as a major symptom of multiple sclerosis. *J. Neurol. Neurosurg. Psychiat.,* **43,** 861–65.

Wolf, J.K., Santana, H.B., and Thorpy, M. (1979). Treatment of 'emotional incontinence' with levodopa. *Neurology (Minneapolis),* **29,** 1435–36.

Yarnell, P.R. (1987). Pathological crying localization. *Ann. Neurol.,* **22 (Suppl. 1),** 133.

# 13

# The Role of Stress
# in Multiple Sclerosis

SHARON WARREN

## WHY STUDY STRESS AND MS?

Interest in a possible relationship between stress and multiple sclerosis (MS) began with the first recorded description of MS. In his diary entitled "The Case of Augustus d'Este, 1822–46," the illegitimate son of Augustus, Duke of Sussex, described symptoms characteristic of the disease that began immediately after the death of a father-figure (Firth, 1941). Based on this case and his experience with several others, Charcot (1877)—the physician who gave MS its name—suggested that emotional shock might play a role in MS etiology.

Early case series provided evidence of an association between stress and MS, but controlled studies have typically been negative or ambiguous. The failure of controlled studies to demonstrate an association may indicate that no significant relationship exists. On the other hand, this failure may be due to the particular methodological difficulties involved in studying stress and MS.

While researchers have taken less interest in stress as an etiological factor recently, patients remain vitally concerned about its effects on disease activity. Since the illness is often characterized by relapsing-remitting symptoms and a variable course, many patients look for ways to minimize exacerbations and disability by altering their lifestyles or environment. While patients are not always able to control events in their lives, the literature suggests that stress reactions are modifiable (Coyne and Lazarus, 1980; Goldberger and Breznitz, 1982). If a relationship between stress and disease activity could be confirmed, then clinicians might be more willing to arrange psychotherapy for patients committed to its possible benefits.

In the past few years, some patients have had another reason for wanting the relationship between stress and MS clarified. Some who believe strongly in the negative effects of stress have launched liability suits against parties whom they blame for unusual stress in their lives, claiming that this has contributed to a decline in their health. Lawyers have begun seeking advice and testimony from experts in the field of stress and MS, but only equivocal evidence of a relationship is available.

## STUDIES OF STRESS AND DISEASE ACTIVITY

Stress research in MS has focused on two aspects: whether stress contributes to the onset of disease and whether it precipitates exacerbations.

### Stress and Onset

Research related to onset dominated early studies, which were primarily based on case series. In general, case series have provided positive support for a relationship between stress and MS.

Moxon (1875) found two patients out of eight who claimed that their symptoms followed an emotional shock with sexual content—the discovery of a husband's affair and the death of a sister in childbirth. Russell (1911), Bramwell (1917), McAlpine (1946), and Adams et al. (1950) also provided evidence that stress occasionally preceded the onset of symptoms in MS.

Two later case series provided more striking support for a relationship between stress and MS. In 1958, Philippopoulos et al. reported case studies in which 35 out of 40 patients described traumatic experiences preceding the onset of their disease. In 1970, Mei-tal et al. found that a psychologically stressful situation immediately preceded onset in 28 out of 32 MS patients.

Case-control studies of a possible relationship between stress and MS have produced conflicting results, but negative findings have predominated. Braceland and Giffin (1950) found no obvious difference between MS patients and neurologic controls when asked whether they associated emotional trauma with the onset of their disease. In 1951 Pratt described a nonsignificant trend in which more MS patients than neurologic controls reported an unusual disturbance or generalized stress within one month before onset of their specific conditions. Baldwin (1952) compared the life histories of 34 patients and 34 neurologic controls; she found that controls had experienced just as many traumatic events as MS patients, but that the MS patients seemed to have had less stability in their lives.

The results of a study by Alter et al. (1968) were ambiguous. They compared MS patients with normal controls for specific types of stressful events at any time prior to onset. Cases and controls differed significantly in their experience of some events, such as difficult wartime experiences and adjustment to postwar immigration, but did not differ on others, such as the death of close family members and friends or periods of unemployment.

Warren et al. (1982) reported the first generally positive relationship between emotional stress and MS. They compared 100 MS patients with 100 hospital controls with primarily neurologic conditions. Significantly more MS patients than controls reported that they were under unusual stress in the two-year period prior to onset. MS patients in this study also described a greater number of stressful life situations or single events than controls did.

## Stress and Exacerbations

A possible link between stress and MS exacerbations has received less attention. Early research, based on case studies, produced negative results. In 1950 Brickner and Simons studied 50 MS patients for evidence that emotional stress had precipitated exacerbations. Only 14% of the patients reported that exacerbations had occurred during, or immediately following, a period of unusual stress. Likewise Pratt (1951) found that only 58 out of 229 exacerbations were preceded by unusual stress in his series of 100 MS patients.

In 1984 Malmgren et al. reported on a prospective study of stress and MS exacerbations that was also negative. From 1976 to 1978, 125 MS patients made a total of 805 visits to the University of California (Los Angeles) MS Research Clinic. Patients were seen at regular intervals and during relapses. At each visit, patients answered a questionnaire about recent exposure to seven types of emotional stress. Relapse rates following unusual stress were compared with relapse rates following visits where no unusual stress was reported, with no significant difference observed.

Research underway at the University of Alberta MS Clinic, however, indicates that there may be a relationship between emotional stress and MS exacerbations. Patients experiencing an exacerbation are being compared with patients in remission on a number of factors that might precipitate a relapse, including trauma, infection, diet, exercise, and pregnancy, in addition to emotional stress. Three scales are being used to assess stress and coping mechanisms: Goldberg and Hillier's General Health Questionnaire (GHQ), a measure of emotional disturbance that includes somatic symptoms, anxiety, social dysfunction, and depression; Lazarus' Daily Hassles and Uplifts Scale; and the Ways of Coping Checklist. To date, 74 age- and sex-matched pairs in exacerbation/remission have been analyzed, and only stress is related to MS exacerbations. More patients in exacerbation than remission score above the median when compared on Goldberg and Hillier's measure of emotional disturbance. More patients in exacerbation also score above the median on Lazarus' Daily Hassles Scale. There is no significant difference, however, between patients in exacerbation/remission in terms of their use of problem- versus emotion-focused coping to deal with stressful events.

## Summary

The role of stress in preciptiating MS onset or exacerbations remains unclear. Since research into a possible relationship between stress and illness intensified approximately 45 years ago, studies have linked emotional stress to a wide variety of diseases. As with MS, however, the findings have frequently been contradictory or weak—with stress virtually never explaining more than 10% of the variance. It may be, as some authors have suggested, that stress merely increases general susceptibility to illness and can be a minor component of any disease (Dodge and Martin, 1970). On the other hand, failure to demonstrate a clear-cut, important relationship between stress and MS may be due to the methodological difficulties involved in studying such a relationship.

## METHODOLOGICAL PROBLEMS IN THE STUDY OF STRESS AND MS

Several methodological problems complicate the study of a possible relationshp between stress and MS, including research design, the measurement of stress, and the question of intervening variables such as coping ability.

### Research Design

When studying the relationship between stress and MS, researchers have typically used one of two research designs: the case series or the case-control method.

The case-series approach is weaker. Without a control group, there is no standard by which to judge the experience of cases. For example, a researcher might be impressed that 75% of his patients report experiencing an emotionally stressful event immediately prior to onset of MS symptoms and interpret this as positive evidence of a relationship. If a group of neurologic controls were also questioned, however, a similar percentage might report experiencing unusual stress prior to onset of their own conditions.

Unlike the case series, the retrospective case-control study does provide a standard of comparison for cases. In this design the researcher identifies a group of individuals who have the disease (cases) and a group who do not (controls). These two groups are compared on the presence of factors thought to be associated with MS onset, to determine whether a statistically significant difference exists.

The case-control design involves other methodological problems, however. One of these is establishing the age at onset in MS patients. It is usually impossible to fix the exact age at which disease activity began in any patient, because MS may remain asymptomatic over long periods of time. Some researchers studying etiology use age at diagnosis, even though equivocal symptoms may have been present for several years. A more appropriate guideline might be the first configuration of MS symptoms severe enough to suggest medical attention, but even this designation complicates the assessment of temporal sequence between supposed cause and effect. If a patient reports that such a configuration occurred at age 25, should questions about stress refer to the period immediately prior to age 25, when in fact the disease process may have begun years before the appearance of clear-cut symptoms? Some clinicians argue that reports of increased stress prior to onset might be due to occult disease, for example, that unnoticed symptoms caused personality changes leading to marital breakdown and family disagreement instead of such stresses precipitating MS. The same issue applies when studying stress and exacerbations whose beginnings may be silent.

In any study of stress and onset, consideration must also be given to the period of time about which controls are questioned. If neurologic controls are selected, should they be asked about stressful events prior to the occurrence of their own disease or prior to the age when MS appeared in cases to whom they are matched? People often dwell on events immediately preceding an illness, which may have caused it, so that their memories of this time tend to be sharper. Also, certain life events may be more common at one age than another. For example, Kanner et al. (1981) have observed that older people considering retirement are often primarily concerned about their economic circumstances, while middle-aged individuals are more likely to report worries associated with family and job responsibilities. Consequently, it might not be appropriate to compare preonset stressors in an MS patient whose disease appeared at age 25 with preonset stressors in a neurologic control whose disease began at 45, particularly because the events associated with different ages tend to vary in the amount of stress they imply (Pearlin and Lieberman, 1977; Hultsch and Plemons, 1979; Brim and Ryff, 1980).

The choice of a comparison group is in itself problematic. Controls with a disease tend to remember more about past events than healthy controls. However, if MS patients are compared with neurologic controls drawn from a single group such as migraine sufferers, and stress happens to be a precipitating factor in that condition, then any relationship between stress and MS would be masked. If a neurologic condition that is known not to be influenced by stress could be identified, then the control group having that diagnosis can be assumed to be representative of the general population with respect to stress. If such a condition cannot be clearly identified, a cross-section of neurologic controls or nonneurologic controls with a variety of illnesses is preferable to a single diagnostic group.

The problem of recall bias in case-control studies has already been alluded to. MS patients often try to identify the cause of their disease. Patients may remember more stressful events prior to onset than healthy controls who have had no reason to review their histories, and MS patients may also exaggerate the impact of those events in retrospect. The same may be true for MS patients in exacerbation who are being compared with patients in remission, although the problem of recall bias is probably aggravated in studies of onset when patients and controls are asked to remember long-past events.

Besides such design issues, researchers studying a possible relationship between stress and MS must deal with problems in the measurement of stress itself.

## Stress Measurement Tools

Experts seem to agree that any event requiring an individual to readjust his or her attitudes or behavior can be stressful, and that coping strategies can buffer the impact of a stressful event. There has been some disagreement, however, about the role of major versus minor events; the relative importance of negative, positive, and neutral events; and whether specific events are more stressful for some people than others. These issues are reflected in the two most widely used stress measurement tools: Holmes and Rahe's Social Readjustment Rating Scale (1967); and Lazarus' Daily Hassles and Uplifts Scale (see Kanner et al., 1981).

Early research attempted to demonstrate a connection between illness onset and the sheer number of changes in an individuals's life. The effects of these events were assumed to be equal and additive; that is, more events were expected to have a greater effect. Major life events were emphasized, regardless of their negative or positive connotations. In developing the Social Readjustment Rating Scale, Holmes and Rahe continued to focus on major events with little distinction between positive and negative changes. They did recognize, however, that the impact of various events might differ. Holmes and Rahe asked a large group of people to list common family, occupational, financial, and personal events that would cause them stress. Respondents were also asked to rank these events in order from least to most stressful and to assign each event a score from 1 to 100, depending on the amount of readjustment they would require. From the items suggested, Holmes and Rahe selected 43 that were consistently listed as stressful and averaged the scores assigned to them by respondents. This resulted in a scale that could measure both the number and weight of stressful events that had occurred in people's lives during a specified time period. For example, the death of a spouse is given the highest possible score of 100; marriage is rated 50; and the lowest score is for a minor violation of the law, rated at 11. Individuals are given a total score based on the sum of the scores assigned to the items they check. These scores are referred to as life change units, and episodes of illness are expected to rise with the total score.

For several years most researchers used Holmes and Rahe's original Social Readjustment Rating Scale or a modified version of it; however, the tool gradually received more scrutiny and criticism. Although Holmes and Rahe supported the contention that positive changes require adapation (and thus could also bring about illness), their measure is heavily weighted toward negative changes. The scale also emphasizes major rather than minor events, largely ignores the possibility that no change could be stressful, and provides no formal option for people to describe stressors that are not included in the list. The Social Readjustment Rating Scale does incorporate some weighting of events, but it assumes that specific events have the same impact on each individual; for example, any person experiencing divorce is assigned 73 life change units, even though for some the circumstances of their divorce might be much more stressful than for others.

Lazarus constructed his Daily Hassles and Uplifts Scales to avoid these criticisms. He argued that the relatively minor stresses and pleasures that characterize everyday life actually have immense adaptational significance and cannot be ignored as a source of stress. Lazarus defines hassles as the irritating, frustrating, and distressing problems that people face in the normal course of living, and he also recognizes that no change may constitute a hassle under certain circumstances; uplifts are life's enjoyable moments. Since no one leads a hassle-free or pleasureless life, he adds that any impact of minor events on health must depend on their frequency or importance to the individual.

The Hassles Scale consists of 117 hassles that were generated by Lazarus and his colleagues, using as their guidelines the areas of health, family and friends, work, the environment, practical considerations, and chance occurrences. Examples include declining physical appearance, not enough time spent with family members, routine on the job, debts, traffic jams, and losing things. The items Lazarus and his staff generated were "pilot-tested" for completeness by a group of Kaiser-Permanente patients, and eventually an open-ended question for respondents to add their own unique hassles was included. Respondents check which hassles they have experienced during the previous three months and indicate their impact on a three-point scale—a score of 1, 2, or 3 corresponding to little, moderate, and considerable impact. Two summary scores can be generated: the number of hassles experienced and their average intensity, which is calculated by dividing the sum of the three-point severity ratings for each checked hassle by the number of hassles experienced.

The counterpart Uplifts Scale, which measures positive experiences, is constructed in a similar fashion. It consists of 135 uplifts generated using the same content area as hassles. Examples include recovering from a minor illness, relaxing with friends, using skills well at work, enjoying nature, and a piece of good luck. As with the Hassles Scale, respondents check uplifts they have experienced in the previous three months and rate their impact on a three-point scale from little through moderate to considerable. Frequency and intensity scores can be generated.

In 1983 Lazarus reviewed the use of life events versus daily hassles for measuring stress. His research team has observed that both hassles frequency and intensity are better predictors of psychological and somatic health than life events. Hassles and life events are only modestly correlated, and although hassles scores make a unique contribution to the variance in health, life events do not. While hassles and uplifts are highly correlated, uplifts alone are not a useful predictor of health outcomes. Lazarus' observations have been published by members of his team (Kanner et al., 1981; DeLongis et al., 1982), and his observations about hassles and psychological symptoms have been supported in independent research (Monroe, 1983).

Despite its apparent advantages in predicting health outcomes, the Hassles Scale is probably less appropriate than the Social Readjustment Rating Scale for examining stress and MS onset. Because patients may be enrolled in a case-control study years after onset, it seems unlikely that they could report hassles as accurately as life events. Prospective studies of stress and onset using either scale are unlikely because of the low MS incidence rate. On the other hand, hassles may be a more appropriate measure of stress prior to exacerbations than life events; if patients are identified in the midst of an exacerbation, their recall of recent hassles may be relatively accurate.

Even if stress can be measured successfully, it is apparent that many people who experience traumatic life changes and severe chronic stress do not become ill—perhaps because of their ability to cope with stressful situations. Studies of stress and MS have typically neglected to examine coping as a possible buffer.

## Coping as an Intervening Variable

Coping is generally viewed as playing a central role in human adaptation to stress, and there is little disagreement over its basic definition. Coping is defined as the management of demands that are perceived as taxing or exceeding an individual's resources.

There is some debate over the number of coping strategies in the human repertoire and the definition of specific strategies such as denial or avoidance. Nevertheless, coping strategies have generally been divided into two broad categories: problem-focused coping involves altering the source of stress; emotion-focused coping implies the regulation of alarming reactions to stressful events (Lazarus and Folkman, 1984).

The most common approach to coping has been to view it as a trait or person-ality style, on the assumption that people are consistent in how they manage their problems. In 1974 Moos reviewed several coping assessment tools and found that all asked individuals what they would usually do in various types of stressful situations. These scales also attempted to assign respondents a coping strategy "label," either a fairly narrow one like avoidance-oriented or a broader classification such as problem- versus emotion-focused coping. On the whole, however, general coping styles have not proven to be good predictors of behavior in specific situations (Cohen and Lazarus, 1973; Lazarus et al., 1974). It might be possible, for example, to classify an individual as primarily problem-focused, but virtually no one is entirely consistent in this respect. Problem-focused coping is often used to manage situations over which people feel they have some control and emotion-focused coping (e.g., denial or avoidance) in unchangeable situations (Pearlin and Schooler, 1978). Since everyone encounters both changeable and unchangeable stressors in the course of daily life, individuals tend to use a variety of coping strategies, depending on the circumstances (Folkman and Lazarus, 1980).

Recently there has been a shift to the assessment of coping as a response to situational demands. This approach considers what a person actually does in a specific encounter, how coping behavior varies from one event to another and over the course of a single event. The Ways of Coping Checklist (Folkman and Lazarus, 1985) is one situation-oriented coping assessment tool that offers an alternative to trait measures. It is a 66-item checklist containing a wide range of strategies people use to deal with taxing events; items are included from the domain of defensive coping (e.g. avoidance, intellectualization, isolation, and suppression), information seeking, problem solving, palliation, inhibition of action, direct action, and magical thinking. These items form eight subscales: one problem-focused; six emotion-focused (wishful thinking, detachment, accentuating the positive, self-blame, tension reduction, and keeping to self); and one subscale that combines both problem- and emotion-focused items (seeking social support). Subjects respond to the items using a four-point Likert scale from 0 = does not apply or not used to 3 = used a great deal. The scale elicits information on how a person deals with a specific stressful encounter. Usually the event is described by the subject in an interview or in a brief written statement, including who was involved, where the event took place, and what happened.

Several researchers have used situation-oriented tools to examine the process of coping with specific events, such as bereavement, divorce, or personal illness, but how people handle any of these situations does not generalize well to other events (Folkman and Lazarus, 1980). To complicate matters, many single events such as illness are multidimensional, in that they include both changeable and unchangeable elements. Consequently, people may use both problem- and emotion-focused strategies to cope with various aspects, and different phases, of a single event (Moos and Tsu, 1977). For example, early on an individual may ignore symptoms of a medical problem, later attempt to cure or control the illness, and eventually "look for the silver lining" when some disability appears inevitable.

Both the process of adjusting to MS and the factors associated with successful adjustment have been studied (Peyser et al., 1980; Brooks and Matson, 1982;

Counte et al., 1983; Dalos et al., 1983; Schiffer, Caine et al., 1983; Schiffer, Ruddick et al., 1983; Maybury and Brevin, 1984; McIvor et al., 1984; Vanderplate, 1984; Zeldow and Pavlou, 1984; Halligan and Reznifkoff, 1985). There may be several reasons why studies of stress and disease activity have neglected coping strategies as a possible mediating factor.

The measurement of coping is in a rudimentary stage, with neither coping style nor situation-oriented measures clearly preferable. Researchers may question how accurately patients and controls would recall their general coping styles, or their response to a specific situation, in studies of stress and MS onset. Current trait measures may not reflect preonset MS coping styles, although cross-sectional research shows that people do not change their styles dramatically over a lifespan (McCrae, 1982; Lazarus and DeLongis, 1983). The value of situation-oriented measurement tools may also be limited in any study of stress and MS onset; cases and controls might have experienced different specific events prior to onset and logically handled them differently—a point that also applies when comparing MS patients in exacerbation versus remission.

The measurement of coping strategies may not even be particularly relevant in studies of stress and MS disease activity. For example, a researcher might observe that more MS patients in remission than exacerbation used problem solving to manage recent life stress and conclude that ineffective coping strategies precipitate exacerbations—a conclusion that implies that problem-focused coping is superior to emotion-focused strategies. Studies indicate that both strategies can be used effectively, however, depending on the stressor involved (Lazarus and Folkman, 1984). In the preceding example, patients in remission may have experienced primarily changeable situations and effectively applied problem-solving strategies. On the other hand, patients in exacerbation may have experienced unchangeable situations and appropriately, but ineffectively, applied emotion-focused coping.

There appear to be no direct measures of successful versus unsuccessful coping. Instead, coping success is often measured indirectly, in that unsuccessful coping is equated with the occurrence of somatic or psychological symptoms. Scales exist to measure somatic symptoms only, psychological symptoms only, or both in combination. Goldberg and Hillier's GHQ (1979) is a typical combination measure, consisting of four subscales: somatic symptoms, anxiety, depression, and social dysfunction. It includes 28 questions on such symptoms as headache, insomnia, nervousness, indecision, worthlessness, pessimism, and isolation. Respondents indicate the extent to which they have experienced these symptoms in the recent past, using a four-point Likert scale (from 0 = not at all to 3 = much more than usual). In 1981 Rabins and Brooks reported that the GHQ is a valid and sensitive instrument for detecting emotional disturbance in MS patients. But can emotional disturbance be used as an indicator of poor coping in studies in which actual disease activity (like MS exacerbations) is the outcome measure; or is emotional disturbance, including somatic symptoms, an outcome measure in itself? Instruments like the GHQ have been used as outcome measures in studies examining the impact of stress on health (Kanner et al., 1981). In fact, Rabins and Brooks used Goldberg and Hillier's scale to measure emotional disturbance as an outcome of having MS. Some direct measures of coping success would be useful, if coping is to be examined as an intervening variable.

## Implications for the Literature

Some discrepancies in the literature on stress and MS may be due to variations in study design and measurement tools. Unlike previous researchers, Warren et al. (1982) asked neurologic controls about events prior to the age when MS occurred in cases to whom they were matched, rather than immediately before the onset of their own illnesses. This approach may combine the benefit of using controls who have reviewed the past for an explanation of their own illnesses with the benefit of comparing cases with controls who were essentially healthy at the point of comparison. If the stressful events that people experience differ from one period to another, this approach also ensures that analogous times in the lives of patients and controls are being examined.

Likewise, the current study by Warren et al. of stress and MS exacerbations is the first to measure daily hassles, an apparently better predictor of health outcomes than life events—which may account for their positive findings.


## DIRECTIONS FOR FUTURE RESEARCH

One of the main threats to internal validity in any study of stress and MS is ambiguity about the direction of causal influence. Because retrospective studies are limited in their ability to establish that stress precedes disease activity, it seems natural to turn to a prospective research design. In this type of study, individuals under unusual stress would be followed along with individuals under no such stress, to determine what proportion of each group developed MS. As previously noted, however, the low incidence rate of MS makes prospective studies of stress and onset unlikely. Prospective studies of stress and relapse are possible, but not necessarily more meaningful as long as overt symptoms are used to monitor exacerbations. Just as the onset of MS is difficult to fix, it is also difficult to identify the exact beginnings of an exacerbation. Until physiological indicators of disease activity replace clinical or subjective measures of relapse, even prospective studies will not be able to establish that stress precipitates exacerbations.

Experimental designs are not out of the question when studying stress and disease activity. Pratt (1951) found a statistically significant difference between the proportion of MS patients in whom a certain emotional stimulus immediately precipitated an exacerbation of symptoms and the proportion of controls who reacted similarly. His work has apparently not been expanded on, possibly because of ethical considerations. An alternate approach to establishing cause with the experimental design, however, is to remove the suspected risk factor. A factor is more likely to be causal if its removal results in a decreased risk of disease; that is, if the association between cause and effect is reversible. Paulley (1977) has observed remission in the somatic symptoms of a group of MS patients undergoing psychotherapy, either to resolve their feelings about past events or to improve ongoing family and social patterns and their attitudes toward them. Confounding can still explain a reversible association; for example, MS patients who are able successfully to reduce stress in their lives may have smaller amounts of an unknown variable (which both causes stress and increases the risk of disease activity) than patients who are unsuccessful. More well-designed experimental studies to test whether stress management lowers exacerbation rates might be valuable in clarifying the relationship between stress and MS.

## IMPLICATIONS OF A RELATIONSHIP BETWEEN STRESS AND MS

When considering the role of stress in MS, it is important to remember that stress may be either a causal factor or a consequence of the disease. LaRocca (1984) suggests that the most accurate model may be a circular one, in which MS produces stress and enhances the impact of other events, in turn precipitating disease activity. The circle's starting point—stress or disease activity—remains unclear.

If stress is involved in MS onset or exacerbations, the relationship may provide clues to a more direct cause such as changes in the immune system. The immune response is evidently involved in MS pathogenesis, and stress is known to have significant effects on the immune system, including the release of corticosteroids, loss of tissue from the thymus, a decrease in circulating T lymphocytes, and the suppression of natural killer cells (Goldberger and Breznitz, 1982). More collaborative research between psychologists and immunologists to monitor concommitant changes in emotional stress, immune response, and disease activity might increase our understanding of both MS etiology and the disease's relapsing-remitting course. Such studies may even suggest mechanisms for the control of disease activity, either through stress management or some other type of intervention.

On the other hand, any relationship between stress and MS may be a reflection of the fact that disease activity causes stress or makes patients more sensitive to unrelated events. Pulton (1977) has noted that because MS patients cannot be isolated from stress, some type of intervention to help individuals cope more effectively might be useful. Past research on psychotherapy or support counseling has been primarily preexperimental in nature. Medical discussion groups (Pavlou et al., 1979), supportive-analytic techniques (Bolding, 1960), the cognitive-behavioral approach (Larcombe and Wilson, 1984), and social support (Spiegelberg, 1980) have all been found to enhance adjustment or reduce depression in MS patients. With the exception of Larcombe and Wilson, however, none of these studies employed a control group, nor did they use any objective pre- or posttest measures to evaluate group effects. In 1985 Crawford and McIvor reported that insight-oriented group psychotherapy was more successful than either social club membership or no treatment in reducing depression among MS patients. More truly experimental studies (like Crawford and McIvor's) are needed to establish the relative merits of psychotherapeutic techniques aimed at helping MS patients to cope.

## REFERENCES

Adams, D.K., Sutherland, J., and Fletcher, W. (1950). Early clinical manifestations of multiple sclerosis. *Br. Med. J.,* **21,** 431–37.

Alter, M., Antonovsky, A., and Leibowitz, V. (1968). Epidemiology of multiple sclerosis in Israel. In: M. Alter and J. Kurtzke, eds., *The Epidemiology of Multiple Sclerosis,* pp. 83–109. Springfield: Thomas.

Baldwin, M.V. (1952). A clinico-experimental investigation into the psychologic aspects of multiple sclerosis. *J. Nerv. Ment. Dis.,* **115,** 299–342.

Bolding, H. (1960). Psychotherapeutic aspects in management of patients with multiple sclerosis. *Dis. Nerv. Syst.,* **21,** 24–26.

Braceland, F.J., and Giffin, M.E. (1950). The mental changes associated with multiple sclerosis. *Proc. Assoc. Res. Nerv. Ment. Dis.,* **28,** 450–55.

Bramwell, B. (1917). The prognosis of disseminated sclerosis. *Edinburgh Med. J.,* **18,** 16–19.

Brickner, R.H., and Simons, D.J. (1950). Emotional stress in relation to attacks of multiple sclerosis. *Res. Publ. Assoc. Res. Nerv. Ment. Dis.,* **28,** 143–49.

Brim, O.G., Jr., and Ryff, C.D. (1980). On the properties of life events. In: P.B. Baltes and O.G. Brim, Jr., eds., *Life-span Development and Behavior,* Vol. 3. New York: Academic Press.

Brooks, N.A., and Matson, R.R. (1982). Social-psychological adjustment to multiple sclerosis: A longitudinal study. *Soc. Sci. Med.,* **16,** 2129–35.

Charcot, J.M. (1877). *Lecons sur les Maladies du Systeme Nerveux.* Paris: Delahaye.

Cohen, F., and Lazarus, R.S. (1973). Active coping processes, coping dispositions, and recovery from surgery. *Psychosom. Med.,* **35,** 375–89.

Counte, M.A., Bieliauskas, L.A., and Pavlou, M. (1983). Stress and personal attitudes in chronic illness. *Arch. Phys. Med. Rehab.,* **64,** 272–75.

Coyne, J.C., and Lazarus, R.S. (1980). Cognitive style, stress perspective, and coping. In: I.L. Kutash and L.B. Schlesinger, eds., *Handbook on Stress and Anxiety,* pp. 144–58. San Francisco: Jossey-Bass.

Crawford, J.D., and McIvor, G.P. (1985). Group psychotherapy: Benefits in multiple sclerosis. *Arch. Phys. Med. Rehab.,* **66,** 810–13.

Dalos, N.P., Rabins, P.V., Brooks, B.R., and O'Donnell, P. (1983). Disease activity and emotional state in multiple sclerosis. *Ann. Neurol.,* **13,** 573–77.

DeLongis, A., Coyne, J.C., Dakof, G., Folkman, S., and Lazarus, R.S. (1982). Relationship of daily hassles, uplifts and major life events to health status. *Health Psychol.,* **1,** 119–36.

Dodge, D., and Martin, W. (1970). *Social Stress and Chronic Illness.* Notre Dame: Notre Dame University Press.

Firth, D. (1948). *The Case of Augustus D'Este.* Cambridge: Cambridge University Press.

Folkman, S., and Lazarus, R.S. (1980). An analysis of coping in a middle-aged community sample. *J. Health Soc. Behav.,* **21,** 219–39.

Folkman, S., and Lazarus, R.S. (1985). If it changes it must be a process: An analysis of emotion and coping during three stages of a college exam. *J. Pers. Soc. Psych.,* **48,** 150–70.

Goldberg, D.P., and Hillier, V.F. (1979). A scaled version of the General Health Questionnaire. *Psychol. Med.,* **9,** 139–45.

Goldberger, L., and Breznitz, S., eds. (1982). *Handbook of Stress: Theoretical and Clinical Aspects.* New York: Free Press.

Halligan, F., and Reznikoff, M. (1985). Personality factors and change in multiple sclerosis. *J. Consult. Clin. Psychol.,* **53,** 547–51.

Holmes, T., and Rahe, R. (1967). The social readjustment rating scale. *J. Psychosom. Med.,* **20,** 458–74.

Hultsch, D.F., and Plemons, J.K. (1979). Life events and life span development. In: P.B. Baltes and O.G. Brim, Jr., eds., *Life-Span Development and Behaviour,* Vol. 2. New York: Academic Press.

Kanner, A.D., Coyne, J.C., Schaefer, C., and Lazarus, R.S. (1981). Comparison of two modes of stress management: Daily hassles and uplifts versus major life events. *J. Behav. Med.,* **4,** 1–39.

Larcombe, N.A., and Wilson, P.H. (1984). Evaluation of cognitive-behaviour therapy for depression in patients with multiple sclerosis. *Br. J. Psychiat.*, **145**, 366–71.

LaRocca, N.G. (1984). Psychosocial factors in multiple sclerosis and the role of stress. *Ann. N.Y. Acad. Sci.*, **436**, 435–42.

Lazarus, R.S. (1983). Puzzles in the Study of Daily Hassles. Presented at Conference on Integrative Perspectives in Youth Development: Person and Ecology, West Berlin.

Lazarus, R.S., Averill, J.R., and Opton, E.M., Jr. (1974). The psychology of coping: Issues of research and assessment. In: G.V. Coelho, D.A. Hamburg, and J.E. Adams, eds., *Coping and Adaptation*, pp. 249–315. New York: Basic Books.

Lazarus, R.S., and DeLongis, A. (1983). Psychological stress and coping. *Am. Psychol.*, **38**, 245–54.

Lazarus, R.S., and Folkman, S. (1984). Coping and adaptation. In: W. Doyle Gentry, ed., *The Handbook of Behavioural Medicine.* New York: Guilford.

Malmgren, R., Detels, R., Visscher, B., Chen, S., and Clark, V. (1984). The Effect of Stress on the Course of Multiple Sclerosis. Presented at 10th Scientific Meeting of the International Epidemiological Association, Vancouver.

Maybury, C., and Brevin, C. (1984). Social relationships, knowledge and adjustment to multiple sclerosis. *J. Neurol. Neurosurg. Psychiat.*, **47**, 372–76.

McAlpine, D. (1946). The problem of disseminated sclerosis. *Brain*, **69**, 233–50.

McAlpine, D., and Compston, N.D. (1952). Some aspects of the natural history of disseminated sclerosis. *Q.J. Med.*, **21**, 135–67.

McCrae, R.R. (1982). Age differences in the use of coping mechanisms. *J. Geront.*, **37**, 454–60.

McIvor, G.P., Riklan, M., and Reznikoff, M. (1984). Depression in multiple sclerosis as a function of length and severity of illness, age, remissions and perceived social support. *J. Clin. Psychol.*, **40**, 1028–33.

Mei-tal, V., Meyerowitz, MD., and Engel, G. (1970). The role of psychological process in somatic disorder: Multiple sclerosis. *Psychosom. Med.*, **32**, 67–85.

Monroe, S.M. (1983). Major and minor life events as predictors of psychological distress: Further issues and findings. *J. Behav. Med.*, **6**, 189–205.

Moos, R. (1974). Psychological techniques in the assessment of adaptive behaviour. In: G.V. Coelho, D.A. Hamburg, and J. Adams, eds., *Coping and Adaptation*, pp. 334–99. New York: Basic Books.

Moos, R., and Tsu, V.D. (1977). The crisis of physical illness: An overview. In: R. Moos, ed., *Coping with Physical Illness*, pp. 1–22. New York: Plenum.

Moxon, W. (1875). Eight cases of insular sclerosis of the brain and spinal cord. *Guy's Hosp. Rep.* (3rd series), **20**, 437–40.

Paulley, J.W. (1977). Psychological management of multiple sclerosis. *Practitioner*, **218**, 100–05.

Pavlou, M., Johnson, P., Davis, F.A., and Lefebre, K. (1979). Program of psychologic service delivery in a multiple sclerosis center. *Prof. Psychol.*, **10**, 503–10.

Pearlin, L. and Lieberman, M.A. (1977). Social sources of emotional distress. In: R. Simmons, ed., *Research in Community Mental Health*. Greenwich: JAI Press.

Pearlin, L. and Schooler, C. (1978). The structure of coping. *J. Health Soc. Behav.*, **19**, 2–21.

Peyser, J.M., Edwards, K.R., and Poser, C.M. (1980). Psychological profiles in multiple sclerosis patients: A preliminary investigation. *Arch. Neurol.*, **37**, 437–40.

Philippopoulos, G.S., Wittkower, E.D., and Cousineau, A. (1958). The etiologic significance of emotional factors in onset and exacerbations of multiple sclerosis. *Psychosom. Med.*, **20**, 458–74.

Pratt, R.T.C. (1951). An investigation of the psychiatric aspects of disseminated sclerosis. *J. Neurol. Neurosurg. Psychiat.*, **14**, 326–35.

Pulton, T.W. (1977). Multiple sclerosis: A social-psychological perspective. *Phys. Ther.,* **57,** 170–73.

Rabins, P., and Brooks, B.R. (1981). Emotional disturbance in multiple sclerosis patients: validity of the General Health Questionnaire. *Psychol. Med.,* **11,** 425–27.

Russell, J.S. (1911). Comment on stress and disseminated sclerosis. In: C. Allbutt, and C. Rolleston, eds., *A System of Medicine,* Vol. 7, p. 809. London: Macmillan.

Schiffer, R.B., Caine, E.D., Bamford, K.A., and Levy, S. (1983). Depressive episodes in patients with multiple sclerosis. *Am. J. Psychiat.,* **140,** 1498–1500.

Schiffer, R.B., Ruddick, R., and Herndon, R. (1983). Psychologic aspects of multiple sclerosis. *N.Y. State J. Med.,* **83,** 312–17.

Speigelberg, N. (1980). Support group improves quality of life. *Assoc. Rehab. Nurses J.,* **5,** 9–11.

Vanderplate, C. (1984). Psychological aspects of multiple sclerosis and its treatment: Towards a biopsychological perspective. *Health Psychol.,* **3,** 253–57.

Warren, S., Greenhill, S., and Warren, K.G. (1982). Emotional stress and the development of multiple sclerosis: Case-control evidence of a relationship. *J. Chron. Dis.,* **35,** 821–31.

Zeldow, P.B., and Pavlou, M. (1984). Physical disability, life stress, and psychological adjustment in multiple sclerosis. *J. Nerv. Ment. Dis.,* **172,** 80–4.

# IV
## Management of
## Neurobehavioral Dysfunction

# Introduction

PAMELA F. CAVALLO

This section presents three approaches to the management of cognitive and affective disturbances in multiple sclerosis (MS). The different approaches do not represent opposing views, but rather share the goal of helping individuals with MS and their families maintain, enhance, maximize, or restore their capacity for social functioning.

Representing the rehabilitation perspective, LaRocca describes a comprehensive care model for MS in Chapter 14. In the past health care systems have been organized to treat people with acute illnesses and temporary physical limitations. People with MS, on the other hand, must confront varied physical and emotional changes that are often lasting, though they fluctuate over the course of the illness. In recent years increasing attention has been paid to the special needs of patients with chronic illnesses. This is particularly critical in a disease like MS, where the life span is normal for most patients. The focus of treatment has shifted from treating the isolated symptom to developing a comprehensive care program to help the individual adapt both physically and emotionally.

Comprehensive care in MS is achieved through the coordinated efforts of different health care disciplines. LaRocca explains the comprehensive care model by using his program at the Albert Einstein College of Medicine as an example. The model requires medical, nursing, and rehabilitative expertise in sharing the case management and coordinating efforts through team conferences, written notes, and informal contact. Other medical specialities lend their expertise via the framework of continuity and coordination provided by the primary care team.

The process often includes family members and is characterized by treatment focusing on symptomatic management and adaptation and an emphasis on education and self-management. Successful intervention requires an understanding of individual and family psychosocial dynamics, clarification for the individual and family of the psychological status, and realistic expectations in planning treatment.

The psychologist plays a central role in addressing the cognitive and emotional issues and in designing and carrying out intervention strategies. The major therapeutic interventions used in the comprehensive care model include individual counseling and psychotherapy, orientation and information groups, psychotherapy groups, and specialized treatment strategies (e.g., stress inoculation therapy). In addition, LaRocca presents a model for the cognitive retraining of MS patients. While cognitive retraining procedures have been used widely in head-injury and stroke populations, there is little information on whether these procedures are being applied to MS patients. Furthermore, we do not know whether these treatments will be effective for MS patients.

Minden and Moes (Chapter 15) suggest a general approach for working with individuals and their families from a psychiatric perspective. They describe a wide range of emotional distress in MS patients: depression, anger, irritability, worry, and discouragement. In addition, many patients experience clinically significant psychiatric conditions, such as bipolar affective disorder and major depression, at a rate that is more common than would be expected.

They also point out that while the cause of psychiatric disorders in MS remains unknown, effective treatments are available for these disorders. The chapter reviews specific and practical management strategies, which include pharmacologic agents, psychotherapy, and cognitive rehabilitation techniques. The authors discuss two different theories concerning cognitive rehabilitation: compensation and recovery of function. The authors suggest that the compensation model may be more useful for people with MS. They describe a comprehensive approach toward developing cognitive retraining programs for people with MS.

In the final chapter Sanford and Petajan describe how the evaluation and treatment of neuropsychological problems in MS can be achieved within the neurologic clinic. They present a model that neurologists can apply to the cognitive and affective problems of MS patients. The chapter concludes with a comment about the need to document problems such as financial difficulties, divorce, and abandonment. In this way legislation may be designed to assist patients and their family members in their struggle with this disease.

# 14

## A Rehabilitation Perspective

NICHOLAS G. LAROCCA

### THE COMPREHENSIVE, MULTIDISCIPLINARY MODEL OF CARE

As a sociomedical experience, multiple sclerosis (MS) has three salient features that make a comprehensive, rehabilitative model of care appropriate. It is chronic; it disables; and it is broad in its effects. The average age of symptom onset is 34; the diagnosis is made between the ages of 20 and 50 in 58% of cases (Baum and Rothschild, 1981). While there are many variations, the course of MS is generally one of slow worsening over an almost normal life span (Kurtzke et al., 1970). For most persons with MS, the physical and emotional challenges are manifold. Limitations in mobility and activities of daily living are the most readily recognized disabilities. Work is often affected: more than 75% of those with MS are unemployed (Kornblith et al., 1986). While the prevalence of MS is not very high, 58 per 100,000 in the United States (Baum and Rothschild, 1981), the cost to the individual and society is large. In 1976 (the latest year for which national statistics are available) the average person with MS lost $4855 in wages and spent $1672 on medical costs (Inman, 1984). MS cuts a deep and wide swath across the lives of those affected. Since any of the myelinated fibers in the central nervous system (CNS) may be damaged by the disease, the variety of problems it causes is very broad. To gait problems may be added sensory disorders, bladder dysfunction, visual loss, fatigue, spasticity, cerebellar ataxia, dysarthria, dysphagia, and psychological changes.

Because the cause and cure of MS continue to elude medical science, an intervention model that does not rely on a cure has, of necessity, evolved (Schapiro et al., 1984). During the past few years a number of major medical centers dealing with MS have adopted a multidisciplinary, comprehensive care model. One of the first centers to use such an approach was the Research and Training Center for MS at the Albert Einstein College of Medicine. This chapter describes the comprehensive care model, using the Einstein program as an example, and discusses the psychologist's role in this model.


## The Evolution of Clinical Care

In this century, clinical medicine has very successfully utilized etiologies, diagnostic criteria, and taxonomies. A careful diagnostic workup identified the disorder in question so that an appropriate cure, based on etiology, could be applied. The consequences of disease were not the major focus of such a model, since a successful cure would generally obviate adverse consequences. Concern about the consequences of illness seemed of lesser importance in acute illnesses that could be classified and cured. In acute illness, time-limited suspension of social roles is accepted (Office of Health Economics, 1977). In chronic illness, especially a chronic disabling illness, the situation is dramatically different, however. When illness and disability are chronic, the permanent nature of limitations necessitates adaptation in social roles rather than their temporary suspension. The continuing problems of the chronically ill are multifaceted, and service needs are therefore greater (WHO, 1980).

Because of the rapidly expanding population of the chronically ill, there has been increased interest over the last few years in understanding the consequences of disease in contrast to the classification of disease or the search for etiology (Office of Health Economics, 1977). The World Health Organization (1980) has even developed a system for conceptualizing the consequences of disease. This system draws on the work of Philip Wood (1980) and classifies the consequences of disease along three axes: impairment, disability, and handicap. Impairment is any loss or abnormality of psychological, physiological, or anatomical structure or function. Disability is any restriction or lack of ability to perform an activity in the manner or within the range considered normal. Handicap is a disadvantage for a given individual, resulting from an impairment or a disability that limits or prevents the fulfillment of a role that is normal for that individual. The traditional focus of clinical care had been the impairment (e.g., pyramidal dysfunction). Disability (e.g., being unable to walk) and handicap (e.g., being unemployed) were either neglected or delegated to others. It is now recognized, however, that effective care in chronic illness must take all three into account (Johnston and Keith, 1983).

Care focused mainly on impairments tended to use a consultative model. Clinical neurologists often had responsibility for such care and might call in consultants from other medical specialties when needed (e.g., urology, psychiatry, plastic surgery). Such care was fragmented, episodic, and highly reactive in nature, however. Preventible problems often appeared, and complications arose unnecessarily. But in recent years the coordination of resources on a continuing basis has replaced the consultative model as the state of the art in the management of chronic disease (see Table 14–1).

**Table 14-1**  Comparison of the Traditional Model and the Comprehensive Care Model in MS

|             | Traditional model | Comprehensive care model |
|-------------|-------------------|--------------------------|
| Orientation | Reactive | Proactive |
| Focus | Impairments | Impairments<br>Disabilities<br>Handicaps<br>Strengths |
| Goals | Cure<br>Symptomatic treatment | Cure<br>Symptomatic treatment<br>Prevention of complications<br>Adaptation to the illness<br>Maximizing strengths |
| Providers | Medical specialists | Multi-disciplinary team |
| System | Consultation | Coordination |
| Time frame | Episodic | Continuous |

## The Concept of Comprehensive Care

Comprehensive care in MS is essentially a rehabilitative model employing concepts and practices long accepted in rehabilitation (Aldes, 1970; Block and Kester, 1970; Brown, 1969). The provision of comprehensive care seeks to maximize an individual's functioning and prevent further deterioration within the limitations imposed by the disease (Block and Kester, 1970; Cailliet, 1968). The comprehensive care model rejects the old, reactive, "call me if you get worse" stance. Instead, the new model assumes a proactive stance, emphasizing symptomatic treatment, prevention of complications, and adaptation through continuity of care by a comprehensive team working in a coordinated fashion. Curing the disease is no longer the only viable goal for the team. Learning to live with both chronic disability and increased risk of morbidity is paramount. Full utilization of a person's potential and maximizing strengths are given high priority. One of the earliest reports to outline the comprehensive model emanated from Rush Presbyterian St. Luke's Medical Center in Chicago (Hartings et al., 1976). Since then, several other descriptions of this model have appeared (Cobble et al., 1988; Maloney et al., 1988; Marsh et al.,1983; Schapiro, 1987; Schapiro et al., 1984; Scheinberg et al., 1983; Scheinberg et al., 1981). The model has been applied so widely that the recently established Consortium of MS Centers now has 40 centers on its rolls. Moreover, the model continues to evolve, with the concepts of wellness and health promotion receiving increasing attention (Cobble et al., 1988).

## THE EINSTEIN PROGRAM

Among the oldest and best known of the comprehensive care centers is the one established by Labe Scheinberg at the Albert Einstein College of Medicine (Schein-

# The Process of Comprehensive Care at the Outpatient Unit

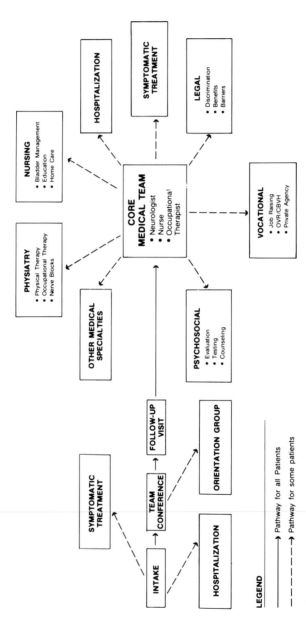

**Figure 14–1** Patients enter comprehensive care at the point of intake. Each patient proceeds through a variety of coordinated steps, some of which are followed for all patients (solid lines) and some of which are optional (broken lines), depending on the needs and wants of the individual.

berg, 1979; Scheinberg and Abissi, 1981; Scheinberg et al., 1981). The program developed at Einstein is used here to illustrate the comprehensive model and the role of the psychologist in it.

## Professional Roles

The program is carried out by a multidisciplinary team that coordinates its efforts through team conferences, written notes, and informal contact. Implementing the comprehensive model is not the exclusive province of any single professional role. At its core, this model requires good medical, nursing, and rehabilitative expertise; however, the team concept results in greater sharing of roles. Neurologist, nurse, physiatrist, and occupational therapist may share responsibility for bladder management. Psychologists, psychiatrists, and social workers address the psychosocial needs of patients and families. Other medical specialties lend their expertise but within a framework of continuity and coordination. Thus all professional roles share the common element of a central focus of case management via the primary care team.

## The Process of Comprehensive Care

As Figure 14–1 illustrates, the process of comprehensive care begins with an intake visit in which several members of the team meet with the patient, and often family members as well. Results of previous diagnostic procedures are reviewed at intake, and unnecessary duplication is avoided. Findings from both the intake assessments and medical record are reviewed by the entire team at a conference. Generally, a treatment plan is formulated within a week. A follow-up visit is standard but may be dispensed with for those who came for only a second opinion or diagnostic consultation. Additional follow-up visits are scheduled on a periodic basis rather than being contingent on acute deterioration in the person's condition. The orientation is one of active coping with a challenging physical condition. The team is there to collaborate with the individual on an active strategy for living with MS. Treatment focusing on symptomatic management and adaptation is instituted as early as the intake visit and continues in keeping with the treatment plan. Education and emphasis on self-management are promoted as early as possible. Periodically, orientation groups are held for newly diagnosed patients. These groups facilitate learning about the disease and sharing experiences in a supportive peer group environment.

Particular emphasis is placed on open communication concerning the diagnosis. With few exceptions, the diagnosis of MS is communicated clearly to the patient and family. Diagnostic euphemisms (e.g., "you have a virus of the spinal cord") are avoided. This approach can spare the patient considerable anguish, uncertainty, and unnecessary diagnostic testing. It also sets the stage for a trusting relationship between the team and the patient.

In keeping with the goal of coordination, the central components of care are offered by staff in the center itself. This includes neurology, nursing, occupational therapy, physiatry, psychiatry, and psychology. Care that can be more conveniently pursued in close proximity to a person's home is referred. Such care includes routine laboratory tests, visiting nurse services, physical therapy, legal services, vocational rehabilitation, and long-term psychotherapy. These decentralized services are provided under the supervision of center professionals, who maintain close, ongoing contact with caregivers.

Most primary care is provided on an outpatient basis. Acute inpatient care is avoided except in those cases where it is absolutely necessary. In contrast, intensive inpatient rehabilitation is extensively utilized, particularly in cases where outpatient approaches are not feasible or when a more intense course of treatment is indicated. Careful follow-up after discharge is designed to maintain and enhance recovery and functional status.

Having examined the workings of the comprehensive care model, we may now look into the role of the psychologist within that model.

## The Role of Neuropsychological Assessment in Treatment Planning

The comprehensive care model emphasizes coordinated assessment and treatment, a high level of family involvement, use of educational principles, and utilization of self-management. Such complex treatment plans necessitate extensive diagnostic studies in several areas, including neurology, nursing, rehabilitation, and psychology. Successful intervention requires an adequate understanding both of relative strengths and of those areas where the individual is most challenged. The psychologist contributes by clarifying major issues concerning psychological status and family relationships.

## Diagnostic Sensitivity in Psychological Screening

Psychological status may be inadequately assessed by the typical neurologic, nursing, and physiatric workup. For example, Peyser et al. (1980) performed neuropsychological testing on 45 MS patients whom an examining neurologist considered mentally normal and found 22 (49%) to have evidence of intellectual impairment. Indeed, in the literature in general, neurologic examination has led to significantly lower estimates of the frequency of intellectual impairment than formal psychological testing (Peyser and Becker, 1984). To avoid underdiagnosis and misdiagnosis of psychological problems, specialized methods and the skills of the psychologist are needed.

## Clarification for the Individual and Family

Significant conflict, confusion, and distress may arise in the family as a result of insufficiently or inappropriately assessing the psychological status. Subtle cognitive problems may be misinterpreted by the family as characterological or attitudinal characteristics. The individual may want for an explanation of mild but significant difficulties with the more challenging aspects of work and family life. A case example is the best way to illustrate these issues.

A 44-year-old securities analyst with a two-year history of MS was referred for psychological testing by his neurologist because of recent problems on the job and at home. His symptoms included gait and balance problems, mild dysarthria, fatigue, loss of appetite, spasticity, and urinary urgency. He was able to walk without assistance, drive, and work a full day, however. On neurologic examination, his intellectual functioning was assessed as normal. He had been having difficulty coping with his work, particularly in organizing and following through on things. Tensions at home had been steadily increasing during the last few months. His wife found it hard to discuss important matters with him and felt he was evasive, indecisive, and unfocused. She attributed these traits to his personality and felt very angry toward him. Testing revealed problems in attention, concentration, verbal recall, visual memory, and word finding. Qualitatively, his thinking was disorganized and not goal-directed. In a feedback session both patient and spouse were somewhat surprised to learn that MS could cause intellectual problems. They had not really considered this as a possible explanation for either family or occupational problems. As a result of this evaluation, the center team reexamined goals and expectations and began to address more closely the adjustment problems of the family.

## Realistic Expectations in Treatment Plans

Ability to execute and benefit from certain treatments may be contingent upon psychological status. Someone dealing for the first time with physical disability and its emotional concomitants may need special support to pursue a time-consuming and challenging retraining program. An individual with serious memory deficits may require special strategies to meet the challenges of self-management of medical care. The psychologist can help to identify both strengths and constraints that may impact on the treatment plans of the team. Again, a case example illustrates the issues.

A 27-year-old laboratory technician with a three-year history of MS was referred to a vocational rehabilitation agency for assistance in retraining. While she used a motorized wheelchair at work, she found the mobility requirements of the job too great for her limitations. She wanted to retrain for a more sedentary occupation such as word processing. The vocational rehabilitation agency sent her to one of their consulting psychologists for an evaluation. At the time of testing, she was in an exacerbation and consequently was extremely depressed and anxious. Testing showed below-average intelligence, concentration problems, difficulty shifting sets, memory deficits, and spatial abnormalities. The recommendation was against any attempt at retraining. The psychology staff at the MS center felt that the evaluation and its conclusions were inappropriate. This woman had been tested at a time when she was distraught because of a serious exacerbation. Moreover, the battery used did not follow generally accepted guidelines for assessment of memory in MS. Three months following the first evaluation, this individual was tested by a psychologist at the MS center using a more appropriate battery which included the selective reminding test, the Wechsler Memory Scale (WMS), and the multiple-choice version of the Benton Visual Retention Test. By this time, the exacerbation had ended and she had made a dramatic improvement emotionally. Results indicated average intelligence and no evidence of neuropsychological deficits. Thus an inadequate earlier assessment had unrealistically lowered expectations for this individual. Greater familiarity with the illness and more sensitivity to its emotional ramifications permitted a more accurate assessment of potential.

## Therapeutic Interventions

Despite the wide utilization of cognitive retraining in stroke and traumatic brain injury, these techniques seem rarely to have been tried with MS patients. Reluctance to recognize the presence of cognitive problems, failure to diagnose such problems, and prejudice against MS as a progressive disorder have retarded development in this area. Instead, therapeutic intervention has often taken the form of disease-modifying agents or counseling aimed at understanding and adapting to MS-related limitations. In a comprehensive care model, addressing psychological issues has a high priority, and the psychologist can play a central role in the design, implementation, and evaluation of intervention strategies. Several strategies are now discussed in the context of the comprehensive care model and the psychologist's place in that model.

## Counseling and Psychotherapy

Cognitive problems in MS are not necessarily the direct result of demyelinative changes. Both depressive and anxious states may compromise functioning in intellectual tasks. It has been this author's experience, however, that memory problems in particular are too frequently attributed to depression. Indeed, in a recent study using the Wechsler Adult Intelligence Test-Revised (WAIS-R), the Wechsler Memory Scale-Revised (WMS-R), and the Minnesota Multiphasic Personality Inventory (MMPI), Gass and Russell (1986) found that depression had a minimal impact on both short-term and long-term memory. Blaming intellectual problems on a more treatable condition such as depression may occur in the service of denial. The psychologist has an important role to play in attempting to identify the contributions of all such factors. Typically, both structural changes and affective state play a role. Counseling and psychotherapy are thus significant in understanding such problems, in adjusting to demyelinative changes, and in alleviating affective contributors to dysfunction. Within the comprehensive care model, a variety of psychotherapeutic approaches have been utilized. Some of the more important are now described.

## Orientation Groups

The comprehensive care program at Rush (Hartings et al., 1976) was one of the first to describe the use of orientation/information groups. At Rush an initial group meeting led by a psychologist and neurologist was used to communicate information on the nature of the disease and to open up discussion of the psychological implications of the illness. This first meeting was followed by a time-limited series of meetings conducted by psychologists and patient leaders.

In a similar vein, the Einstein program has for some years offered information/orientation groups for newly diagnosed patients and family members (LaRocca et al., 1987). Often, the newly diagnosed patient has spent many months or years with frightening and unpredictable symptoms, followed by a harrowing and expensive diagnostic odyssey. Because MS is little known to the general public, few of the newly diagnosed know what to expect. Moreover, many feel they have been entrusted with a terrible secret whose revelation to family, friends, and associates could unleash pity, ostracism, and worse. Self-image is under siege, and the future looks clouded and bleak.

Orientation/information groups can be held over the course of several weeks or compressed into an all-day workshop. The psychologist can act as leader, with a physician or nurse participating for an hour or so to provide answers to specific medical questions. With the cushion of peer support, the members of the group can explore new information, compare notes, and express feelings with others who share similar experiences. Even the reticent group member may benefit by learning that it is all right to talk about the illness and the feelings it brings. Such communication may then be approached more easily in the future. At the time of diagnosis, not everyone is ready to talk about the illness and its ramifications. In such instances, orientation and information seeking can be delayed until the moment is right.

## Psychotherapy Groups

Many of the advantages of the group format just described carry over to psychotherapy as well. In group psychotherapy with psychiatric patients, Yalom and Rand (1966) found that groups with higher degrees of compatibility showed greater cohesiveness, a characteristic related to successful outcome. In MS groups, cohesion is quickly established as people compare notes concerning case histories, symptoms, treatments, and the like (Pavlou et al., 1978). As a result, intimacy can be achieved relatively rapidly. The group can then proceed to a productive exploration of painful feelings, adaptive strategies, relationships, and fantasies concerning the future. Even very sensitive topics such as bladder dysfunction and memory problems can be dealt with in the safe environment created by a supportive peer group.

Only two controlled studies have examined the efficacy of group treatment in MS. Crawford and McIvor (1985) found that depression improved following long-term psychodynamic group therapy. Larcombe and Wilson (1984) also found improvement in depression using short-term cognitive-behavioral group therapy. It would thus appear that there is both theoretical and empirical support for the utilization of group therapy in MS.

## Individual Treatment

Individual psychotherapy also has an important place in a comprehensive model (Kalb et al., 1987). For many patients, discussion of the illness with a group of others with MS is overwhelming. A course of individual therapy may pave the way toward sharing with others. In addition, there are situations in which individual therapy may be chosen on clinical grounds, for example, when the normal grief reaction following diagnosis or an exacerbation develops into depression. Individual treatment may also be indicated when the stress related to MS aggravates preexisting problems.

Therapy with individuals who have MS raises many special issues. Persons with

MS have been told that they have a physical disability. For some, entry to psychotherapy may imply that they are emotionally disabled as well. An alternative model (Kalb et al., 1987) views therapy as an important tool in the process of constructively adapting to MS and learning to live with its ramifications. This model implies that the psychotherapist utilize a strategy that Kalb et al. (1987) have called "intermittent psychological support." For example, Hartings et al. (1976) described how the Rush program was designed to allow patients to "plug in" to psychological services on a periodic basis in times of unusual stress or symptom exacerbation.

There is empirical support for such a model. Several studies have shown that changes in the disease are related to psychological distress (Brooks and Matson, 1982; Dalos et al., 1983) and depression (Cleeland et al, 1970; Surridge, 1969). A study completed at the Einstein Center and summarized in Table 14–2 further confirmed these findings (LaRocca et al., 1988). Patients who were more neurologically impaired or more disabled in activities of daily living did not show more negative affect, demoralization, or lower self-esteem. In contrast, patients who were in an exacerbation did have a more negative psychological status. This and the studies reported above indicate that it is not the severity of the illness that is most important in psychological status, but rather the occurrence of changes in symptoms. Thus the psychotherapist must be prepared for periodic flare-ups in illness-related stress requiring a new round of therapeutic contacts.

The first controlled study of individual therapy in MS was recently completed by Dr. Frederick Foley at the Einstein Center (Foley et al., 1987). Table 14–3 summarizes the results of that study. Forty MS patients were randomly assigned to one of two 6-week treatment conditions: stress inoculation training (SIT) or current available care (CAC), essentially a modified waiting-list placebo condition. The SIT condition included cognitive-behavioral psychotherapy and progressive deep-muscle relaxation training. At posttest, patients in the SIT condition were significantly less depressed, anxious, and distressed than the control group and were utilizing more problem-focused coping strategies than the control patients. It thus appears that even a short course of individual therapy can have demonstrably positive effects for persons with MS.

**Table 14-2**   Correlation between Psychological Measures and Disease Characteristics in MS Patients ($N = 94$)

|              | Affect balance[a] | Demoralization | |
|--------------|:-----------------:|:------:|:-----------:|
|              |                   | Total[b] | Self-esteem[a] |
| EDSS         | −.04              | .02    | −.02        |
| ISS-M        | .10               | −.07   | .10         |
| Exacerbation | −.24*             | .25**  | −.20*       |

Reprinted from LaRocca et al. (1988).
*$p < .05$; **$p < .01$
EDSS—Expanded Disability Status Scale
ISS-M—Incapacity Status Scale-Modified
[a]Higher scores indicate more positive perceptions
[b]Higher scores indicate more negative perceptions

**Table 14–3**  Comparison of Stress Inoculation Training and Current Available Care in MS Outpatients

| | SIT | | | | CAC | | | | | |
| | Pretest | | Posttest | | Pretest | | Posttest | | | |
| Measure | M | SD | M | SD | M | SD | M | SD | F(1,34) | q |
|---|---|---|---|---|---|---|---|---|---|---|
| BDI | $24.4_a$ | 13.0 | $13.2_b$ | 10.5 | $21.7_a$ | 15.0 | $21.6_a$ | 14.2 | 18.54 | 6.5 |
| STAI-S | $51.8_a$ | 15.6 | $37.2_b$ | 13.8 | $54.6_a$ | 16.9 | $50.5_a$ | 13.0 | 6.54 | 6.5 |
| STAIT | $53.6_a$ | 12.8 | $46.2_b$ | 13.1 | $54.5_a$ | 13.1 | $51.9_{ab}$ | 13.4 | 3.31 | 4.2 |
| Hassles | $88.1_a$ | 44.0 | $57.5_b$ | 37.6 | $90.2_a$ | 49.5 | $89.2_a$ | 67.1 | 5.78 | 5.2 |
| PFC | $12.6_a$ | 4.7 | $16.2_b$ | 4.8 | $12.2_a$ | 5.7 | $11.8_a$ | 4.6 | 7.39 | 6.0 |

Reprinted from Foley et al. (1987).
Note. SIT = stress inoculation training; CAC = current available care; BDI = Beck Depression Inventory; STAI-S = State-Trait Anxiety Inventory, State; STAI-T = State-Trait Anxiety Inventory, Trait: Hassles = Hassles Scale Intensity Score; PFC = Problem-Focused Coping from the Ways of Coping Checklist. Means with different subscripts differed significantly at $p < .01$. Duncan $q$ scores listed compare posttest scores.

## Cognitive Retraining

Among the intellectual deficits that may accompany MS, memory problems are probably the most common and the most disabling (Rao, 1986). There have been few if any attempts to apply cognitive retraining techniques in MS, despite promising results in the treatment of memory problems following closed head injury (Grafman, 1984), stroke (Gasparrini and Satz, 1979), and temporal lobectomy (Jones, 1974).

Schacter and Glisky (1986) have distinguished two major approaches to the treatment of memory problems: compensatory strategies and restorative strategies. Compensatory strategies do not attempt to improve memory function per se but instead utilize methods to compensate for lost function in everyday activities. This approach relies on external aids such as lists, labeling of the home, and cuing. In contrast, restorative strategies seek to improve memory function directly, on the assumption that the brain has some capacity for recovery of function (O'Connor and Cermak, 1987). Many restorative methods rely on the teaching of either visual or verbal organizational strategies to enhance memory function. In one such approach, subjects visually couple objects with a peg list of numbers (Patten, 1972). Most such approaches are hard to carry over to everyday life, however, since they entail artificial strategies and actually increase the cognitive effort required for remembering.

An alternative approach aimed at the direct restoration of memory function employs graded practice in any of a variety of memory tasks, building on preserved memory function (Schacter and Glisky, 1986). Such strategies often utilize computers for presentation, feedback, and scoring. Recently, the Einstein Center received funding from the National Multiple Sclerosis Society to initiate a study of memory remediation using a computer-mediated program of graded practice in list learning. This project will entail a placebo controlled trial in a sample of MS patients with significant memory problems. Many such studies will be needed to determine which if any of the available treatment strategies are of value.

## The Psychologist's Relationship to Other Team Members

Within the comprehensive care model, the psychologist may assume several complementary roles. As a member of the primary care team, the psychologist may lend assessment skills in the areas of intellect, affective status, and family and social life. As a consulting specialist, the psychologist may be called in to perform intensive evaluation when the psychological status is unclear and to render specialized treatment for those in need. The psychologist may be the only member of the team with formal training in research methods. In the role of researcher, the psychologist can contribute to the team's formulation of research questions, operationalization of key concepts, and execution of research designs.

## Integral Member of the Team

Psychosocial issues need to be considered in the care of each and every patient. As an integral member of the team, the psychologist provides important expertise in this area. While a formal psychological screening or interview with each patient may rarely be feasible, the psychologist's input in treatment planning and follow-up is essential. Particularly at the time of diagnosis, the psychologist may be needed to assist in dealing with the shock, uncertainty, and grief that may ensue.

## Consulting Specialist

Within the comprehensive model, the psychologist generally serves as both integral team member and consulting specialist. The psychologist is called on to perform specialized assessment and treatment for patients challenged in the areas of intellectual functioning, affective state, and family adjustment. The impact of the psychologist as consulting specialist can be enhanced, however, if the psychologist also serves as a full member of the team. As a member of the team, the special skills and knowledge of the psychologist can benefit from more extensive lines of formal and informal communication, a better understanding of the process of care, and the opportunity for more complete follow-up and feedback.

## Researcher

The psychologist is often the only member of the team trained as a professional researcher. In contrast to basic scientists or statisticians, the psychologist may also possess the skills and commitment of a service provider. The psychologist is thus in a unique position to help provide a bridge between the often-conflicting demands of patient care and scientific method. This role is particularly crucial in the area of clinical research designed to illuminate questions of efficacy and cost-benefit. Increasingly, neurologists, nurses, and other team members have received training in research and, like the psychologist, pursue the dual goals of care and inquiry. In this more complex model, the comprehensive team focuses on research, training, and patient care. The psychologist in such a team not only provides research skills, but may also serve to encourage the utilization of multivariate models that adequately incorporate psychosocial issues in medical research.

## CONCLUSIONS

The comprehensive care model has as its goals symptomatic treatment, prevention of complications, facilitation of adaptation, promotion of health, and maximization of human potential. These goals are pursued by an integrated, multidisciplinary team providing continuity of care. Many of the most crucial issues facing the model are psychological in nature. Such issues include adjustment, personal fulfillment, family relationships, social contacts, stress, grief, depression, and intellectual functioning. Using specialized skills, the psychologist has a critical role to play in the team's concerted response to the broad consequences of MS and the potential of each individual.

## ACKNOWLEDGMENTS

The author gratefully acknowledges the invaluable assistance of David Masur, Ph.D., Frederick Foley, Ph.D., Labe C. Scheinberg, M.D., and the late Seymour R. Kaplan, M.D., without whose help this chapter could not have been completed.

The preparation of this chapter was supported in part by grants from the National Institute on Disability and Rehabilitation Research (G008006808, G008300040, and H133B80018) and the National Multiple Sclerosis Society (RG1135-A-4, RG1941-A-1, & RG1459-A-7).

## REFERENCES

Aldes, J.H. (1970). Rehabilitation of multiple sclerosis patients. *J. Rehab., 33,* 10–22.

Baum, H.M., and Rothschild, B.B. (1981). The incidence and prevalence of reported multiple sclerosis. *Ann. Neurol, 10,* 420–28.

Block, J.M., and Kester, N.C. (1970). Role of rehabilitation in the management of multiple sclerosis. *Mod. Treat., 7,* 930–40.

Brooks, N.A., and Matson, R.R. (1982). Social-psychological adjustment to multiple sclerosis: A longitudinal study. *Soc. Sci. Med., 16,* 2129–2135.

Brown, J. (1969). Recent studies in multiple sclerosis: Inferences on rehabilitation and employability. *Mayo Clin. Proc., 44,* 758–65.

Cailliet, R. (1968). Rehabilitation in multiple sclerosis. In: S. Licht, ed., *Rehabilitation and Medicine,* pp. 446–59. Baltimore: Waverly Press.

Cleeland, C., Mathews, C., & Hopper, C. (1970). MMPI profiles in exacerbation and remission of multiple sclerosis. *Psychol. Rep., 27,* 373–74.

Cobble, N.D., Wangaard, C., Kraft, G., and Burks, J.S. (1988). Rehabilitation of the patient with multiple sclerosis. In: J.A. Delisa, D. Currie, B. Gans, P. Gatens, J.A. Leonard, and M. McPhee, eds. *Principles and Practices of Rehabilitation Medicine,* pp. 612–34. Philadelphia: Lippincott.

Crawford, J.D., and McIvor, G.P. (1985). Group psychotherapy: Benefit in multiple sclerosis. *Arch. Phys. Med. Rehab., 66,* 810–13.

Dalos, N.P., Rabins, P.V., Brooks, B.R., O'Donnell, P. (1983). Disease activity and emotional state in multiple sclerosis. *Ann. Neurol., 13,* 573–77.

Foley, F.W., Bedell, J.R., LaRocca, N.G., Scheinberg, L.C., and Reznikoff, M. (1987). Efficacy of stress-inoculation training in coping with multiple sclerosis *J. Consult. Clin. Psychol.*, **55**, 919–22.

Gasparrini, B., and Satz, P. (1979). A treatment for memory problems in left hemisphere CVA patients. *J. Clin. Psychol.*, **1**, 137–50.

Gass, C.S., and Russell, E.W. (1986). Differential impact of brain damage and depression on memory test performance. *J. Consult. Clin. Psychol.*, **54**, 261–63.

Grafman, J. (1984). Memory assessment and remediation. In: B.A. Edelstein and E.T. Couture, eds., *Behavioral Assessment and Rehabilitation of the Traumatically Brain Damaged*, pp. 151–189. New York: Plenum Press.

Hartings, M.F., Pavlou, M.M., and Davis, F.A. (1976). Group counseling of MS patients in a program of comprehensive care. *J. Chron. Dis.*, **29**, 65–73.

Inman, R. (1984). Disability indices, the economic costs of illness, and social insurance: The case of multiple sclerosis. *Acta Neurol. Scand.*, **70** (Suppl. 101), 46–55.

Johnston, M. and Keith, R. (1983). Cost-benefit of medical rehabilitation: Review and critique. *Arch. Phys. Med. Rehab.*, **64**, 147–54.

Jones, M.K. (1974). Imagery as a mnemonic aid after left temporal lobectomy. *Neuropsychologia, 12*, 21–30.

Kalb, R., LaRocca, N., and Kaplan, S. (1987). Sexuality. In L. Scheinberg ed., *Multiple Sclerosis: A Guide for Patients and Their Families;2d ed., pp. 177–95. New York: Raven Press.*

Kornblith, A.B., LaRocca, N.G. and Baum, H.M. (1986). Employment in individuals with multiple sclerosis. *Int. J. Rehab. Res.*, **9**, 155–65.

Kurtzke, J., Beebe, G., Nagler, B., Nefzger, M., Auth, T., and Kurland, L. (1970). Studies on the natural history of multiple sclerosis. *Arch. Neurol.*, **22**, 215–25.

Larcombe, N.A., and Wilson, P.H. (1984). An evaluation of cognitive behavior therapy for depression in patients with multiple sclerosis. *Br. J. Psychiat.* **145**, 366–71.

LaRocca, N.G., Kalb, R.C., and Kaplan, S.R. (1987). Psychological issues. In: L.C. Scheinberg, and N.J. Holland, eds., *Multiple Sclerosis: A Guide for Patients and Their Families*, 2d ed., pp. 197–213. New York: Raven Press.

LaRocca, N.G., Scheinberg, L.C., and Kaplan, S.R. (1988). Disease characteristics and psychological status in multiple sclerosis. *J. Neurol. Rehab.*, **1**, 171–78.

Maloney, F.P., Burks, J.S., and Ringel, S.P., eds. (1985). *Interdisciplinary Rehabilitation of Multiple Sclerosis and Neuromuscular Disorders.* New York: Lippincott.

Marsh, G., Ellison, G., Strite, C. (1983). Psychosocial and vocational rehabilitation approaches to multiple sclerosis. *Ann. Rev. Rehab.*, **3**, 242–67.

O'Connor, M., and Cermak, L.S. (1987). Rehabilitation of organic memory disorders. In: M. Meier, A. Benton, and L. Diller, eds., *Neuropsychological Rehabilitation, pp. 260–79,* New York: Guilford Press.

Office of Health Economics. (1977). *Physical Impairment: Social Handicap.* London: Office of Health Economics.

Patten, B.M. (1972). The ancient art of memory-usefulness in treatment. *Arch. Neurol.*, **26**, 28–31.

Pavlou, M.M., Hartings, M.F., and Davis, F.A. (1978). Discussion groups for medical patients: A vehicle for improved coping. *Psychother. Psychosom.*, **30**, 105–15.

Peyser, J.M., and Becker, B. (1984). Neuropsychological evaluation in patients with multiple sclerosis. In: C.M. Poser, eds., *The Diagnosis of Multiple Sclerosis* pp. 143–58. New York: Thieme Stratton.

Peyser, J.M., Edwards, K.R., Poser, C.M., and Filskov, S.B. (1980). Cognitive function in patients with multiple sclerosis. *Arch. Neurol.*, **37**, 577–79.

Rao, S.M. (1986). Neuropsychology of multiple sclerosis: A critical review. *J. Clin. Exp. Neuropsychol.,* **8,** 503–42.

Schacter, D.L., and Glisky, E.L. (1986). Memory remediation: restoration, alleviation and the acquisition of domain-specific knowledge. In: B. Uzzell, and Y. Gross, eds., *Clinical Neuropsychology of Intervention,* pp. 257–82. Boston: Kluwer Publishing.

Schapiro, R.T. (1987). *Symptom Management in Multiple Sclerosis.* New York: Demos Publications.

Schapiro, R.T., van den Noort, S., and Scheinberg, L.C. (1984). The current management of multiple sclerosis. *Ann. N.Y. Acad. Sci.,* **436,** 425–34.

Scheinberg, L.C. (1979). Studies in the long term psychosocial problems of patients with multiple sclerosis. *Int. J. Rehab. Res.,* **2,** 540–42.

Scheinberg, L.C., and Abissi, C. (1981). Multiple sclerosis: Diagnosable and treatable. *Resident and Staff Physician, April,* 75–81.

Scheinberg, L.C., Giesser, B., and Slater, R. (1983). Management of the chronic MS patient. *Neurology and Neurosurgery Update Series,* **4,** 1–8.

Scheinberg, L.C., Holland, N.J., Kirschenbaum, M., Oaklander, A., and Geronemus, D. (1981). Comprehensive long-term care of patients with multiple sclerosis. *Neurology,* **31,** 1121–23.

Surridge, D. (1969). An investigation into some psychiatric aspects of multiple sclerosis. *Br. J. Psychiat.,* **115,** 749–64.

Wood, P.H. (1980). Appreciating the consequences of disease: The international classification of impairments, disabilities and handicaps. *WHO Chronicle,* **34,** 376–80.

World Health Organization. (1980). *International Classification of Impairments, Disabilities, and Handicaps.* Geneva: World Health Organization.

Yalom, I.D., and Rand, K. (1966). Compatibility and cohesiveness in therapy groups. *Arch. Gen. Psychiat.* **15,** 267–75.

# 15

# A Psychiatric Perspective

SARAH L. MINDEN AND ELISABETH MOES

In this chapter we present a general approach for addressing the emotional and cognitive disorders of neurologically impaired patients. In addition, we discuss a number of diagnostic and management issues that are specific to patients with multiple sclerosis (MS) and their families. The chapter includes detailed sections on the use of antidepressant medication and cognitive rehabilitation strategies in MS patients. We do not review studies that address the nature, prevalence, and etiology of emotional and cognitive disorders in MS patients, since such information has been presented in previous chapters in this volume.

## DIAGNOSIS OF EMOTIONAL DISORDERS

Since different psychiatric disorders respond to different treatment approaches, accurate diagnosis is essential. A thorough psychiatric evaluation includes an assessment not only of symptoms, but also of how MS has affected the patient's work, social, and family life; the quality of the patient's support system and how the patient uses it; and the specific meaning the illness has for the patient. It is important to learn about previous psychiatric problems and treatment and family history of affective disorders. The clinician should ascertain the contribution to the present difficulties made by situational factors, biology, and the patient's personality and coping capacity. Patients should undergo a complete medical evaluation, including history, review of systems and current medication, physical examination, and laboratory tests as indicated.

## Normal Adjustment

Normal adjustment to MS involves a process that varies in duration and intensity with each person, but almost all patients and many family members go through it. This process is similar to that which dying patients experience, as described by Kubler-Ross (1969) and others. In MS, however, the timing of the different stages is tied to the course of the illness: denial may be prolonged, and anger and grief may not emerge until a patient's limitations begin to interfere with daily life, perhaps not for many years after the first symptoms. When clinicians are familiar with these stages, they can more correctly distinguish pathological from normal reactions.

On hearing the diagnosis many people are shocked. This is often followed by denial, which may lead people to seek a second opinion or fail to keep appointments, follow medical advice, or accept help and information. Generally the denial lifts as people are ready and able to face their situation. Many then become angry: "Why me? It's not fair." This stage is uncomfortable for both patients and caregivers but passes more quickly when the angry feelings are accepted as understandable. Grief follows, as people allow themselves to feel for what they have lost and may continue to lose. Patients who were stable for many years and then deteriorated fairly quickly may be surprised by the intensity of their reactions: their apparently "good" adjustment simply was a factor of having few problems to deal with. When grief is allowed to follow its normal course, people often experience a lifting of the sadness, a new-found vitality, and an enthusiasm for re-engaging in life. They have learned how to exchange the old ways of finding satisfaction in their lives for new ones that allow for their particular limitations.

## Depression

Depressive symptoms, sadness, tearfulness, irritability, hopelessness, and withdrawal, are experienced by everyone at some time in their lives and, when time-limited and only moderately intense, represent a normal response to the losses associated with MS (Minden et al., 1987). A patient may lose not only the capacity for normal physical function, but also his or her roles in family and society, usual work and leisure activities, and relationships. This in turn may threaten a person's sense of being a worthwhile, competent, and autonomous adult and deprive life of purpose and meaning.

Depressive syndromes, on the other hand, involve a sustained period of depressed mood or loss of interest with associated symptoms of such severity that work and social life are adversely affected. Persons suffering from major depression may experience significant changes in appetite, sleep disturbance, and psychomotor retardation or agitation. They may feel worthless and become preoccupied with thoughts of death; some become actively suicidal. While major depressions characteristically are discrete episodes of change in mood and level of functioning, dysthymia is a chronic, persistent depressive disorder lasting at least two years. Bipolar disorder is diagnosed when, in addition to depression, patients have experienced episodes of mania. These distinct periods of "abnormally and persistently elevated, expansive, or irritable mood" are characterized by decreased need for sleep, pressured speech, flight of ideas, distractibility, and inflated self-esteem. Patients may become hyperactive and engage in activities indicative of impaired judgment such as shopping sprees and sexual indiscretions. Patients' histories typically reveal impaired occupational and social functioning and possibly psychiatric hospitalizations. Hypomanic episodes are less severe and do not produce such disruptions of daily life. Cyclothymic disorder involves at least two years of numerous hypomanic and minor depressive episodes with no more than two months without symptoms. When the clinical picture does not fully reflect these syndromes but instead indicates a maladaptive reaction to a recent, identifiable psychosocial stressor, the clinician should consider the diagnosis of adjustment disorder with depressed or anxious mood (American Psychiatric Association, 1987).

Certain standard criteria used to diagnose major depression can be confused with symptoms of MS. Diminished ability to think or concentrate may be a symptom of depression (pseudodementia) or of true cognitive impairment. While formal neuropsychological testing is important, it is not infallible, and in some cases only repeated assessment, a trial of antidepressant medication, and careful follow-up may clarify the diagnosis (Caine, 1981; McAllister, 1983). Fatigue is also a symptom common to MS and major depression. Fatigue due to MS is typically related to exertion or heat, worsens as the day progresses, and is relieved by rest. Patients complain that they want to do something, but they simply are too tired or need to rest (Freal et al., 1984). By contrast, fatigue due to depression is more constant throughout the day or worse in the morning and associated with disinterest and lack of motivation. Finally, pathological laughing and weeping, likely the result of bifrontal disease, represents a transient affective display that does not accurately reflect the patient's inner feeling state. While these reactions may be triggered by sad or funny thoughts, patients generally recognize that there is no real reason to be laughing or crying. Amitriptyline has proven to be an effective treatment (Schiffer et al., 1985).

In some patients depression may be masked by other, more prominent symptoms—multiple somatic complaints, chronic pain, anger, irritability, or anxiety—and patients may deny that they feel depressed. In addition, obsessive-compulsive symptoms, delusions, and hallucinations may be associated with severe depressive disorders. It is important to remember that depression may be caused by a large number of medications and medical conditions, including cancer, endocrinopathies, and cardiovascular disease. All patients should have a thorough medical evaluation to rule out these causes.

Information about a patient's psychiatric history and the family's psychiatric history can help establish the diagnosis. A patient who has had a previous depressive episode is more likely to have another. Similarly, patient's with bipolar disorder will have a history of mania or hypomania. A family history of depression and related disorders suggests the diagnosis: bipolar disorder occurs at a much higher rate in first-degree relatives than in the general population, and unipolar depression may also be associated with depression, alcoholism, and sociopathy in the family.

## Suicide

Suicide is not uncommon in MS (Kahana et al., 1971), and many patients have suicidal thoughts. Clinicians should ask patients directly if they have thought that life is not worth living or considered ending it all. Contrary to popular belief, asking about suicide does not put the idea into someone's mind, and patients with suicidal ideas generally acknowledge them. Research has shown that the majority of suicide victims are seen by their physicians within a few months of death. If there is any indication of suicidal thinking or preoccupation with death, the clinician should inquire about details of a plan and any past attempts and outcome and then determine the seriousness of the patient's intent to die. Hopelessness about the future and the feeling that there is no one or nothing to live for are important determinants of suicidal wishes. Pathological illness behavior such as refusal to take medication or severe anorexia may indirectly express suicidal impulses. While suicide is essentially unpredictable, risk factors for completed suicide include male gender, older age, physical illness, alcoholism, and social isolation. A patient with cognitive impairment may have little intent to die, but poor judgment may turn a suicidal gesture into a fatality. When there is a clear intent or a potentially lethal plan and if there is no adequate support system to engage and monitor the patient, immediate psychiatric referral is indicated. In evaluating the suicidal patient, the clinician's judgment is the key diagnostic tool (Bassuk and Birk, 1984).

## Anxiety

Like depression, anxiety may be a normal response to learning the diagnosis of MS and to major changes in functional capacity and life circumstances. While uncomfortable, normal anxiety is time-limited and responds to support, clarifying misapprehensions, and realistic reassurance. Anxiety requires more aggressive treatment when it persists for many weeks, produces severe discomfort, interferes with daily life and relationships, or reaches psychotic proportions. Panic attacks are marked by a sudden onset of various symptoms which include shortness of breath, dizziness, palpitations, shaking, sweating, choking, nausea, numbness and tingling, chest pain, and fear of dying or going crazy (American Psychiatric Association, 1987). It is important to distinguish anxious and irrational avoidance of certain places and situations (e.g., agoraphobia) from the realistic concerns of a patient with MS (e.g., fear of being in a crowded place in a patient who is incontinent or ataxic).

## Organic Mental Disorders

Although demyelination may play a role in the biology of the mood disorders outlined, current knowledge is too limited to indicate how it does so. Therefore, we think it is reasonable to assign the diagnosis of organic mental disorder to patients with symptoms of delirium (Matthews, 1979), dementia (Young et al., 1976), and the behavioral and personality changes characteristic of frontal and temporal lobe disease. Delusions and hallucinations in patients who have no previous psychiatric history and who do not meet the criteria for schizophrenia may also arise as a result of structural brain disease (Awad, 1983; Geocaris, 1957). Although not common, acute confusion may be the major presentation of an exacerbation and may respond to ACTH or corticosteroids. We have seen patients with encapsulated delusions who have had evidence of temporal lobe dysfunction on electroencephalogram (EEG).

ACTH and prednisone may precepitate depression, hypomania, mania, and psychosis in susceptible individuals (Cass et al., 1966; Falk et al., 1979; Minden et al., 1988). Treatment generally requires only cessation of the drug, although some patients may need additional antipsychotic medication. Patients at risk are those with histories of major depression and first-degree relatives with depression or alcoholism (Minden et al., 1988). If treatment with these medications is essential, the clinician might consider using lower doses or lithium carbonate during treatment (Falk et al., 1979).

### Family Problems

MS affects the whole family. Not only are family members called on to provide emotional and practical support for the patient, but they, too, must deal with disappointment, uncertainty and loss, and major shifts in roles. Family members who need to assume additional responsibilities or give up activities outside the home may feel angry and, in turn, guilty. They may be torn between wishes to care for the person with MS and to pursue their own interests. Peters and Esses (1985) found less cohesion, more disorganization, and more conflict in MS families than in others, while we have found that some MS families have difficulty with roles, problem solving, and emotional responsiveness when compared with other disabled patient groups (D. Bishop and S. Minden, unpublished data). In addition, financial problems are common: only 30% of patients are fully employed 10–15 years after onset of MS symptoms (Colville, 1983; Poser et al., 1981), and a survey in 1976 found that the average household lost 44% of its income because of decreased earnings and high medical expenses (Biometry and Field Studies Branch, National Institute of Neurological and Communicative Disorders and Stroke, 1984).

The clinician should inquire directly about how the family is coping and look for signs of conflict and symptoms of depression in all members. Special attention should be given to how the children are functioning. In some MS families children are dysphoric and anxious and have behavioral and interpersonal problems (Arnaud, 1959; Braham et al. 1975). They may show their unhappiness only indirectly, through difficulty in school, withdrawal from friends, and behaving badly at home.

## GENERAL PRINCIPLES IN THE MANAGEMENT OF EMOTIONAL DISORDERS

### The Patient-Doctor Relationship

The key to successful management of both affective and cognitive disorders is a stable, ongoing relationship between patient and doctor. In such a relationship a patient or family member should feel able to talk about the emotional stresses of the illness and to seek help for painful and disruptive emotional symptoms. Similarly, a physician should know the patient well enough to detect emotional difficulties early and offer assistance. Sustaining such an association may be a difficult task at times. The length of time it may take to diagnose MS (on average, from four to nine years after symptom onset [Gorman, et al., 1984; Scheinberg et al., 1984]) contributes to patients' frustration with their physicians' inability to tell them what is wrong. During this period, many patients feel misunderstood by caregivers, and when attention is focused on symptoms like anxiety and depression, they feel devalued and criticized. As a result, basic trust in the ability of the physician to respond empathically may be eroded.

Many physicians, anticipating negative reactions, delay telling patients the diagnosis or use confusing euphemistic terms such as demyelinating disease, myelitis, chronic viral infection of the nervous system (Scheinberg et al., 1984). By contrast, a survey of 100 MS patients found that 88% wanted to be told the correct diagnosis by their neurologists, and 52% wanted to be told as soon as the diagnosis was suspected. Patients wanted clear, detailed explanations of the disease process in language they could understand with sufficient opportunity to discuss the implications for themselves and their families (Gorman et al., 1984). Since many people are overwhelmed at first, information should be repeated at subsequent visits and questions asked to check comprehension (Gans, 1983). Power and Sax (1978) found that honest and complete sharing of information by the physician enhanced the ability of both patient and family to cope with the illness. When a physician sees a patient who feels mistreated by past caregivers, it is important to empathize with the anger and hurt without assigning blame. In time, even patients who have had unfortunate experiences may come to understand the difficulties of diagnosis and accept the normal limitations of caregivers.

Honesty includes telling the patient that there is much the physician cannot know: what the course and outcome will be or what will arrest the disease. At the same time, realistic reassurance is important—it engenders hope, which in turn facilitates the work of doctor and patient toward the common goal of improving the patient's functioning. False reassurance, however, can be destructive (Kessel, 1979). A clinician can offer hope by pointing out, for example, that most people do not become severely handicapped, by emphasizing strengths rather than weaknesses, and by treating aggressively whatever is corrigible. Unhappy news may be tempered by a caregiver's genuine concern to be helpful, sensitivity to an individual patient's and family's circumstances, and empathic tolerance of their emotional reactions. The clinician can convey support by directly suggesting that a patient might be worried about some things and by inviting the patient to talk about them. Asking patients to describe their daily lives in detail not only provides an accurate picture of a person's day-to-day functional capacity, but also shows that the clinician cares about the patient as a person. Open and direct communication is important not only at the time of diagnosis, but throughout the course, particularly when there is deterioration in functional capacity, when cognitive deficits become apparent, or when major life decisions such as change in employment or nursing home placement are being considered.

## Discussing Intellectual Deterioration

While severely impaired patients may not acknowledge their cognitive deficits (Shiffer and Slater, 1985), less affected patients and family members may be very aware of changes in mental functioning and emotional control. They find it confusing and frustrating to have caregivers deny that MS can produce these problems. Patients and families report feeling relieved when their perceptions are confirmed and, in spite of their sadness and concern, many use the opportunity to begin planning for the future. Families function better when they understand that a patient's forgetfulness or difficult behavior is not his or her "fault" but just as much a product of the disease as is having trouble walking. While we encourage clinicians to talk frankly to patients and families, it is crucial to be sensitive to how frightened most people are of losing their mental acuity. Noting deficits should be balanced by pointing out strengths and offering rehabilitation opportunities.

## Discussing Emotional Problems

Many people still believe that depression and other emotional difficulties are "moral" problems, thinking, for example, that they result from a lack of effort by the depressed person or a lack of caring by the other people around. This distorted picture may lead people to feel too ashamed to seek treatment and may create anger and resentment within families. It can be corrected by telling both patients and families from the beginning that it is likely that they will feel anxious and depressed at times, that most people do, and that help is available. The clinician can also point out that many depressions are biologic disorders and that treatment is generally effective.

## Talking with the Family

It is useful to establish a relationship with a patient's spouse or parents. They can help evaluate a patient's mood and functional capacity and can serve as allies in treatment and rehabilitation programs. Family members may also need encouragement to seek help for themselves. Parents often look for guidance in talking with their children about MS. Children need to know that they can ask questions and have them answered truthfully. They should know that their parent is not going to die, that they did not cause the MS, and that they cannot catch it or pass it on to someone else (Minden and Frankel, 1987).

## Referral for Emotional Problems

While some physicians prefer to manage the emotional disorders of their patients themselves (Schiffer, 1987), most choose to refer their patients with significant problems to a psychiatrist for evaluation and treatment. Psychologists, psychiatric social workers, or psychiatric nurses can be helpful to patients with adjustment difficulties and marital and family dysfunction. It is best if the patient sees a mental health professional who is familiar with MS. Attention should be paid to how the patient is told about the referral, since many people are ashamed of emotional problems: they fear they may be considered "crazy" or that their physician is trying to "get rid of" them. It is useful to address these misapprehensions directly. The referring physician should tell the patient clearly what symptoms have prompted the referral and talk about the consultant's expertise in helping with these kinds of problems. The patient should know in advance what to expect: that the initial meeting usually lasts about one hour and that the mental health clinician will inquire about current and past emotional symptoms, family, work, and social life, and may suggest additional meetings or medication. The patient should be reassured by knowing that information pertinent to his or her care may be shared, but that everything else will be kept confidential.

## SPECIFIC TREATMENTS FOR EMOTIONAL DISORDERS IN MS

The sections that follow present specific suggestions for treatment of emotional disorders in MS patients; they apply to family members as well. Clinicians vary considerably in their interest in and experience with psychiatric problems, so that we have tried to balance elementary with more sophisticated material. Clinicians also have their own preferences in terms of medication and psychotherapeutic techniques. Although we have tried to present an overview of treatment approaches, what we have written inevitably reflects our own clinical experience and practice. Readers should also draw on other sources and their own experiences. In particular, the discussion of medication should be supplemented by specific psychopharmacology resources.

### A Comprehensive Approach

Emotional disorders are multifaceted problems that require multidimensional treatment. The combination of psychotherapy and antidepressant medication has been shown repeatedly to be more efficacious for treating depression than either treatment alone (Weissman, 1979). The evidence suggests that medication has an earlier impact on depressive symptoms, although it still takes about eight weeks to become apparent, while the beneficial effect of psychotherapy, especially on social functioning, will be evident some weeks after that (NIMH Treatment of Depression Collaborative Research Program, 1986; Weissman, 1979). Medication should not be prescribed without careful monitoring for positive and adverse effects. Many patients are apprehensive about taking medication, and the availability of a concerned physician to answer questions and evaluate symptoms not only represents good treatment, but also will enhance compliance. Most patients have difficulty at some time in adjusting to their disease and will benefit from talking with a concerned caregiver.

Ultimately, patients choose their own treatment: some will refuse medication or be unable to take it because of undesirable side effects; others will refuse psychotherapy because of the time and expense involved, unfounded fears of uncovering disavowed feelings and thoughts, or limited understanding of the process.

Clinicians should support any impulse toward reasonable treatment that a patient expresses, even if it is not what he or she would recommend; in time many patients "come around" to accept a more effective treatment program.

## Individual Psychotherapy

A variety of psychotherapeutic theories and techniques exist for understanding and treating emotional disorders. These include long- and short-term psychoanalytic psychotherapy, behavioral therapy, interpersonal psychotherapy, and cognitive therapy (Glass et al., 1980; Laracombe and Wilson, 1984; Rush, 1982). The psychoanalytic psychotherapies seek character change and resolution of interpersonal problems (as opposed to simple symptom relief) through acquiring insight into the origins of unresolved inner conflicts. Both interpersonal psychotherapy and cognitive therapy are short-term (12–16 sessions), structured interventions that have been designed specifically to relieve symptoms in nonpsychotic, depressed outpatients. Interpersonal psychotherapy is based on psychoanalytic principles and techniques but focuses on resolving current difficulties in interpersonal relationships (Klerman et al., 1984), while cognitive therapy (Beck et al., 1979) seeks to correct negative concepts of the self, the world, and the future. Behavior therapists use a variety of techniques to train depressed patients in social skills and cognitive restructuring (Kovacs, 1980) and to desensitize patients to anxiety-provoking situations. Which technique is selected depends on a variety of factors, including the therapist's training and the patient's goals, psychological capacities, and economic resources. Outcome studies of psychotherapy have emphasized the importance of "fit" between patient and therapist, particularly their positive regard for each other, and the patient's motivation.

Regardless of the techniques used, psychotherapists working with MS patients should consider the following. First, MS patients typically seek help when they experience psychological pain, often at the time of an exacerbation, a life crisis precipitated by the illness, or when there has been a significant deterioration in functional capacity. When their illness is stable and life is relatively predictable, MS patients are, understandably, less motivated to engage in treatment. While therapists generally work at helping patients remain in treatment, they may find that in the case of MS patients, allowing them to come and go as they wish will strengthen the therapeutic alliance, enhance the patient's sense of control, and make it more likely that the patient will seek out the therapist when other problems arise. Second, while certain themes arise in the psychotherapy of most MS patients—loss of function, roles, and self-esteem; conflict over dependence; apprehension about the future—each person is an individual who assigns his or her own meaning to the illness and its consequences as a result of personal and developmental experiences. Third, in order to empathize with the patient's situation and convey to the patient a genuine wish to understand what it is like to have MS, the therapist should learn in detail what daily life is like for the patient. No aspect of living is unimportant. How long does it take the patient to get out of bed in the morning? How does the patient bathe, dress? How often does the patient go out? Where? With whom? How? Through such inquiry, affects will be mobilized and problem areas identified.

Finally, cognitive deficits are not a contraindication to psychotherapy. Even patients who appear to have little concern and appreciation for their physical and cognitive handicaps may experience distress about other areas of their lives. With time and an attentive therapist, many do talk about what they have lost and how difficult life is for them. Surridge made an important observation when he noted that many patients whom he had originally considered euphoric, when interviewed a second time were rediagnosed as depressed (Surridge, 1969). Moreover, since language and comprehension are rarely affected in MS, and since memory deficits are not often profound, even the most severely affected MS patients are able to engage in conversation about the problems they struggle with.

## Group Psychotherapy

Many MS patients prefer and benefit from group therapy with other MS patients. Groups include those led by a professional therapist, self-help groups without a leader, and groups led by a person with MS. Local chapters of the National Multiple Sclerosis Society (NMSS) often sponsor these groups and hold educational meetings that can have a similar therapeutic effect. Groups provide people with social interaction, emotional support, information and practical advice, as well as hope and inspiration. There is good evidence that therapeutic groups improve patients' abilities to cope with the illness and may reduce depression and contribute to a greater sense of control (Crawford and McIvor, 1985). The suggestion of "someone who has been there" carries great weight with most people (Crawford and McIvor, 1985; Hartings et al., 1976; Pavlou et al., 1978). Some patients resist involvement with group activities because they fear seeing people who are more disabled than themselves. This is often a concern early in the course of the illness, which may reflect psychological denial, and it generally passes with time.

## Couple and Family Therapy

Couples and families, including young children, often find it useful to talk with a mental health clinician about their worries. If family dysfunction is severe—bitter marital conflict, an alienated healthy spouse, a neglected patient, a troubled child—couple or family therapy is the treatment of choice. Therapists may help families understand the reasons for the current problems, develop shared activities, minimize blame and guilt, and maximize appreciation of each individual's needs and wishes. Therapy also provides a model and stimulus for ongoing discussion about MS within the family.

## Medication

Medication may be very effective for patients with major depression, bipolar disorder, generalized anxiety, panic attacks, or psychosis. Little is known about the outcome of treatment for these disorders in MS patients or if the disease process alters the pharmacokinetics or brain effects of psychoactive medications. One well-designed study found the desipramine was more effective than placebo for major depression in MS patients and that at 150 mg per day side effects were minimal (Schiffer et al., 1987). Until more research is done in this area, clinicians should be conservative, follow standard regimens, and draw on their own and colleagues' experience.

**Heterocyclic Antidepressants.** A large number of antidepressants have been developed since the 1950s. There are two major classes, the heterocyclics (formerly, tricyclics) and monoamine oxidase inhibitors or MAOIs. The more recently developed drugs appear to have fewer adverse effects, although they are no more effective than the original ones.

MS patients, of course, are susceptible to any of the usual adverse effects of antidepressants. Special attention should be paid to the anticholinergic effects, particularly the possibility of urinary retention and infection and decreased gastrointestinal motility in patients with preexisting bladder and bowel problems. Blurred vision may result from ciliary muscle relaxation, but generally, tolerance develops after the first few weeks of treatment; this symptom may be difficult for a patient whose vision is already compromised. Some have recommended using 1% pilocarpine nitrate eyedrops for a short time if necessary (Schoonover, 1983). Other troublesome anticholinergic effects include dry mouth and tachycardia which usually resolve fairly quickly, as well as retarded ejaculation and pathological sweating in the distribution of the superior cervical ganglion. Patients with persistent dry mouth may develop mouth infections and dental caries; severe cases may respond to a lower dose or 25 mg of bethanechol chloride, up to three times per day if not contraindicated. Anticholinergic effects are additive with antipsychotic and antiparkinson drugs, sedative-hypnotics, and antihistamines. The antidepressants with the most powerful anticholinergic effects include amitriptyline, imipramine, and trimipramine, while amoxapine, nortriptyline, and maprotiline are moderately anticholinergic. The least anticholinergic preparations are desipramine, protriptyline, and trazodone (Schoonover, 1983).

MS patients should be warned about symptoms of light-headedness and the chance of falling because of postural hypotension. They should be instructed to change position slowly, and patients with significant symptoms should have lying and standing blood pressure evaluated one-half hour after a dose. The heterocyclics are contraindicated in patients with narrow-angle glaucoma, recent myocardial infarction, and preexisting bundle-branch block (Glassman and Bigger, 1981), and they should be discontinued if there are persistent significant alterations in blood pressure, arrhythmias, fainting, heart failure, or other evidence of cardiac compromise. Doxepin, desipramine, amoxapine, maprotiline, and trazodone appear to produce the fewest cardiac effects, while amitriptyline seems to cause the greatest number of problems; nortriptyline, protriptyline, and imipramine have been responsible for a moderate number of cardiotoxic reactions (Schoonover, 1983). The clinician should carefully monitor other medications to avoid undesirable synergistic effects.

In treating MS pateints it is important to note that many of the heterocyclics produce sedation (especially amitriptyline, trimipramine, doxepin, and trazodone). The least sedating are desipramine and protriptyline (Schoonover, 1983). Heterocyclics also can lower the seizure threshold. They may lead to psychomotor slowing, clouded thinking, and difficulty concentrating, as well as dizziness, muscle weakness, fatigue, and a variety of neurologic symptoms that mimic those of MS

(Schoonover, 1983). Since amoxapine has dopamine-blocking properties and can produce extrapyramidal reactions, it may not be the best choice for MS patients. Heterocyclics may induce mania, psychosis, or confusion in some patients.

**Monoamine Oxidase Inhibitors.** The MAOIs generally are used as a second-line medication for depressions that have not responded to heterocyclics. Life-threatening hypertension may develop at high doses or when an MAOI is taken with a sympathomimetic drug, food with a high tyramine content, or inappropriately with a heterocyclic antidepressant. Patients must be carefully instructed about which foods and medications to avoid as well as about symptoms of a hypertensive crisis and what to do should they occur. If a patient cannot reliably follow the prescribed diet, he or she should not take these medications. Patients considered for MAOI treatment should be evaluated by a psychiatrist.

**Lithium Carbonate.** Lithium is effective for preventing manic, hypomanic, and depressive episodes in patients with bipolar disorder. It is not an effective treatment alone for acute episodes. It has also been used in MS patients to prevent manic and hypomanic reactions to ACTH (Falk et al., 1979; Kemp et al., 1977). Lithium requires careful pretreatment and ongoing evaluation of renal, cardiac, and thyroid status along with frequent assessment of blood levels. MS patients may be troubled by such side effects as polyuria and polydipsia, gastrointestinal symptoms, action tremor, muscle weakness, mental dullness, impaired memory and concentration, and fatigue (Schoonover, 1983). Indeed, a variety of neurologic symptoms can occur at therapeutic levels (Gelenberg, 1983), and the usual signs of toxicity may be confused with an MS exacerbation (Mehta, 1976; Peselow et al., 1981; Solomon, 1978).

**Initiating and Monitoring Treatment with Antidepressants.** Before initiating pharmacologic treatment the clinician should ensure that there are no contraindications to taking the medication, including current or planned pregnancy, and rule out possible drug interactions. Patients should be educated thoroughly about the risk of overdose and potential side effects and told explicitly what to do in each case.

Patients generally respond to pharmacologic treatment when they have vegetative signs (anorexia, weight loss, insomnia), diurnal mood variation with worse mood in the morning, psychomotor retardation or agitation, autonomous and pervasive symptoms, an acute onset, and a family history of depression and responsiveness to medication (Schoonover, 1983). A specific medication is chosen because it was previously effective for the patient or for a biologic relative; produces few unwanted effects; offers specific actions such as sedation for an agitated patient or stimulation for a lethargic patient; or affects a neurotransmitter system different from that of a previously ineffective drug. For example, significant norepinephrine uptake-blocking is produced by desipramine, maprotiline, nortriptyline, protriptyline, and amoxapine, while trazodone produces significant serotonin uptake-blockade. Imipramine, doxepin, and trimipramine have moderate uptake-blocking effects on both neurotransmitters (Schoonover, 1983).

To minimize unwanted effects and to detect them early, treatment of MS patients should begin with small doses that are increased gradually, for example, 25 mg of desipramine daily for three days, then 50 mg daily for three days, and so on until depressive symptoms begin to remit, side effects develop, or the recommended maximum dose is achieved. Clinicians should consult standard references for appropriate doses of each medication. In MS patients it is wise to follow plasma levels to find the lowest possible dose that reaches therapeutic range. Bladder and bowel function, mental and neurologic status, and orthostatic changes in blood pressure should be followed closely. Patients with cardiac risk factors should have initial and periodic EKGs and consultation with a cardiologist. Patients with a tendency to urinary retention should be monitored closely for symptoms and undergo diagnostic catheterization and urinalysis if needed. The full daily dose is generally given at bedtime to minimize motor and mental slowing and to take advantage of sedating effects; some patients, however, may have fewer side effects with divided doses. Patients who are suicidal should receive small amounts of medication at a time, or the prescription should be handled by a family member (Schoonover, 1983).

The physician should either see the patient frequently or maintain telephone contact during the initiation phase to watch for adverse effects and minimize anxiety. Patients may be helped to continue medication by educating them about what to expect, thoroughly evaluating their complaints, and providing reassurance when indicated. They should know from the beginning that it is impossible to predict which drug will be effective, that it may be necessary to try several, and that it will take at least three weeks after a therapeutic dose has been established before depressive symptoms diminish. In addition, they should be told to expect resolution of sleep and appetite difficulties before change in their mood.

If after three weeks there is no response to a drug in therapeutic range or at the maximum recommended dose, another antidepressant with different pharmacologic properties should be tried. If there is no improvement with the second trial, the clinician should rethink the diagnosis, obtain a consultation with a psychiatrist or psychopharmacologist, and consider electroconvulsive therapy or an MAOI. In switching to an MAOI, there should be a drug-free interval of two weeks.

When the patient has a satisfactory response, the antidepressant should be continued for 6–12 months to cover the usual duration of a depressive episode. The drug should be discontinued gradually to avoid withdrawal symptoms; it can be restarted should depressive symptoms return. For patients with chronic depression, maintenance heterocyclic treatment at lower doses (e.g., 25–50 mg daily) or lithium may be indicated.

Lithium carbonate is the treatment of choice for patients with bipolar disorder, although carbamazepine may be useful for patients who cannot tolerate the side effects of lithium. Patients often require additional treatment with a heterocyclic during depressive episodes and an antipsychotic when manic. Combined treatment with an antidepressant and an antipsychotic is indicated for psychotic depressions. Patients who are currently psychotically depressed or manic should be treated by a psychiatrist. Patients with a history of mania or who take lithium but are not followed by a psychiatrist should be referred to a psychiatrist for treatment if they become depressed.

**Anti-Anxiety Medication.** The benzodiazepines are useful for patients with generalized anxiety disorder, while the treatment of choice for panic attacks is a heterocyclic or an MAOI. Because of the potential for the benzodiazepines to produce psychological and physiological dependence, they should be prescribed for time-limited periods during a crisis or other time of stress and anxiety. Anti-anxiety medication is most appropriate when symptoms interfere with a patient's usual capacity to function and when the anxiety is the result of an indentifiable stressor. When patients know from the beginning that medication will be available when they need it, but that it would not be in their best interest to take it when they do not need it, the risk of dependency is minimized. Excessive reliance on medication can interfere with developing lasting coping skills; however, no patient should be deprived of relief from painful symptoms. MS patients in particular may be troubled by sedation, ataxia, and impaired intellectual functioning with the benzodiazepines, but these are dose related and generally resolve quickly (Minden, 1987).

Choice of drug depends on physician familiarity, previous effectiveness for a given patient, and half-life. Long-acting drugs like diazepam, chlordiazepoxide, clorazepate, and prazepam are given once daily, while those with a shorter duration of action such as oxazepam and lorazepam may be taken at intervals throughout the day (Gelenberg, 1983). Medication should be started at the lowest possible dose, increased until symptoms abate or side effects become troublesome, and then gradually discontinued. Withdrawal states have been reported in 10–15% of patients following abrupt discontinuation of these drugs: they may occur after high doses taken for short periods or after standard doses taken for long intervals. Withdrawal symptoms begin earlier and may be more severe in benzodiazepines with short half-lives. It may be difficult to distinguish between withdrawal symptoms and return of the original anxiety symptoms.

Drugs like the barbiturates and meprobamate have a narrow margin of safety between therapeutic and lethal doses and should be avoided.

**Other Treatments.** Electroconvulsive therapy (ECT) is indicated for patients who require immediate relief of life-threatening or incapacitating depression and mania, who have had a good response in the past, or who are unable to take medication. Relative contraindications to ECT include a recent myocardial infarction, active pulmonary inflammation, central nervous system (CNS) tumors, raised intracranial pressure, and anesthetic risk. Confusion and short-term memory loss may occur but are minimized with unilateral electrode placement (Schoonover, 1983).

Psychiatric hospitalization is indicated for those with suicidal ideas, intense suffering, and an inability to care for oneself, for clarifying a diagnosis or for a trial of medication under observation. It is useful when outpatient treatment has failed and when destructive modes of interacting within a family need interrupting.

Respite care, arranged through the local MS society or independently, can help patients and families cope better. When seen as a positive step toward improved functioning, it can be used to interrupt family conflict, restore the energy of a burdened spouse, or give a shut-in patient a change of scene.

## DIAGNOSIS OF COGNITIVE DISORDERS IN MS

A comprehensive neuropsychological evaluation should precede treatment of cognitive dysfunction. It serves to establish a baseline and guide the design of treatment. The evaluator should identify areas of preserved ability and strengths that can be used in the rehabilitation process and identify and prioritize the problems targeted for intervention. Treatment of cognitive dysfunction must be tailored to the specific capabilities of each patient. No intervention can be applied to everyone or benefit all patients.

Cognitive functions are both hierarchical and interactive. Through the assessment process the clinician can determine which areas have been directly affected by the disease and which are secondarily affected. For example, poor performance on a story recall task may be due to a specific breakdown in one of several memory processes or to attentional lapses, word-finding problems, distractibility, poor motivation, or anxiety, any of which may interfere with recounting the story. These and other functions need to be evaluated carefully so that the time, effort, and money spent on rehabilitation are not wasted by addressing the problem at the wrong level. Accurate delineation of problem areas will also save patients, family, and staff from needless frustration and disappointment.

Patients with MS may present particular challenges to assessment because of upper extremity weakness and visual deficits. The impact of medication, fatigue, and depression must also be considered in interpreting the results of testing.

In addition to the administration of neuropsychological tests, the evaluation should involve in-depth interviews of the patient and family members. Although current assessment tools are increasingly sophisticated in design, various capacities are best evaluated through systematic questioning and direct observation. These functions include the ability to initiate activities, set goals, structure tasks, and use good judgment in social situations and in problem solving; awareness of deficits; and responsiveness to feedback. Important background information that has been forgotten, denied, or overlooked by the patient may be provided by a family member. The evaluator must also determine if the family is available to participate in the rehabilitation process and if it has the emotional and intellectual resources to do so.

## GENERAL PRINCIPLES OF MANAGEMENT AND SPECIFIC TREATMENTS FOR COGNITIVE DISORDERS IN MS

Neuropsychologists are increasingly called upon to apply their understanding of cognitive functioning and their assessment skills to rehabilitation. To date, most of the work in this area has been done with stroke or head-injury patients. While it may be premature to generalize from results obtained with these groups to populations with different patterns of deficits and prognoses, there are some strategies that are likely to be useful to MS patients.

There are currently two different theories concerning cognitive rehabilitation. On the one hand is the view that treatment should help the patient compensate for functions that are irretrievably lost (Miller, 1980). On the other is the view that recovery of function is possible (Wilson, 1987). Unfortunately, studies that have reported improved functioning do not show whether it is based on the use of alternative cognitive skills or on recovery of damaged mechansims. These contrasting models, of compensation and of recovery (Diller, 1987), dictate different treatment approaches: learning new strategies for performing lost functions (e.g., use of a notebook for a memory-impaired individual) or using prosthetic devices (e.g., a calculator for an acalculic patient) or practice of functions that are impaired to aid recovery. For MS patients the model of learning to compensate for lost functions may be more useful.

While outlining specific interventions for each type of deficit that can arise in MS is beyond the scope of this chapter, a basic approach to developing cognitive retraining programs for MS patients follows.

### Individualized Program

A rehabilitation program should reflect the needs and capacities of an individual patient. After designing an individualized treatment plan based on the initial evaluation, it is important to adapt the elements and goals of the program to each patient's evolving capacities, limitations, and rate of improvement. Capitalizing on a patient's strengths will help engage him or her in the program and may lead to more rapid improvement. It is useful for patient and family to plot daily and weekly graphs that monitor the patient's progress (e.g., number and types of tasks completed during the day, frequency with which assistive devices are used) and to indicate periods of greatest and least productivity during the day. If internal and environmental factors are also recorded, it becomes possible to determine which factors limit or facilitate improvement (e.g., fatigue, the presence of a family member). The effects of medication should be monitored closely.

### Motivation

Motivation is important for both behavior change and improving cognitive functioning. A person must feel it is worthwhile to change for his or her own reasons. Successful outcome is rarely its own reward. Behavioral reinforcement techniques can be vital components in the effective remediation of cognitive deficits. Patient and therapist should set short-term goals together, and even minor improvements should be rewarded frequently. This is particularly important for patients with memory dysfunction, apathy, difficulties setting goals and structuring tasks, and depression. Graphs showing improvement are a tangible reminder of both procedure and its success. Various methods for identifying and delivering incentives are discussed in the extensive literature on behavior modification (Campbell and Stanley, 1963; Craighead et al., 1976; Goldfried and Davidson, 1976; Kazdin, 1977; Wilson, 1987; Wood, 1987).

## Simplicity

It is important to limit the scope of an intervention to what is feasible and not try to change too many things at once. In setting priorities it is important to attend to the hierarchical and interactive relationships among cognitive functions, which functions the patient wants most to improve, and which tasks will be easiest to accomplish. For example, if the neuropsychological evaluation had identified an attentional deficit underlying problems in other areas, the difficulties with attention should be targeted for change, rather than trying to make changes in all areas simultaneously.

Similarly, limitations of patients must be recognized. Techniques used to enhance memory in unimpaired people that depend on elaborate cognitive strategies (e.g., finding words to rhyme with items on a shopping list) and those that were developed for individuals with unusual memory needs (such as actors who must memorize long speeches and police officers who must recognize faces of criminals) are not suitable for patients with memory problems. Treatments that require significant mental effort on the part of the patient, particularly MS patients who fatigue easily, are also unlikely to be successful. Simpler, more common strategies—writing information in a notebook or calendar—are more effective because of their ease and familiarity. Rather than teaching a particular imagery procedure or rehearsing a schedule, time might be better spent if the patient has a watch with an alarm that rings every half hour and is trained to check a notebook when the alarm sounds. When physical limitations make writing impossible, someone else can write the information; for visually impaired patients, a prerecorded cassette tape can be used (special switches are available for patients with poor motor control).

## Relevance

Orientation, memory for daily events, and a sense of accomplishment are enhanced by routines that provide structure and consistency and that are relevant to a particular patient's own experience. It has been observed that caregivers respond to memory-impaired people by limiting the amount of information about family and world events they receive. Perhaps they are concerned that the patient will become more confused with too much information, or that since the information will be forgotten, there is no need to bother talking about it. Whatever the reason, the effect is to remove the kinds of markers of time that we all use to order our lives and place events in context. It is no surprise that a patient who is treated in this way will become increasingly confused and forgetful. Current-events groups that present information in small chunks, offer repetition, and encourage discussion can help alleviate this problem. More personal information relating to family news can be recorded by a family member on a monthly basis on a loop cassette tape (as used for telephone answering machines) and played and replayed at frequent intervals. This also helps patients feel emotionally connected to, and supported by, their families.

Problem-solving sessions with a therapist to help deal with difficulties encountered in everyday life such as paying bills, arranging transportation, and performing work and household duties are important to patients. These sessions are essential for patients with impairment of the executive functions of the frontal lobes. Sessions should focus on pinpointing the problem, setting manageable goals, and structuring a step-by-step solution. While ideally a family member may be trained to take on this role, periodic supervision from a neuropsychologist is essential. If there are issues around changes in roles such as relinquishing responsibilities to a spouse, it may be less emotionally stressful to the family to have the therapist conduct the treatment alone.

## Evaluating Outcome

Since rehabilitation work with MS patients is relatively new, each clinician should evaluate the effectiveness of any intervention using objective measures and specific outcome criteria. Therapists should have an operational definition of the behavior targeted for intervention; determine the frequency of the behavior prior to intervention; and specify exactly what the intervention consists of, how often it is to be delivered, by whom, and under what circumstances (e.g., time of day, location), and how changes in performance are to be recorded. Simple increases or decreases in the targeted behavior do not, in and of themselves, imply that the intervention has been successful or unsuccessful until alternative explanations for the change have been carefully considered and ruled out. The methodology developed for single-subject studies in behavior modification provides a useful guide to operationalizing performance and interventions.

## SUMMARY AND CONCLUSION

The concepts and approaches outlined in this chapter have proved successful in understanding and treating emotional and cognitive disorders in individual MS patients. Other strategies may also be of value. What is needed now is rigorous evaluation of various treatments using substantial numbers of patients, well-matched controls, standardized diagnostic and treatment procedures, and testable outcome criteria. Perhaps even more important is the need to recognize that treatment of these disorders is possible, highly desired by patients and families, and gratifying to those who work with MS patients.

In dividing this chapter into emotional and cognitive disorders we did not intend to imply a precise separation between these aspects of psychological life. Indeed, a patient's emotional state can have a significant impact on cognitive performance, and intellectual deficits may both precipitate and mimic disorders of mood. Cognitive rehabilitation will be very difficult to accomplish in a depressed patient. Emotional and cognitive disorders in MS cannot be understood outside the context of an individual who has, in addition to a progressive, disabling neurologic condition, a personality and a life independent of the illness and who is a vital part of a family and social system.

## REFERENCES

American Psychiatric Association (1987). *Diagnostic and Statistical Manual of Mental Disorders,* Third Edition, Revised Washington: American Psychiatric Association.

Arnaud, S.H. (1959). Some psychological characteristics of children of multiple sclerotics. *Psychosom. Med.,* **221,** 8–21.

Awad, A. (1983). Schizophrenia and multiple sclerosis. Single case study. *J. Nerv. Ment. Dis.,* **171,** 323–24.

Bassuk, E., and Birk, A. (1984). *Psychiatric Emergencies.* New York: Plenum.

Baum, H.M., and Rothschild, B.B. (1981). The incidence and prevalence of reported multiple sclerosis. *Ann. Neurol.,* **10,** 420–28.

Beck, A.T., Rush, A.J., Shaw, B.F., and Emery, G. (1979). *Cognitive Therapy of Depression.* New York: Guilford.

Biometry and Field Studies Branch, Intramural Research Program, National Institute of Neurological and Communicative Disorders and Stroke (1984). *Multiple Sclerosis. A National Survey.,* NIH Publication No. 84-2479.

Braham, S., Houser, H.B., Cline, A., and Posner, M. (1975). Evaluation of the social needs of nonhospitalized chronically ill persons. 1. Study of 47 patients with multiple sclerosis. *J. Chron. Dis.,* **28,** 401–19.

Caine E.D. (1981). Pseudodementia. Current concepts and future directions. *Arch. Gen. Psychiat.,* **38,** 1359–64.

Campbell, D.T., and Stanley, J.C. (1963). *Experimental and Quasi-experimental Designs for Research.* Chicago: Rand McNally College Publishing Co.

Cass L.J., Alexander, L., and Enders, M. (1966). Complications of corticotropin therapy in multiple sclerosis. *J.A.M.A.,* **197,** 105–11.

Colville, P.L. (1983). Rehabilitation. In: J.F. Hallpike, C.W.M. Adams, and W.W. Tourtelotte, eds. *M.S. Pathology, Diagnosis, and Management,* pp. 631–54. Baltimore: Williams and Wilkins.

Craighead, E.W., Kazdin, A.E., and Mahoney, M.J. (1976). *Behavior Modification. Principles, Issues, and Applications.* Boston: Houghton Mifflin.

Crawford J.D., and McIvor G.P. (1985) Group psychotherapy: benefits in multiple sclerosis. *Arch. Phys. Med. Rehabil.,* **66,** 810–13.

Diller, L. (1987). Neuropsychological rehabilitation. In: M. Meier, A. Benton, and L. Diller, eds. *Neuropsychological Rehabilitation.* New York: Guilford.

Falk, W.E., Mahnke, M.W., and Poskanzer, D.D. (1979). Lithium prophylaxis of corticoptrophin-induced psychosis. *J.A.M.A.,* **241,** 1011–12.

Freal, J.E., Kraft, C.H., and Coryell, J.K. (1984). Symptomatic fatigue in multiple sclerosis. *Arch. Phys. Med. Rehabil.,* **65,** 135–38.

Gans, J.S., (1983). Psychosocial adaptation. *Seminars Neurol.,* **3,** 201–11.

Gelenberg, A.J. (1983). Serious toxicity from lithium. *Biol. Ther. Psychiat.,* 7, 21–22, 24.

Geocaris, K. (1957). Psychotic episodes heralding the diagnosis of multiple sclerosis. *Bull. Menn. Clin.,* **21,** 107–16.

Glass, G.V., Smith, M.L., and Miller, T.I. (1980). *The Benefits of Psychotherapy.* Baltimore: Johns Hopkins University Press.

Glassman A.H., and Bigger, J.T. (1981). Cardiovascular effects of therapeutic doses of tricyclic antidepressants. *Arch. Gen. Psychiatry,* **38,** 815, 820.

Goldfried, M.R., and Davison, G.C. (1976). *Clinical Behavior Therapy.* New York: Holt, Rinehart, and Winston.

Gorman, E., Rudd, A., and Ebers, G.C. (1984). In: C.M. Poser, D.W. Paty, L.C. Scheinberg, W.I. McDonald, and G.C. Ebers, eds. *The Diagnosis of Multiple Sclerosis*, pp. 216–22. New York: Thieme-Stratton.

Hartings, M.F., Pavlou, M.M., and Davis, F.A. (1976). Group counseling of MS patients. *J. Chron. Dis.,* **29,** 65–73.

Kahana, E., Leibowitz, U., and Alter, M. (1971). Cerebral multiple sclerosis. *Neurology,* **21,** 1179–85.

Kazdin, A.E. (1977). *The Token Economy.* New York: Plenum.

Kemp, K., Lion, J.R., and Magram, G. (1977). Lithium in the treatment of a manic patient with multiple sclerosis: a case report. *Dis. Nerv. Syst.,* **38,** 210–11.

Kessel, N. (1979). Reassurance. *Lancet,* **1**(8126), 1128–33.

Kubler-Ross, E. (1969). *On Death and Dying,* New York: Macmillan.

Klerman, G.L., Weissman, M.M., Rounsaville, B.J., and Chevron, E. (1984). *Interpersonal Psychotherapy of Depression.* New York: Basic Books.

Kornblith, A.B., LaRocca, N.G., and Baum, H. (1986). Employment in individuals with multiple sclerosis. *Int. J. Rehab. Research,* **9,** 155–65.

Kovacs, M. (1980). The efficacy of cognitive and behavior therapies for depression. *Am. J. Psychiat.* **137,** 1495–1501.

Laracombe, N.A., and Wilson, P.H. (1984). An evaluation of cognitive-behavior therapy for depression in patients with multiple sclerosis. *Br. J. Psychiat.,* **145,** 366–371.

Matthews, W.B. (1979). Multiple sclerosis presenting with acute remitting psychiatric symptoms. *J. Neurol. Neurosurg. Psychiat.,* **39,** 1008–13.

McAllister, T.W. (1983). Overview: Pseudodementia. *Am. J. Psychiat.,* **140,** 528–33.

Mehta, D.B. (1976). Lithium and affective disorders associated with organic brain impairment (Letter to the editor). *Am. J. Psychiat.,* **133,** 236.

Miller, E. (1980). Psychological intervention in the management and rehabilitation of neuropsychological impairments. *Behavior Ther. Res.,* **18,** 529–35.

Minden, S.L. (1987). Anxiety. In: W.T. Branch, Jr., ed., *Office Practice of Medicine,* 2nd ed., pp. 1324–37. Philadelphia: W.B. Saunders.

Minden, S.L., and Frankel D. (1987). *Plaintalk. A Booklet about Multiple Sclerosis for Family Members.* Waltham: Massachusetts Chapter National Multiple Sclerosis Society.

Minden, S.L., Orav J., and Reich, P. (1987). Depression in multiple sclerosis. *Gen. Hosp. Psychiat.,* **9,** 426–34.

Minden, S.L., Orav, J., and Schildkraut, J.J. (1988). Hypomanic reactions to ACTH and prednisone treatment for multiple sclerosis. *Neurology,* **38,** 1631–34.

NIMH Treatment of Depression Collaborative Research Program. Presented at American Psychiatric Association Meeting, Washington, D.C., May 1986.

Pavlou, M., Hartings, M., and Davis, F.A. (1978). Discussion groups for medical patients. *Psychother. Psychosom.,* **30,** 105–15.

Peselow, E.D., Fieve, R.R., Deutsch, S.I., and Kaufman, M. (1981). Coexistent manic symptoms and multiple sclerosis. *Psychosomatics,* **22,** 824–25.

Peters L.C., and Esses, L.M. (1985). Family environment as perceived by children with a chronically ill parent. *J. Chron. Dis.,* **38,** 301–8.

Poser S., Bauer, H.J., Ritter, G., Friedrich, H., Beland, H., and Denecke, P. (1981). Rehabilitation for patients with multiple sclerosis. *J. Neurol.,* **224,** 283–90.

Power, P., and Sax, D. (1978). The communication of information to the neurological patient: some implications for family coping. *J. Chron. Dis.,* **31,** 57–65.

Rush, A.J. (1982). *Short-Term Psychotherapies for Depression.* New York: Guilford.

Scheinberg, L.C., Kalb, R.C., LaRocca, N.G., Giesser, B.S., Slater, R.J., and Poser, C.M. (1984). The doctor-patient relationship in multiple sclerosis. In: C.M. Poser, D.W.

Paty, L.C. Scheinberg, W.I. McDonald, G.C. Ebers, eds. *The Diagnosis of Multiple Sclerosis,* pp. 205–15. New York: Thieme-Stratton.

Schiffer, R.B. (1987). The spectrum of depression in multiple sclerosis: An approach for clinical management. *Arch. Neurol., 44,* 596–99.

Schiffer, R.B., Herndon, R.M., and Rudick, R.A. (1985). Treatment of pathological laughing and weeping with amitriptyline. *N.E.J.M., 312,* 1480–82.

Schiffer, R.B., and Slater, R.J. (1985). Neuropsychiatric features of multiple sclerosis, recognition and magnagement. *Seminars Neurol., 5,* 127–33.

Schiffer, R.B., Wineman, N.M., and Guttormsen, S. (1987). Desipramine in the treatment of multiple sclerosis. Presented at the Symposium on Mental Disorders, Cognitive Deficits, and Their Treatment in Multiple Sclerosis, Odense, Denmark, Nov. 18–21.

Schoonover, S.C. (1983). Depression, In: E.L. Bassuk, S.C. Schoonover, and A.J. Gelenberg, eds., *The Practitioner's Guide to Psychoactive Drugs,* pp. 19–77. New York: Plenum.

Solomon, J.G. (1978). Multiple sclerosis masquerading as lithium toxicity. *J. Nerv. Ment. Dis., 166,* 663–65.

Surridge, D., (1969). An investigation into some aspects of multiple sclerosis. *Br. J. Psychiatry, 114,* 749–64.

Weissman, M.M. (1979). The psychological treatment of depression. Evidence for the efficacy of psychotherapy alone, in comparison with, and in combination with pharmacoptherapy. *Arch. Gen. Psychiat., 36,* 1261–69.

Wilson, B.A. (1987). *Rehabiliation of Memory.* New York: Guilford.

Wood, R.I. (1987). *Brain Injury Rehabilitation: A Neurobehavioral Approach.* Rockville, Md.: Aspen Publishing.

Young, A.C., Saunders, J., and Ponsford, J.R. (1976). Mental change as an early feature of multiple sclerosis. *J. Neurol. Neurosurg. Psychiat.* **39,** 1008–13.

# 16

## Effects of Multiple Sclerosis on Daily Living

MARY EVE SANFORD AND JACK H. PETAJAN

The failure of health care professionals to acknowledge the presence of cognitive and affective problems in multiple sclerosis (MS) patients may impede the adjustment process to this disease and create additional stress for MS patients as well as their families and friends. The patient is often blamed for his failure to perform. It is common to hear as a litany of rationalizations for the failure to perform comments such as "If she would only get enough rest," "Pay attention," "Take his medicine," "Get enough exercise," "Stop trying to do so much."

The social consequences of such stresses on a young mother or father can be significant. Failure to perform at home (e.g., lack of attention to children, inability to keep up with household tasks) may lead to unfortunate acting out in children. The MS patient may lose his or her job while appearing to have minimal neurologic impairment. Such problems are confronted on a regular basis in the MS clinic.

The disclosure of cognitive problems and affective disorder in greater than 50% of MS patients does not surprise clinicians who interact with MS patients on a daily basis. It is common knowledge among neurologists that MS patients seem to have a greater than usual share of personal and social problems. Some physicians have preferred not to deal with this group of patients because of the chronic social distress that may surround their lives. Yet as late as 1980, MS was reported in the clinical literature as not causing any cognitive deficits (Slater and Yearwood, 1980).

The majority of MS patients experience only mild to moderate neurologic disability and are employed (Slater and Yearwood, 1980). Among those patients attending an MS clinic, however, a much smaller percentage are likely to be employed, owing to the presence of greater disease involvement (Colville, 1982).

Furthermore, it is among this group that cognitive problems may be more prevalent. Until recently, it has not been adequately appreciated that patients with relatively benign disease may experience cognitive deficit (Lyon-Caen et al., 1986). Also, clinicians managing newly diagnosed patients or those with benign disease have not focused attention on cognitive or affective problems for fear of creating unwarranted anticipatory anxiety in the patient and family. It is our view that an understanding of the potential cognitive and affective problems can result in reduced tension between the patient and his or her family and associates.

It is helpful to consider the impact of cognitive and affective problems in relation to the following categories of patients: (1) those with normal affect, mild neurologic deficit and ability to cope with family or occupational responsibilities; (2) those with altered affect, characterized by easy laughing and crying, elation, euphoria, and/or depression, and without apparent cognitive deficits; and (3) those with both affective and cognitive problems manifested as circumstantiality, impaired recent memory, poor judgment (common sense), and usually an abundance of social problems. Our clinical experience tells us that most patients fall into the first two categories and that probably fewer than 25% suffer overt impairment of mental status. There is a lack of accurate data on how cognitive and affective problems are distributed in the entire MS population since most studies involve groups of patients attending MS clinics. What is known is that our past estimates of the prevalence of these problems in the MS population have been low and that for many reasons they have often been overlooked in the individual MS patient (Lyon-Caen et al., 1986; Peyser et al., 1980; van den Burg et al., 1987).

## COMMON EMOTIONAL RESPONSES TO MS

In many ways the various emotional reactions to MS are similar to those seen in other chronic illnesses. Apprehension or anxiety is not uncommon, both initially and during exacerbation, stemming from a sense of losing control over body functions and personal destiny. Apprehension also occurs from concerns about the nature of the illness itself, its uncertain course, medication effects, impact on work, family, and friends, and frustrations about physical limitations and accompanying difficulties with activities of daily living. It is not uncommon for these fears to be expressed as anger and frustration. With time, these feelings usually subside. Grieving for lost capacities should also be understood and explained as a normal part of the adjustment process for patients and families alike. Guilt feelings about not being able to carry on with one's preillness activities and responsibilities are not uncommon. Patients and family members should be helped to understand that this reaction only complicates an already difficult situation.

Despite psychological distress, most MS patients generally cope well at home and in the workplace (Brooks and Matson, 1977). The premorbid personality and the social structure surrounding the patient are crucial to satisfactory adjustment. A trusting relationship with a physician, a supportive family and friends, and membership in a supportive social organization characterize those patients who cope well (Brooks and Matson, 1982). One study demonstrated that patients who were more depressed perceived family and friends as providing less social support than those who were less depressed (Riklin et al., 1984). Those patients who are alone and distrustful appear to experience more depression and alienation.

As noted elsewhere in this volume (e.g., see Chapter 12), depression has been recognized as a relatively common concomitant of MS. It is typically viewed as a natural emotional reaction to an unpredictable, progressive illness. Clinical reports suggest that depression worsens during periods of disease activity and improves during periods of disease remission (Cleeland et al., 1970; Dalos et al., 1983). According to Schiffer (1987; Chapter 12), patients who experience depression with an exacerbation respond less well to all forms of therapy directed at treating the depression, because the depression is a direct result of the disease process itself. He has further suggested that when depression occurs in association with a clinical exacerbation, treatment should be the same as for other symptoms of MS, reserving more specific antidepressant therapies for those patients with less active disease. If Schiffer is correct and the depression of some MS patients results directly from the demyelinative process, some interesting questions can be raised regarding the structural and neurochemical bases for depression in general.

Denial is a common coping mechanism early in the course of any chronic illness. This mechanism can be effective if the disease is mild and does not interfere with proper treatment. Denial will allow the patient to compartmentalize problems for a period of time so that he or she can focus on other aspects of life. Problems begin to occur as the disease progresses and the patient refuses to use necessary aids (e.g., repeated falling from refusing to use a cane or a wheelchair). Such patients exhibit an inability to accept help and expressions of concern from family and friends (Brooks and Matson, 1977). Their inflexibility in response to physical disability results in even greater impairment of performance. Denial of disability can also occur in the patient with moderate to severe cognitive disturbance. In these cases, denial actually represents reduced personal insight and awareness in response to diffuse brain involvement.

## CONSEQUENCES OF COGNITIVE/AFFECTIVE PROBLEMS ON ACTIVITIES OF DAILY LIVING

The impact in daily life of cognitive and affective problems has two aspects. First is the problem itself, such as an impairment of recent memory, which can impede accomplishing ordinary daily tasks such as those required in homemaking or work. When this occurs in a young person without an obvious neurologic deficit, the second aspect of the problem becomes evident: family and associates may be unable to understand that such a problem could occur or be able to grasp its severity. Only through failure to perform and the resulting distress to all concerned do the patient and others become aware that a problem exists. Diminished self-esteem ensues. Anger, frustration, and resentment may develop in the patient and his or her family and associates.

The following case histories are typical in our clinic:

A young mother raising a number of small children finds that she is unable to organize her daily activities. She becomes unable to cope with the demands of her children and finally gives up. Her husband comes home from work and finds her sitting and staring into space while the children run about unattended. The house is in disarray. The evening meal has not been prepared. The young woman can only explain that she is tired. Subsequent neuropsychological testing reveals significant memory and problem-solving deficits. The husband, seeing his wife up and about and appearing strong, cannot understand her inability to perform despite repeated explanations to the contrary. The marriage ends as the woman's cognitive problems become worse and the husband finds himself unable to manage his home and hold down a job.

A young woman with a promising law career who graduated at the top of her class finds that she is unable to manage all the details necessary in the preparation of a legal brief. Her colleagues are even more aware of her difficulties. Her neurologic examination is normal. She is bright and alert, clearly above average intellectually. Neuropsychological testing reveals isolated deficits in memory and visuospatial concept formation. Despite her assets and the very minor degree of dysfunction, she is forced to leave the law firm and abandon her career.

A school teacher and father of four develops a slowly progressive gait disorder over many months and finally requires a cane. At the same time, gradual deterioration of mental status occurs. He begins to experience problems with recent memory, judgment, and impulsive acting out. He remains fluent but confabulates considerably. This is discovered during numerous follow-up evaluations associated with a clinical drug trial. Despite his severe deficits, he successfully interviews for a job as school counselor and expresses the desire to pursue this career change. His intelligent wife, who also holds a responsible position with a utilities company, becomes acutely aware of her husband's problems. Stress rises to an intolerable level at home as he becomes abusive toward his children. Nursing home placement finally occurs when he is found to be responsible for an automobile accident that results in injury to himself and two of his children. Because of his verbal facility and manipulative behavior, however, he returns home to create additional problems. The patient's parents remain adamant in the belief that their son is "normal" and that his wife is simply trying to get rid of him. In such situations the magnitude of the interpersonal stresses cannot be exaggerated. It is the unexpected presence of severe cognitive or affective problems in a young person that is the source of the primary stress. This is further confounded by the prevalent view that MS is only a "neurologic" disease that does not affect how people think or feel, that is, that it does not affect the "mind."

## ASSESSMENT OF DAILY LIVING PROBLEMS IN MS

The Sickness Impact Profile (SIP) has been used in our clinic to quantify the impact of MS on daily living activities (Gilson et al., 1975). This self-administered test characterizes the effects of illness on physical and psychosocial activities. It is a standardized questionnaire composed of 136 items in 12 different categories of physical and psychosocial functioning. Each item describes a specific dysfunctional behavior, and respondents are asked to check only the items describing present dysfunction due to their illness. The test takes about 20 minutes to complete. Scores are calculated using predetermined weights based on estimates of the relative severity of each dysfunctional item. Reliability and validity of the SIP have been carefully tested.

The SIP was administered to 102 MS patients randomly selected from the MS clinic at the University of Utah Medical Center during weekly visits to the clinic over a two-year period. Sixty-two females and forty males participated. Seventy-eight were married, twenty-two divorced, and two were single. Average years married were 9.1 (SD = 11.6), average years since diagnosis were 8.28 (SD = 5.84), but years since first symptoms were 13.0 (SD = 7.3). Forty-four percent had a Kurtzke Extended Disability Status Score (EDSS) of 0–4 (mild), ten percent of 4–6 (moderate), and forty-six percent of 6–9 (severe involvement). Seventy-nine patients had a chronic-progressive form of the disease, while twenty-three had the remitting-relapsing form.

Because it was known that MS patients manifest a variety of cognitive and emotional difficulties that might affect the perception of dysfunction, 60 randomly chosen spouses of patients were also asked to assess their MS-afflicted spouses using the SIP. These individuals were told that the investigators were interested in the spouse's as well as the patient's views of the illness and its effects on daily living. No collaboration between the two was possible, since the test was administered simultaneously in separate locations.

Table 16–1 shows the means and standard deviations in each category for the 102 patients. In each category scores range from 0 to 100, with higher scores indi-

**Table 16–1**  A Comparision of Dysfunction in Arthritis, Cancer and MS Patients Using the SIP

| SIP Categories | Mean SIP Score for General Population N = 624 | | Mean SIP Score for 183 CANCER Patients | | Mean SIP Score for 79 RHEUMATOID ARTHRITIS Patients | | Mean SIP Score for 102 MULTIPLE SCLEROSIS Patients | |
|---|---|---|---|---|---|---|---|---|
| | $\overline{X}$ | $\sigma$ | $\overline{X}$ | $\sigma^*$ | $\overline{X}$ | $\sigma$ | $\overline{X}$ | $\sigma$ |
| Total SIP Score | 3.6 | (5.3) | 10.5 | | 15.6 | (9.0) | 27.6 | (15.6) |
| *Category I: Physical dimension* | | | 10.0 | | 14.0 | (10.0) | 17.7 | (12.2) |
| Ambulation | 3.1 | (7.0) | 13.8 | | 21.0 | (13.8) | 28.0 | (16.7) |
| Body care and movement | 1.0* | | 8.0 | | 12.7 | (10.1) | 20.1 | (17.4) |
| Mobility | 2.7 | (7.3) | 11.0 | | 10.4 | (12.1) | 15.8 | (19.3) |
| *Category II: Psychosocial dimension* | | | 8.0 | | 11.3 | (9.6) | 24.4 | (19.1) |
| Emotional behavior | 3.8 | (9.6) | 10.1 | | 13.2 | (12.9) | 22.5 | (22.9) |
| Social interaction | 5.2* | | 10.2 | | 11.7 | (11.6) | 21.5 | (19.0) |
| Alertness behavior | 4.0 | (8.7) | 5.0 | | 13.0 | (17.8) | 27.9 | (28.9) |
| Communication | 1.1 | (3.6) | 1.5 | | 6.9 | (8.5) | 15.2 | (14.9) |
| *Independent Categories* | | | | | | | | |
| Work | 8.5 | (19.4) | 25.1 | | 46.5** | (31.4) | 37.6 | (31.4) |
| Sleep and rest | 7.2 | (13.2) | 21.0 | | 17.6 | (14.9) | 25.9 | (18.6) |
| Eating | 1.6 | (3.3) | 6.2 | | 3.5 | (5.5) | 4.3 | (6.6) |
| Household management | 5.4 | (12.5) | 20.1 | | 26.3 | (21.0) | 29.1 | (22.3) |
| Recreational pastimes | 10.2 | (15.8) | 24.5 | | 26.7 | (19.3) | 30.4 | (23.8) |

*$\sigma$ not available

**These are estimated scores. Due to revisions in the earlier version of the SIP, strict comparable scores are not available for these categories.

cating greater dysfunction. Comparison data are from a normative sample and two
chronic illness groups, metastatic cancer ($n$ = 183) (Sanford and Swenson, 1978)
and rheumatoid arthritis ($n$ = 79) (Deyo et al., 1982).

The MS patients were found to be more dysfunctional in 13 of 15 daily living
areas than the other two patient groups. In the category of daily work, rheumatoid
arthritis patients were most dysfunctional, and in the category of eating, cancer
patients were most dysfunctional. A comparison of MS and rehumatoid arthritis
patients revealed the former to have a significantly higher total SIP score ($p$ <.005)
(See Table 16–1).

A comparison of scores for chronic-progressive and remitting-relapsing patients
revealed all 15 scores to be higher for the chronic-progressive group, with 8 of the
15 scores being significantly ($p$ <.05) higher (see Table 16–2). In the psychosocial
categories three of the five dysfunctional scores (total psychosocial scores, social
interaction, and communication) were also higher, but not significantly so, for the
chronic-progressive group in comparison with those with remitting-relapsing
disease.

In the five independent categories (work, sleep and rest, eating, household management, and recreation pastime), all means were higher for the chronic-progressive MS patients than for the remitting-relapsing patients, with values for work,
eating, and household management being statistically significant. As expected, a
comparison of SIP scores between patients with Kurtzke scores of 0–4 and 6–10

**Table 16–2**   Comparison of Chronic Progressive and Relapsing-Remitting Patients on the SIP

| SIP Categories | Mean (SD) SIP Score for 79 Chronic-Progressive Patients | | Mean (SD) SIP Scores for 23 Relapsing-Remitting Patients | | Significance Level |
|---|---|---|---|---|---|
| | X̄ | σ | X̄ | σ | |
| Total SIP Score | 29.6 | (15.4) | 19.9 | (13.1) | .005 |
| *Category I:* | | | | | |
| Physical dimension | 20.3 | (12.0) | 8.6 | (7.4) | .001 |
| Ambulation | 31.9 | (15.7) | 15.0 | (13.2) | .001 |
| Body care and movement | 23.0 | (17.8) | 10.5 | (10.9) | .001 |
| Mobility | 18.6 | (20.3) | 5.4 | (9.4) | .001 |
| *Category II:* | | | | | |
| Psycho-social dimension | 24.8 | (19.3) | 22.2 | (17.6) | — |
| Emotional behavior | 21.9 | (21.7) | 22.7 | (25.5) | — |
| Social interaction | 22.2 | (19.2) | 18.4 | (17.8) | — |
| Alertness behavior | 27.2 | (27.8) | 28.6 | (29.4) | — |
| Communication | 16.4 | (15.6) | 11.9 | (11.5) | — |
| *Independent Categories* | | | | | |
| Work | 40.4 | (31.4) | 26.3 | (27.8) | .05 |
| Sleep and rest | 26.5 | (17.7) | 21.9 | (19.7) | — |
| Eating | 4.7 | (6.9) | 2.4 | (5.0) | .10 |
| Household management | 32.8 | (23.3) | 15.5 | (9.7) | .001 |
| Recreational pastimes | 31.9 | (23.1) | 24.1 | (24.7) | — |

**Table 16-3**  DSS versus SIP

| SIP | DSS | | |
|---|---|---|---|
| | 0-4 | 6-10 | Significance Level |
| Total SIP | 23.5 ± 16.2 | 32.0 ± 14.7 | 0.02 |
| Ambulation | 19.3 ± 12.8 | 36.5 ± 16.9 | 0.001 |
| Mobility | 9.8 ± 14.6 | 23.5 ± 22.3 | 0.001 |
| Body movement | 10.7 ± 10.9 | 30.1 ± 17.9 | 0.001 |
| Physical dimension | 11.2 ± 8.3 | 24.8 ± 12.5 | 0.001 |
| Alertness behavior | 32.7 ± 33.5 | 20.9 ± 21.4 | 0.05 |
| Home management | 19.8 ± 18.4 | 38.2 ± 23.9 | 0.001 |
| Work | 29.5 ± 29.7 | 47.2 ± 30.6 | 0.01 |
| Eating | 2.8 ± 5.3 | 5.8 ± 7.8 | 0.05 |

(Table 16-3) revealed significantly more dysfunction in all areas in patients with high disability.

When the mean SIP score of the 60 patients and their randomly chosen spouses were compared, there were no significant differences in 14 of the 15 scores. In the category of daily work, spouses rated MS patients as somewhat more dysfunctional ($p < .10$). This difference may depend as much on the spouse's desire for performance as on the ability of the MS patient to assess his or her level of dysfunction accurately (Table 16-4).

**Table 16-4**  Comparison of Perceived Problems with Daily Living Activities in 60 MS Patients and Spouses

| SIP Categories | Mean (SD) SIP Score for 60 patients | | Mean (SD) SIP Score for 60 spouses | |
|---|---|---|---|---|
| | $\overline{X}$ | $\sigma$ | $\overline{X}$ | $\sigma$ |
| Total SIP Score | 27.6 | 15.6 | 28.8 | 13.9 |
| *Category I* | | | | |
| Physical dimension | 17.7 | 12.2 | 18.6 | 12.2 |
| Ambulation | 28.1 | 16.7 | 26.7 | 15.5 |
| Body care, movement | 20.1 | 17.4 | 21.6 | 19.1 |
| Mobility | 15.8 | 19.3 | 17.6 | 18.2 |
| *Category II* | | | | |
| Psycho-social dimension | 24.4 | 19.1 | 23.5 | 16.2 |
| Emotional behavior | 22.5 | 22.9 | 22.3 | 17.9 |
| Social interaction | 21.5 | 19.0 | 22.8 | 19.1 |
| Alertness behavior | 27.9 | 28.5 | 27.9 | 27.5 |
| Communication | 15.2 | 14.9 | 12.9 | 13.7 |
| *Independent Categories* | | | | |
| Work[a] | 37.6 | 31.3 | 46.9 | 30.9 |
| Sleep and rest | 25.9 | 18.6 | 27.8 | 19.1 |
| Eating | 4.2 | 6.6 | 4.5 | 8.2 |
| Household management | 29.1 | 22.3 | 29.3 | 21.3 |
| Recreational pastimes | 30.4 | 23.8 | 29.8 | 21.8 |

[a] $p < .10$.

In summary, the data demonstrate that these MS patients were significantly impaired in most areas of daily living and that their perception of impairment was apparently quite accurate, in spite of cognitive problems in some of the patients. Comparison of the level of dysfunction of these MS patients with the two other illness groups revealed the MS patient to be as impaired if not more so in most areas. The impact of MS on daily living is not adequately appreciated, nor are the significant effects of such symptoms as fatigue, lack of attention, memory deficit, and impaired personal organization on the ability to perform.

In a recent survey of 656 MS patients (Kraft et al., 1986), 250 variables covering symptoms, diagnosis, adjustment, service use, and service need were examined. Medical needs, with the exception of bladder management and physical therapy, were perceived as well met, while counseling and vocational needs were less well met. The need for counseling and vocational guidance was not related to the level of disability, but rather to the age of the patient and recency of onset.

In can be concluded that psychosocial problems occur in MS patients with great frequency, independent of the degree of disability. Because the disease develops most commonly in young adults, psychosocial problems surrounding employment, family relationships, sexual partners, educational plans, and so on are very common. Establishing the diagnosis itself in the absence of any disability whatsoever can create emotional turmoil and cast into disarray carefully laid plans for the future. Patients perceive that help in these areas is not being given and that it is an issue separate from the disease itself.


## PROBLEMS IN THE DISCOVERY OF COGNITIVE/AFFECTIVE PROBLEMS IN THE CLINIC

For a number of reasons, cognitive and affective problems appear to be underdiagnosed in the MS population. To assess the ability of physicians to identify the cognitive and emotional problems of the MS patient, we obtained physician's assessments of 236 patients with chronic-progressive MS. These assessments were compared with patient self-reports of cognitive/affective disturbance on interview and the patients' responses to pencil-and-paper tests of cognitive/affective disturbance. All patients were being evaluated as part of a double-blind clinical trial to assess the efficacy of cyclosporin-A. Physician and patient self-report data were obtained as part of the Minimal Record of Disability (Slater and Scheinberg, 1985), which grades severity of involvement as normal, mild, moderate, or severe. Three standardized tests of cognitive and affective state were administered: the Folstein Mini Mental State (MMS) (Folstein et al., 1975), the Beck Hopelessness Scale (Beck et al., 1974), and the State Anxiety Inventory (Speilberger et al, 1970).

Results indicated that physicians and patients reported no cases of severe depression, while the scores on the Beck Hopelessness Scale suggested that 8.5% of patients were severely depressed. Similarly, the State Anxiety Inventory revealed moderate and severe anxiety in 6.7% and 4.7% of patients, respectively, while neither physicians nor patients acknowledged the presence of significant anxiety. On the Folstein MMS, 14% of patients had a moderate to severe cognitive deficit, while only 3% and 9% of the patients were reported to have cognitive deficit by neurologic examination or self-report, respectively. This study revealed that both physicians and patients underestimate the prevalence and severity of depression, anxiety, and cognitive problems.

## STRATEGIES FOR DISCOVERING COGNITIVE/AFFECTIVE PROBLEMS IN MS PATIENTS

Recognizing that cognitive and affective problems are commonly overlooked in the usual clinical setting compels us to develop better techniques for their detection. While the presence of significant neurologic deficit should suggest that such problems might exist, it must be emphasized that the patient with little or no deficit may have a disproportionate degree of cognitive or affective problems. As mentioned, even the usual inquiry concerning affective state may not yield adequate information. Furthermore, the usual clinical assessment of cognitive function does not have sufficient sensitivity for detection of the features of subcortical dementia that impair accessing and association of stored information.

Clinicians caring for MS patients must be aware of these problems and their impact. It should be considered essential to obtain psychological data on new patients, those in the crisis of exacerbation, those experiencing especially distressing symptoms resulting in disability, and those experiencing pain.

Once the decision is made to obtain psychological data, the next step is to obtain a measure of affective state. After assuring confidentiality, the patient might take such a test before being examined. The Beck Hopelessness Scale (Beck et al., 1974), the General Health Questionnaire (GHQ) (Goldberg, 1978), and the Profile of Mood States (McNair et al., 1984) are a few of the convenient, reliable measures of mood that are available. The score can be obtained at once and if responses so indicate, further inquiry can follow.

Assessment of cognitive status is more difficult, since the usual mental status examination, given as a component of the neurologic examination, often does not detect cognitive abnormality. The decision to evaluate cognition may be based on the following considerations: (1) need for baseline level of function, (2) patient inquiry or demand, (3) occupational factors such as poor work performance, employee or colleague complaints, patient awareness of on-the-job difficulties, or need for career planning, (4) interpersonal adjustment problems or failure to meet expectations of others, (5) need to assess competence for various levels of independent living, (6) requirement by rehabilitation or disability service agencies, and (7) assessment of response to specific therapies.

Tests of cognition can be presented to the patient as a routine component of the neurologic examination, as measures of higher cortical function. The patient as well as the physician should understand that such tests do not ascertain the presence of "craziness" or disturbed perceptions of reality, but rather, that they measure the patients ability to register, recall, and associate various kinds of information, all of which are functions dependent on complex connections between various brain regions, especially cortex to cortex. Such tests may be explained as a more elaborate version of tests already taken. Most patients accept these tests with equanimity and good humor if they are presented in like manner. An example of a comprehensive neuropsychological evaluation is presented in Chapter 4. The Cognitive Function Study Group of the National Multiple Sclerosis Society has also developed a briefer cognitive test battery (1–2 hours) that was designed specifically to evaluate the problems found in MS patients (Peyser et al., in press).

## ASSISTANCE FOR PATIENTS WITH COGNITIVE AND AFFECTIVE PROBLEMS

If a cognitive or affective problem has been defined, having a methodology for addressing the problems is helpful. The following discussion suggests a method for arriving at a treatment plan.

### Definition of the Problem(s)

If a problem (e.g., depression, anxiety, memory deficit) has been recognized in the patient, then the nature of the problem should be discussed with the patient. It is essential to describe these problems in a nonthreatening, nonpejorative manner. With the patient's consent, it is advisable to inform significant others of the nature and severity of the problem by discussing the manifestations of a specific problem with a spouse or relative. This time is not wasted. Most often such explanations will need to be repeated, along with reassurance and advice about how specific problems might be managed. The importance of patient, sympathetic, and understanding associates cannot be overstated.

The explanation of a neuropsychological problem, whenever possible, should be conveyed to the patient. It is best to discuss such problems in the light of basic information about the pathophysiology of MS. For example, the process of demyelination slows and may block the conduction of nerve impulses. As a consequence, it may be difficult to retrieve and associate certain kinds of information. Just as a computer stores information in various files, each one with its own specific label, the brain stores information in crystallized memory in various locations, depending on the modality of input. The recall of information or the solution of problems requiring access to different kinds of information may require different strategies as well as more time in the MS patient. In some cases information is retrieved after long delays, or problems are solved by circuitous routes. It is somehow reassuring to know that the information is most often still there, even though it is less accessible. The islands of information lost and the total failure to register seen in such disorders as Alzheimer's or Pick's diseases are not common in MS. It is essential to explain to all concerned that the patient is not "going crazy," a commonly expressed concern in our experience, but that the patient may have to develop different strategies for carrying out certain mental functions.

### Negotiation of Specific Solutions

**Medication.** Severe depression generally responds to antidepressant medication. The usual considerations directing the use of such medications must be applied to the MS patients: Is there a personal history of depression that antedates the diagnosis of MS? Is there a family history of depression? Are there episodes of hyperactivity or mania? Has the patient experienced the loss of a loved one? After diagnosis of the type of depressive disorder (see Chapters 12 and 15) and its possible relation to the existence of MS, it may be decided to use medication. However, the various manifestations of MS, such as neurogenic bladder, spasticity, or paresthesias, may also be affected by the treatment. Urinary retention may be induced by the anticholinergic affects of a tricyclic antidepressant. Weakness may be enhanced in someone already on a spasmolytic drug such as baclofen, while paresthesias may become more tolerable as a salutary side effect of the medication (Young and Delwaide, 1981a,b; Klawans and Weiner, 1981a,b).

Anxiety disorders may antedate MS. Anxiety is a symptom of a variety of neurotic disorders, but it may also represent a dysautonomic manifestation of MS itself. Severe anxiety is also responsive to a variety of drugs. As mentioned above, anxiety may not be acknowledged during the interview, but symptoms of anxiety may be elicited during the neurologic examination. The most commonly prescribed anxiolytic agents are members of the benzodiazepine family (e.g., diazepam). These drugs are quite effective at first but usually require dose adjustment upward as the drug effect is attenuated over time. Varying degrees of addiction may develop with long-term use, so if such use is indicated, rapid withdrawal of drug is usually associated with severe anxiety, tremor, depression, and sometimes more serious effects such as grand mal seizure (Klawans and Weiner, 1981b). The response to treatment is usually dramatic. The addition of an anxiolytic drug to other drugs used in the treatment of spasticity may be synergistic. Rarely, anxiolytic drugs may induce a profound state of depression or sedation.

**Psychotherapy.** Depressed patients with intact cognition have been shown to respond to cognitive behavior therapy (Larcombe, 1984), a substantial component of which is the provision of factual information about MS to patients so that they may acquire a more realistic view of the disease. Cognitive behavior therapy is best accomplished with patients who have a comparable degree of deficit and have essentially normal cognition. Patients may have a stereotypic view of MS as an illness uniformly producing disability or early demise. They may find themselves engaged in negative future forecasting about the rest of their lives or make erroneous assumptions about how important others view the diagnosis or disability. Such problems are most common in the newly diagnosed or minimally involved patients. Interaction with a sympathetic therapist who has basic information about MS can be helpful.

The patient with significant cognitive impairment is less responsive to psychotherapy, and supportive therapy to the patient and family may be more important. The therapist can play an important role in defining the cognitive/affective issues that disable the patient. This can greatly reduce the frustration and anger experienced by family members that ultimately feed back on the patient.

**Support Groups.** It has been established that the sharing of problems and their solutions among MS patients benefits both the recipient and the giver of information (Pavlou et al., 1979). Opinions vary as to what constitutes the ideal composition of such groups. It is our opinion that it is necessary to avoid mixing those with severe cognitive deficit and those with normal mentation if the intent of the group is to achieve solutions to difficult situational problems. Inappropriate questions, circumstantial thinking, inability to listen to and understand the comments of others, and ideas of reference as components of dementia in some participants can prevent altogether the successful operation of a group. Furthermore, the perception of mental abnormality in other MS patients by those much less involved can be frightening. Groups gathered for the purpose of recreation, general emotional support, and education, however, can be quite heterogeneous.

Support groups that include family members are especially beneficial for those families in which there are patients with cognitive impairment. Family members may also form groups for sharing their own adjustment problems. A therapist or other professional facilitator who is informed about MS should manage such groups to prevent them from becoming sessions of shared agony without resolution or hope.

**Situational (Environmental) Management.** The patient's living situation may require change. Application of adaptive aids (e.g., installation of wheelchair ramps, bathroom handlebars) may reestablish a sense of control for the patient. Spending some time each day or several times per week at a "respicenter" or "achievement" center may give both the patient and family time to recover from interpersonal stresses that derive from unfilled expectations.

The interpersonal environment of the patient is even more important than the physical environment. An MS patient may be better off without a psychologically or physically abusive spouse. It is common to see frustration in the spouse deprived of "child care" emerge as anger, sometimes violent, against the MS patient. It is quite likely that abuse of the disabled MS person is underreported.

At times hospitalization is indicated for extremely stressful situations that may precede or accompany exacerbations. Justification for hospitalizations is usually possible because of associated medical problems or frank exacerbation. Separation of the patient from a stressful environment, even for a short time, can be of immense benefit.

**Utilization of Community Resources.** Medical social workers, local chapters of the MS society, and welfare agencies may provide information about available community resources. Among the resources available are visiting nurses, housekeeping services, child care, family and marital counseling, funds for persons with specific disabilities, child support, and food services. The designations of various agencies and the overlap of responsibilities between federal and state agencies is confusing for all concerned. Investigation of the patients insurance or disability benefits can take many hours. It has been our experience that the legally accepted definition of disability very often does not fit the MS patient. This is generally true of federal guidelines for the Social Security Administration. The MS patient with severe impairment of mental status but able to walk without assistance may be denied benefits although unable to function in the workplace. A skilled medical social worker can be of great assistance in this vital area of management.

## Formulation of the Treatment Contract

Since MS is a chronic illness that impacts on individuals in a variety of settings, no single solution to a problem is applicable to all individuals. This statement holds for all levels of treatment. No treatment or method of management can succeed without the concurrence of all those involved. The physician must clearly define the consequences of failure to comply. If agreement cannot be reached on one method, others may have to be developed. Following discussion and agreement, it is helpful to provide all persons concerned with a list of the items in the treatment plan. These must be recorded in the patient's record.

## Follow-up Evaluation and Adjustment of Management

Changes in the management plan may be necessary as new problems develop or recovery takes place. Roles assumed by family members may have to be relinquished or altered as disability status changes. These changes may be more difficult to bring about than the adjustment of the patient himself. At times, family members may assume quite destructive care-taking roles that serve to maintain the patient in a passive, dependent relationship.

Follow-up visits for patients with chronic-progressive disease and significant disability may be widely spaced. It may be assumed by the physician that because treatment directed at the disease is not usually applied, follow-up visits at frequent intervals are not necessary. In most cases, follow-up visits should be scheduled every four–six months or at the very least, annually.

## COMMENT AND SUMMARY

While the neurologic examination and assessment of disability does include an evaluation of cognitive and affective state, it is apparent that only severe involvement is usually detected. This leaves undetected a large number of patients with significant psychological dysfunctions that may impair performance both at home and in the workplace. Considerable distress may occupy the lives of these patients. Their dysfunction and associated distress are for the most part comparable to, or greater than, that experienced by patients with such disorders as metastatic cancer and rheumatoid arthritis. An overview of community resources as well as public and professional awareness of these problems reveals a substantial vacuum of both knowledge and resources. Because the problems have not been clearly defined and, in fact, have been kept from public notice, with MS defined as a neurologic disorder not affecting the "mind," community resources are most often not suited to the needs of these patients. For example, nursing homes are most often designed for the elderly. It is customary for young MS patients requiring recuperative care or rehabilitation to refuse to go to nursing homes. Care centers for young MS patients, preferably with associated child care facilities so that they might serve as patient day care centers, are sorely needed.

Financial support for patients and dependent families often occurs as a result of divorce or abandonment of a young woman with minor children rather than out of any consideration for her illness. Further documentation of such conditions may help in the formulation of appropriate legislation designed to assist these families and to provide day care for patients and their children.

It is recommended that the clinician caring for MS patients utilize a plan to detect affective or cognitive problems that may contribute to psychosocial dysfunction. If appropriate, it is suggested that the affective state be ascertained first through use of a brief, paper-and-pencil test. This permissive and safe testing mode appears most likely to yield valid results. Detection of potentially treatable depression and/or anxiety is of great practical importance. Assessment of cognitive status may be undertaken on the suggestion of the patient himself or herself for purposes of employment or to ascertain disability for financial compensation. The decision to carry out testing of cognitive status under the direction of a neuropsychologist must be based on careful consideration of how the information is to be used.

## REFERENCES

Beck, A.T., Weisman, A., Lester, D., and Trexler, L. (1974). The measurement of pessimism: The Hopelessness Scale. *J. Consult. Clin. Psychol.,* **40,** 861–65.

Brooks, N.A., and Matson, R.R. (1977). Adjusting to multiple sclerosis: An exploratory study. *Soc. Sci. Med.,* **11,** 245–50.

Brooks, N.A., and Matson, R.R. (1982). Socio-psychological adjustment to multiple sclerosis. *Soc. Sci. Med.,* **16,** 2129–35.

Cleeland, C.S., Matthews, C.G., and Hopper, C.L. (1970). MMPI profiles in exacerbation and remission of multiple sclerosis. *Psychol. Rep.,* **27,** 373–74.

Colville, P.L. (1982). Rehabilitation. In: J.F. Hallpike, C.W.M. Adams, and W.W. Tourtellottes, eds., *Multiple Sclerosis,* pp. 631–54. Baltimore: Williams and Wilkins.

Dalos, N.P., Rabins, P.V, Brooks, B.R., and O'Donnell, P. (1983). Disease activity and emotional state in multiple sclerosis. *Ann. Neurol.,* **13,** 573–77.

Deyo, R.A., Inui, T.S., Leininger, J., and Overman, S. (1982). Physical and psychosocial function in rheumatoid arthritis: Clinical use of a self-administered health status instrument. *Arch. Intern. Med.,* **142,** 879–82.

Folstein, M.F., Folstein, S.E., and McHugh, P.R. (1975). Mini-Mental State: A practical method for grading the cognitive state of patients for the clinician. *J. Psychiat. Res.,* **12,** 189–98.

Gilson, B.S., Gilson, J.S., and Bergner, M. (1975). The Sickness Impact Profile: Development of an outcome measure of health care. *Am. J. Public Health,* **65,** 1304–10.

Goldberg, D.P. (1978). *Manual of the General Health Questionnaire.* New York: National Foundation for Educational Research Publishing.

Klawans, H.L., and Weiner, W.J. (1981a). Affective disorders. In: *Textbook of Clinical Pharmacology,* pp. 181–98. New York: Raven Press.

Klawans, H.L., and Weiner, W.J. (1981b). Anxiety. In: *Textbook of Clinical Pharmacology,* pp. 215–24. New York: Raven Press.

Kraft, G.H., Freal, J.E., and Coryell, J.K. (1986). Disability, disease duration and rehabilitation service needs in multiple sclerosis: Patient perception. *Arch. Phys. Med. Rehab.,* **67,** 164–68.

Larcombe, N.A., and Wilson, P.H. (1984). An evaluation of cognitive-behaviour therapy for depression in patients with multiple sclerosis. *Br. J. Psychiat.,* **145,** 366–71.

Lyon-Caen, O., Jouvent, R., Hauser, S., Chaunu, M.-P., Benoit, N., Widlocher, D., and Lhermitte, F. (1986). Cognitive function in recent onset demylinating diseases. *Arch. Neurol.,* **43,** 1138–41.

McNair, D.M., Lorr, M., and Droppelman, L. (1984). *Profile of Mood States, Manual.* San Diego, Calif.: Educational and Industrial Testing Service.

Pavlou, M., Johnson, P., and Davis, F. (1979). A program of psychologic service delivery in a multiple sclerosis center. New York: National Multiple Sclerosis Society.

Peyser, J.M., Edwards, K.R., Poser, C.M., and Filskov, S.B. (1980). Cognitive function in patients with multiple sclerosis. *Arch. Neurol.,* **37,** 577–79.

Peyser, J.M., Rao, S.M., LaRocca, N.G., and Kaplan, E. (in press). Guidelines for neuropsychological research in multiple sclerosis. *Arch. Neurol.*

Riklin, M., McIvor, G.P., Reznikoff, M. (1984). Depression in multiple sclerosis as a function of length and severity of illness, age, remissions and perceived social support. *J. Clin. Psychol.,* **40,** 1028–33.

Sanford, M.E., and Swenson, J.R. (1978). *Assessment of Daily Living Problems in Utah Cancer Patients.* Unpublished manuscript.

Schiffer, R.B. (1987). The spectrum of depression in multiple sclerosis. *Arch. Neurol.,* **44,** 596–99.

Slater, R.J., and Scheinberg, L.C. (1985). *Minimal Record of Disability for Multiple Sclerosis.* New York: National Multiple Sclerosis Society.

Slater, R.J., and Yearwood, A.C. (1980). Facts, faith and hope. *Am. J. Nursing,* **50,** 276–81.

Spielberger, C.D., Gorsuch, R.L., and Lushene, R.E. (1970). *STAI Manual for the State-Trait Anxiety Inventory.* Palo Alto, Calif.: Consulting Psychologists Press.

Van den Burg, W., van Zomeren, A.H., Minderhoud, J.M., Prange, A.J.A., and Meijer, N.S.A. (1987). Cognitive impairment in patients with multiple sclerosis and mild physical disability. *Arch. Neurol.,* **44,** 494–501.

Young, R.R., and Delwaide, P.J. (1981a). Drug therapy: Spasticity, Part I. *N. Engl. J. Med.,* **304,** 28–33.

Young, R.R., and Delwaide, P.J. (1981b). Drug therapy: Spasticity, Part II. *N. Engl. J. Med.,* **304,** 96–99.

# Index

Demyelination. *See also* Lesions
  definition, 16
  description of lesion, 16
  effects on oligodendrocytes, 15, 27–27, 30
  sclerosis (scarring), 19
Depression. *See* Affective disorders
Diagnosis, 5–11. *See also* Computerized tomography; Magnetic resonance imaging
Diplopia, 6–7
Disability Status Scale (DSS). *See* Kurtzke disability scales
Dizziness. *See* Vertigo
Double vision. *See* Diplopia
Dysarthria, 8, 91, 96
  lesions producing, 8
  in subcortical dementia, 91
  swallowing difficulties, 8

EEG. *See* Electrophysiological studies
Electrophysiological studies
  EEG, 64
  evoked potentials, 10, 64
Emotional disorders. *See* Affective disorders
Epidemiology of MS, 5
Etiological hypotheses. *See* Lesions, pathogenesis of
Euphoria. *See* Affective disorders
Evoked potentials. *See* Electrophysiological studies
Exacerbations
  annual rate, 12–13
  correlation with cognitive dysfunction, 146
  definition, 6
Executive functions, 67–68, 96
  abstract reasoning, 67
  behavioral fluency, 67
  concept formation, 67
  correlation with MRI findings, 67, 126–27
  interaction with disease course, 67
  planning and organizational skills, 67
Expanded Disability Status Scale (EDSS). *See* Kurtzke disability scales
Experimental allergic encephalomyelitis (EAE), 25–26, 32–33, 49
  lesions on MRI, 49
  therapeutic implications, 33

Fatigue, 67
Frontal-subcortical dysfunction, 65, 67, 96, 164–65
  frontal lobe release signs, 164
    correlation with cognitive dysfunction, 164–65

Huntington's disease, 88, 92, 97, 107, 113–14. *See also* Subcortical dementia

Intelligence, 64–65, 70, 96
  correlation with MRI findings, 126–27
  interaction with disease course, 65, 138
  interaction with duration of illness, 65, 96, 137–38
  interaction with physical disability, 65, 96
  interpretative problems in MS population, 66
  longitudinal studies, 64–65, 137–47
  methodological issues, 65
  verbal-performance IQ discrepancy, 64
  role of sensorimotor dysfunction, 64
IQ. *See* Intelligence

Korsakoff's syndrome, 113
Kurtzke disability scales, 112
  correlation with activities of daily living, 256–57
  correlation with cognitive dysfunction, 164–65
  correlation with frontal lobe release signs, 164
  correlation with memory disturbance, 112
  limitations, 165

Language functions, 66–67, 96
  aphasia, 66–67, 70, 96
  correlation with MRI findings, 126–27
  frontal-subcortical tracts, 67
  interaction with disease course, 66
Learning. *See* Memory disturbance
Lesions, 19
  acute, 24–26
    on CT, 39
    on MRI, 48–49
  changes in blood vessels, 22
  chronic, 22–24
  fibrillary gliosis (scarring), 16, 21, 23–24
  inflammation in acute stages, 16, 26
  lack of correlation with anatomical boundaries, 22
  location in cerebrum, 20–21
  natural history, 16, 20–21
  pathogenesis of, 25–30
  relative sparing of axons in, 16, 22
  remyelination, 30–32
  shadow plaques, 30
  temporal profile on MRI, 54–55

Magnetic resonance imaging, 8–10, 37, 40–55, 64, 73–74, 94–95, 122–30, 166
  annual rate of new lesions, 12, 54
  disease course, 54–55